THE HANDBOOK OF GENETIC COMMUNICATIVE DISORDERS

THE HANDBOOK OF GENETIC COMMUNICATIVE DISORDERS

Edited by

Sanford E. Gerber

Adjunct Professor
Department of Speech and Hearing Sciences
Washington State University

Emeritus Professor
Department of Speech and Hearing Sciences
University of California, Santa Barbara

Former Visiting Professor
Department of Communication Disorders
Eastern Washington University

Academic Press
San Diego New York Boston
London Sydney Tokyo Toronto

This book is printed on acid-free paper.

Academic Press
a Harcourt Science and Technology Company
525 B Street, Suite 1900, San Diego, California 92101-4495
http://www.academicpress.com

Academic Press Limited
Harcourt Place, 32 Jamestown Road, London NW1 7BY, UK
http://www.academicpress.com

Library of Congress Catalog Card Number: 00-111521

International Standard Book Number: 0-12-280605-0

PRINTED IN UNITED STATES OF AMERICA
01   02   03   04   05   06   SB   9   8   7   6   5   4   3   2   1

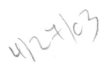

CONTENTS

1

INTRODUCTION

SANFORD E. GERBER

2

DELINEATION OF GENETIC COMPONENTS OF COMMUNICATIVE DISORDERS

GLENN E. GREEN AND RICHARD J. H. SMITH

3

PRENATAL AND POSTNATAL CRANIOFACIAL DEVELOPMENT

SYLVAN E. STOOL

4

MORPHOGENESIS AND GENETICS OF INNER EAR DEVELOPMENT AND MALFORMATION

DOROTHY A. FRENZ, JUAN REPRESA, AND THOMAS R. VAN DE WATER

5

GENETIC DEAFNESS

ROBERT J. RUBEN

6

GENETIC LANGUAGE DISORDERS

JULIE WILLIAMS AND JIM STEVENSON

7

GENETICS IN CRANIOFACIAL DISORDERS AND CLEFTING: THEN AND NOW

ROBERT J. SHPRINTZEN

8

STUTTERING AND GENETICS: OUR PAST AND OUR FUTURE

SUSAN FELSENFELD AND DENNIS DRAYNA

9

CONCEPTS IN BEHAVIORAL GENETICS AND THEIR APPLICATION TO DEVELOPMENTAL AND LEARNING DISORDERS

JEFFREY W. GILGER

10

GENETIC PRIVACY AND ETHICAL, LEGAL, AND SOCIAL ISSUES

SHARON DAVIS

11

TREATMENT AND PREVENTION

SANFORD E. GERBER

FOREWORD

Without doubt, the single area in which practicing clinicians lack current and clinically relevant training and information is genetics; and, more specifically, the role of genetics in communicative disorders. Over the past 15 years, I have noted this to be the case in my interactions with audiences throughout the United States and around the world. The question I regularly receive from practicing clinicians is "Can you help me find a readable book on genetics, one that contains information that I can put into practice right away?" Up to this time, there was no single source I could refer them to. You now hold the answer in your hands. Clinically relevant, empirically sound, and eminently readable is how I would describe the information contained in *The Handbook of Genetic Communicative Disorders*.

Sandy Gerber, a long-time advocate for persons with special needs, has compiled an impressive array of contributors. As a whole, they deal with a wide range of issues regarding genetics. Each author is a master clinician, and under the editing of a master editor, a most helpful book has emerged. The material contained in *The Handbook of Genetic Communicative Disorders* should prove to be a valuable resource for clinicians for years to come.

A review of the contents reveals coverage of a wide range of issues of interest to rehabilitation professionals. Issues regarding hearing impairment and deafness are discussed in several chapters. Each chapter provides the reader with basic and more advanced information to assist in gaining a better understanding of the role of genetics in determining the etiology of hearing loss and management of persons with hearing impairment.

The role of genetics in communicative disorders is covered in several additional chapters. Of particular interest is the information regarding behavioral genetics in communicative disorders. I know of nothing comparable and highly recommend it. The chapters that describe the role of genetics in craniofacial disorders and development provide the reader with a comprehensive and yet clinically germane discussion. In addition, the chapter on ethical, legal, and social implications will provide the reader with much valuable information and suggestions for dealing with these issues. In the context of changing health-care funding, this chapter will prove most illuminating and helpful. Further, many clinicians, regardless of employment setting, do not have a clear understanding of referral suggestions when the input of a geneticist is needed. Many practicing clinicians are unwilling to trust their instincts and thus remain uncertain of how to best determine if a referral to the geneticist is warranted.

The final chapter, written by Dr. Gerber, discusses current practice regarding treatment and prevention of genetic disorders. The field of genetics is changing rapidly, particularly in the clinical application of advanced research. This chapter affords the reader an opportunity to better understand how current research translates into everyday practice, a most valuable resource.

As you can surmise, I am quite excited about this text and the potential it has to upgrade the practicing clinician's knowledge base regarding the practical side of genetics. I have known Sandy Gerber for a number of years. He is a clinician's clinician, and his passion for the subject matter contained in this text is evident throughout. I highly recommend this text as a permanent part of every clinician's professional library. I know I will use it frequently in my clinical practice.

Louis Rossetti
Oshkosh, Wisconsin

CONTRIBUTORS

Sharon Davis (199), The Arc of the United States, Silver Spring, Maryland 20910

Dennis Drayna (151), National Institute on Deafness and Other Communicative Disorders, Rockville, Maryland 20850

Susan Felsenfeld (151), Department of Speech–Language Pathology, Duquesne University, Pittsburgh, Pennsylvania 15282-2231

Dorothy A. Frenz (69), Department of Otolaryngology, Department of Anatomy and Structural Biology, Albert Einstein College of Medicine, Yeshiva University, Bronx, New York 10461

Sanford E. Gerber (1, 213), Department of Speech and Hearing Sciences, Washington State University, Spokane, Washington 99201

Jeffrey W. Gilger (175), Human Biology Program and the Department of Speech–Hearing–Language Sciences and Disorders, University of Kansas, Lawrence, Kansas 66045

Glenn E. Green (11), Department of Surgery, Pediatrics, and Speech and Hearing Sciences, University of Arizona, Tucson, Arizona 85724

Juan Represa (69), Department of Otolaryngology, University of Valladolid, Valladolid, Spain 47005

Louis Rossetti (xiii), Department of Communication Disorders, University of Wisconsin, Oshkosh, Wisconsin 54901

Robert J. Ruben (89), Departments of Otorhinolaryngology, and Pediatrics, Montefiore Medical Center, Albert Einstein College of Medicine, Bronx, New York 10467-2490

Robert J. Shprintzen (129), Communication Disorder Unit, Center for Genetic Communicative Disorders and Center for the Diagnosis, Treatment, and Study of Velocardiofacial Syndrome, Department of Otolaryngology & Communicative Science, State University of New York Upstate Medical University, Syracuse, New York 13210

Richard J. H. Smith (11), Molecular Otolaryngology Research Laboratory, Departments of Otolaryngology and Genetics, University of Iowa, Iowa City, Iowa 52242

Jim Stevenson (113), Department of Psychology, University of Southampton, Southampton, S017 1BJ, United Kingdom

Sylvan E. Stool (31), Department of Otolaryngology, The Children's Hospital of Denver, Denver, Colorado 80218

Thomas R. Van De Water (69), Department of Neuroscience and Department of Otolaryngology, Albert Einstein College of Medicine, Yeshiva University, Bronx, New York 10461

Julie Williams (113), Department of Psychological Medicine, University of Wales College of Medicine, Cardiff, Wales, CF14 4XN, United Kingdom

PREFACE

I was surprised and pleased when Academic Press, in the person of Mark Zadrozny, asked me to put together this volume. I was also rather intimidated. I am not a geneticist, although I have long been interested in the topic, as it is necessarily involved in my teaching and writing. Given that I am not a geneticist, I declined authorship but offered to edit a volume in which the contributors are experts—and they are.

As I note in the first chapter, most of us in the disciplines of audiology and speech–language pathology are rather newcomers to these understandings. That's unfortunate, and the most general goal of this book is to get us closer to where I think we should be. I hope we have succeeded.

Anyway, I have a prejudice. No. I would rather call it an interpretation of the facts. We cannot be free of our genes. Indeed, there are many patients in whom the etiology of a communicative disorder is not determined, but that doesn't mean that there isn't one. The National Institutes of Health, on its webpage (March 2, 2000), observed that "virtually all diseases have a genetic component."

In a survey that I did some years ago (Gerber, 1990), it was found that nearly 45% of the incidence of congenital deafness is known to be of genetic origin. That's not a surprise; most other reports have noted similar proportions. For example, Dallapiccola and colleagues (1996) claimed that half of the incidence of congenital deafness is of genetic origin. Many such surveys have also reported a large number described as etiology unknown. That, too, is not a surprise. However, if 45% of those whose etiologies we do know are genetic, it seems to me that 45% of those whose etiologies we do not know must also be genetic. There are many examples. Alport syndrome, the combination of Bright's disease and sensorineural deafness, has been found in the *COL4A5* gene on the X chromosome. Similarly, the genes have been located and identified for Usher syndrome, Waardenburg syndrome, Stickler syndrome, and many others.

Here is another issue: what is the role of genetics in so-called acquired disorders? We know, for example, that about half of children exposed prenatally to rubella turn out to be deaf (Bordley *et al.*, 1967). Why only half? What about the other half? It strikes me as sensible to assume that either or both of two things must occur: one, those who are affected have some genetic predisposition to be so affected; or, two, those who are not affected have some genetic resistance to those effects. The late D. W. Smith (1982) had observed that "the genetic background may have a profound influence on the likelihood of a given environmental teratogen causing malformation" (p. 554).

Here is another example: the Native American population has had a 33-fold greater incidence of hepatitis A than in the population at large and as much as 24 times the incidence of pneumococcal disease. Why? Clearly, there must be some kind of genetic predisposition even when one accounts for environment.

Actually, I hope to find the answers to many of these issues in this book. Of course, one reason I continue to edit volumes like this is that this is my form of continuing education. I learn a lot from doing this, and I enjoy it. I hope that my readers also learn and enjoy.

There is quite a collection of contributors here, and I am honored that they have agreed to participate. Some of them are old friends, some are new friends, and one is a former student. I invited them because I believe them to be the best experts in their chosen areas of study. Nevertheless, I am the editor, so I am to be blamed where damage was done to the expression of their knowledge and they are to be credited when I got it right. Actually, this is the first collection of its kind (as far as I know). There are some excellent volumes on genetic deafness (e.g., Ruben *et al.*, 1991; Martini *et al.*, 1996), on genetics of speech and language disorders (e.g., Ludlow & Cooper, 1983; Rice, 1996), and more recently on syndromal communicative disorders (e.g., Shprintzen, 1997). But I believe that this is the first to cover communicative disorders broadly and to include the biologists with the clinicians. I hope that the reader agrees that this is valuable.

The book divides into three parts after my introduction. The next chapters consider the underlying biology in some way. Richard Smith and Glenn Green from the University of Iowa, in Chapter 2, look into how we know all that we know. They talk about twin studies, sibling studies, consanguineous families, the use of animal models and candidate genes, and linkage analysis. Genetics is a statistical as well as a biological study.

The next two chapters tell us what happens to express those genes. In Chapter 3, Sylvan Stool of The Children's Hospital of Denver describes both prenatal and postnatal development of the craniofacial complex, as it needs to be understood by the speech–language pathologist. Dorothy Frenz of the Albert Einstein College of Medicine and her colleagues, in Chapter 4, describe the morphogenesis of the auditory system, including tissue origins and interactions and how they are developmentally expressed. This chapter also relates specific gene mutations to various areas of the inner ear.

The next chapters deal with the disorders themselves. Robert Ruben, distinguished professor of otolaryngology and pediatrics at the Albert Einstein College of Medicine, takes off from Chapter 4 in Chapter 5 with an explication of genetic deafness. It is from Bob that I learned the term "fate mapping" to describe what happens.

Speech and language are not the same thing, and may be disordered in different ways. In Chapter 6, our British colleagues Julie Williams and Jim Stevenson discuss genetic language disorders. These are, or seem to be, developmental problems that underlie what gets expressed or understood. Clefts of the palate or of the lip are not isolated anomalies. These are complex disorders. In Chapter 7, Robert Shprintzen (SUNY Health Science Center at Syracuse) examines how our knowledge of genetics has impacted the study of craniofacial disorders and, therefore, care delivery. Stuttering has been, in many ways, an ongoing mystery. Sue Felsenfeld (now at Duquesne University) and Dennis Drayna (of NIDCD), in Chapter 8, examine how studies of the genetics of stuttering have moved us a giant step toward solution of this mystery. Finally, in Chapter 9, on neurogenic disorders, we look at how the study of genetics has impacted some more mysteries: autism, for example, and dyslexia. In this chapter, Jeffrey Gilger of the University of Kansas describes for us a rather new approach to genetics: behavioral genetics. How do our genes get involved in such a complicated process as the learning of language and in such problems as autism or dyslexia?

The last chapters take up matters that are brought about by all of the above. So we have these disorders that more and more often are seen to be of genetic origin. What do we do about it? How does it matter? Who should know about this? Advances in genetics have led to questions about genetic privacy. In Chapter 10, Sharon Davis, who directs research for The Arc of the United States, raises issues of genetic privacy and genetic discrimination. These are real issues and come increasingly to our attention. Anyway, can we fix them? The advances in genetic treatment occupy a great deal of media attention. Finally, the last chapter is mine. Chapter 11 asks "Can we treat or (better) prevent genetic disorders?" In this chapter, I make the case that we often can, and so we should.

All in all, we have covered a great deal. I have been assisted in this effort by some colleagues. Professor Don Lightfoot of the Eastern Washington University biology department kept me from making serious errors in my discussion of genetic treatments. My students, colleagues, and friends Jonnell Block and Katherine Couture were of great help in organizing and identifying the references and the figures. It is my hope that all of our readers will be not only informed but will also have their clinical practice enhanced with this knowledge. It's complicated, it's exciting, and can be extremely useful.

Sanford E. Gerber
Spokane, Washington

REFERENCES

Bordley, J. E., Brookhouser, P. E., Hardy, J., & Hardy, W. G. (1967). Observations on the effect of prenatal rubella in hearing. In F. McConnell & P. H. Ward (Eds.), *Deafness in childhood* (pp. 123–141). Nashville: Vanderbilt University Press.

Dallapiccola, B., Mingarelli, R., & Read, A. P. (1996). Methods of identifying hearing loss genes. In A. Martini, A. Read, & D. Stephens (Eds.), *Genetics and hearing impairment* (pp. 33–47). San Diego: Singular.

Gerber, S. E. (1990). Review of a high risk register for congenital or early-onset deafness. *British Journal of Audiology, 24*, 347–356.

Ludlow, C. L., & Cooper, J. A. (Eds.) (1983). *Genetic aspects of speech and language disorders.* New York: Academic Press.

Martini, A., Read, A., & Stephens, D. (Eds.) (1996). *Genetics and hearing impairment.* San Diego: Singular.

National Institutes of Health (2000). National Genome Research Institute. www.nih.gov, March 2.

Rice, M. L. (Ed.) (1996). *Toward a genetics of language.* Mahwah, NJ: Erlbaum.

Ruben, R. J., Van De Water, T. R., & Steel, K. P. (Eds.) (1991). *Genetics of hearing impairment.* New York: The New York Academy of Sciences.

Shprintzen, R. J. (1997). *Genetics, syndromes, and communication disorders.* San Diego: Singular.

Smith, D. W. (1982). *Recognizable patterns of human malformation.* Philadelphia: Saunders.

1

INTRODUCTION

SANFORD E. GERBER

Department of Speech and Hearing Sciences
Washington State University
Spokane, Washington

I. SOME BACKGROUND

Forty-two million Americans have some type of communicative disorder; 28 million of them have some degree of hearing impairment. Among any 1000 people, 95 report being hearing impaired; undoubtedly there are still more who do not report or who deny their hearing impairments. Speech or language disorders affect 14 million Americans, of whom 2 million stutter and another million have aphasia. Children, of course, can have communicative disorders from birth. How many of the congenital disorders are genetic? What proportion of late-onset or early-onset disorders has been inherited? One percent of live births have single gene mutations, and over 10% of the population are at risk for late-onset genetic disorders. As many as 3 to 4% of all children are born with genetic disease or anomaly, and as many as 10% will have problems of genetic origin by the age of 1 year (Jung, 1989). About 7 in every 1000 births are affected by a chromosomal

The Handbook of Genetic Communicative
Disorders

1

disorder (Gerber, 1998). Three children in every 1000 births are hearing impaired. These are matters that need to be addressed in order to enhance and improve our professional skills and to treat our patients. After all, etiology links to prognosis. What are the prognoses for genetic communicative disorders? Can they be treated?

Where are we—the hearing and speech clinicians—in all of this? Certainly, we are latecomers. Shprintzen (1997) commented that we have been left behind. Other disciplines, he noted, have incorporated clinical and molecular genetics into their practice and education, but we have been slow to do so. Our curricula contain very little—usually nothing at all—about genetics, genetic bases of communicative disorders, and communicative problems themselves as genetic disorders. This is unfortunate. It is unfortunate because it can limit our clinical skills and, therefore, the benefits that could be available to our patients. As Sparks (1982) reminded us, children with genetic disorders do receive treatment from speech clinicians in schools, clinics, and other institutions. For example, Friedreich disease (or Friedreich ataxia) is an example of a genetic disease in which there are characteristic prosodic and segmental properties (Brancal & Ferrer, 1998). Adults with genetic communicative disorders also receive our services. In 1998, the American Speech–Language–Hearing Association (ASHA) surveyed 600 of its members to learn the extent to which we are (or are not) knowledgeable about genetics, genetic disorders, or genetic treatments. The results showed that 30% of those professionals surveyed had had no background or education in genetics, and fewer than 20% reported having had any formal course work (Willig *et al.*, 2000).

As we enter the twenty-first century of the Common Era, we recall that genetics has been a twentieth-century science. It is only in the last decades of the twentieth century, however, that novel advances have gotten the attention of the public media—for example, the fact that a sheep was cloned in the 1990s. Genetic breakthroughs and new discoveries are announced weekly, if not daily, in the press. Some of these are especially relevant to the study, diagnosis, and treatment of communicative disorders, such as the discovery of the genes for Usher syndrome, Duchenne muscular dystrophy, and some forms of breast cancer. A gene that underlies Rett syndrome has now been identified (Baker, 1999). We now know, for example, that the gene for Stickler syndrome is on the 12th chromosome; the gene for the velocardiofacial syndrome is on the 22nd; Usher syndrome (in its various forms) has been mapped to chromosomes 1, 3, 10, 11, and 14; Waardenburg syndrome to chromosome 2; and so on and on. Gene mutations on the 22nd chromosome are known to contribute to palatal clefts. Dyslexia seems to be located on the 6th, among others (see Chapter 6).

In an earlier book (Gerber, 1998), I had remarked that, prior to the twentieth century, our understanding of what came to be called genetics was more mystical than biological, even though the work of genetics' ancestor, Gregor Mendel, was done in the nineteenth century (1865). (By the way, Mendel seems to have been unaware of Charles Darwin.) Earlier writers—that is, before Mendel or Darwin—had talked about an *aura seminalis*, or a preexisting homunculus, or that development arises *de novo* (i.e., from nothing), although even Hippocrates had observed common traits within families.

Along came Mendel, growing peas, but no one seemed to notice or care until the start of the twentieth century. Thompson (1986) made the same observation. She said that it took 35 years for anyone to notice Mendel's work. Today, she added, genetics has achieved significance both for the basis of medicine and for clinical practice. Kelly (1986) also mentioned that it wasn't until the second half of the twentieth century when genetic disorders assumed increased significance to the health sciences. In 1910, Morgan observed that genes are organized on chromosomes, but it wasn't until 1942 that it was proposed that genes are made of DNA. By 1987, genes for muscular dystrophy, cystic fibrosis, Huntington disease, and breast cancer were isolated.

Grobstein (1988), in a wonderful book, pointed out that genetic diagnosis adds stress to increased significance. It is clear that we have entered the age of genetics, even if somewhat delayed. Nuland (2000), for example, predicts a time "when pharmacologic agents will be tailored to the genetic characteristics of specific diseases and even specific patients" (p. 130).

Mendel articulated three laws, and they remain the basis for the study of genetics. First is the law of *unit inheritance*, that is, the parents' traits are not simply blended somehow in the offspring, although this had been the common view before his work. Second, he observed *segregation*: a single pair of genes is not found in the same gamete (germ cell) but instead they segregate and pass to different gametes. And third, he noted that different gene pairs assort to different gametes independently of each other: the law of *independent assortment*. However, Mendel's laws indicate that each chromosome of a pair has an equal chance of being passed on; maybe, maybe not. Statistically, then, about half of the offspring of a given mating would express the traits of one parent and the other half would express the trait of the other parent. Now we know about segregation disorder, in which this half-and-half statistic is not realized. In one study of insects, only 3 to 5% of offspring expressed the characteristics associated with one parent (Ganetzky, 2000). Life isn't always simple and doesn't always follow statistical predictions.

II. WHAT IS THE PROBLEM?

Are communicative disorders genetic? How do we know? Hearing impairments and craniofacial anomalies are the clearest instances. As pointed out in the Preface, much of congenital deafness is genetic. For example, as many as half of the incidence of nonsyndromal hearing impairment is due to mutations in the GJB2 gene that encodes for an essential inner ear protein (McGuirt & Smith, 1999). This is true also of the incidence of early-onset and even of late-onset hearing impairment. Konigsmark (1971) had introduced the term "heredo-degen-erative" deafness. An illustration: We had followed the fourth deaf child of deaf parents. It was clear that she was not deaf at 1 week of age, less clear at 3 weeks, clear by 3 months that she was hearing impaired, and she had the poorest hearing of all four children by the time she was 7 years old.

Also, we sometimes use the inherently paradoxical term "early presbycusis," early old hearing; but indeed there is such a thing. Gates *et al.* (1999) found that up to 55% of the presbycusis phenotype is inherited. Another obvious example of a late-onset hearing impairment is otosclerosis. Otosclerosis is dominantly inherited, but is rarely seen clinically before the third decade of life. Shprintzen (1997) considered that virtually all instances of human disability and disease have a genetic component, although it may not be direct or immediately obvious. He was speaking primarily of craniofacial anomalies, but his comment applies rather generally. It was 1939 when Severina Nelson reported that stuttering runs in families; and, later, she and her colleagues showed that stuttering is concordant in twins (Nelson *et al.*, 1945). In fact, many years later, it was shown that stuttering is concordant in more than 80% of monozygotic twins but in only 10.5% of dizygotic twins (Godai *et al.,* 1976). Ingham, in 1987, reported that at least 75% of cases of stuttering are inherited.

Clefts of the lip with or without clefts of the palate may be of genetic origin, or may be produced by environmental factors or chromosomal anomalies. They are often multifactorial or, as many geneticists believe, caused by a single mutant gene with allelic restriction (Peterson-Falzone, 1989).

Language problems are not yet as clear, but there is evidence forthcoming (e.g., Lahey & Edwards, 1995; Spitz *et al.*, 1997; Tomblin & Buckwalter, 1998). Rice (1996) noted that there is not yet concrete evidence of a connection between one's genes or some combination of genes and one's grammatical abilities, but we should expect to find a genetic contribution of some sort. More recently, Zoll (1999) has suggested that genetic language disabilities may be linked to the 7q31 gene. A former colleague once made an interesting observation. She said that she was working with a child who had a significant language delay. The child's father couldn't spell. She, and I, submit that this is not just a coincidence. Wolff *et al.* (1996) have reported this also.

Dyslexia, also a language problem, is known to be inherited (Regehr & Kaplan, 1988; Wolff *et al.*, 1995). And so on and on. Hallahan and Kauffman (1997), in their excellent text, observed that familiality studies have shown that persons whose first-degree relatives have learning disabilities have an increased risk of having them, too. Of course, there is undoubtedly more than one genetic cause of learning disabilities, that is, genetic heterogeneity (Hallahan *et al.*, 1996). Still, there is greater concordance among monozygotes than among dizygotes, that is, these disorders occur more often in identical twins than in fraternal twins. Now there is some evidence that autism is inherited and the defective gene is located on chromosome 7 or chromosome 13 (Barrett *et al.*, 1999). Phonological language disorders, also, have been shown to be more common among children whose parents had such disorders than among controls (Felsenfeld *et al.*, 1995).

To be sure, we may be unable to discover the genetic properties of any one patient's disorder, but that doesn't mean that there are none. Some years ago, I did a survey of a large number of reports about the incidence of congenital deafness (Gerber, 1990). On the average, these reports show that about 43% of the incidences of congenital deafness are inherited. However, many of these reports include a category of etiology unknown. It seems to me that if 43% of the known incidents are genetic then about 43% of the unknown incidents must also be genetic. The problem is, as Kapur (1996) noted, the lack of prevalence data on congenital hearing impairment. Some 40% of prevalence is unknown, and this is due to the delay in diagnosis. Yet, he cited one study in which it was found that 24% of cases of congenital deafness were of recessive origin.

III. SOME LANGUAGE

To read what follows, we must all speak the same language. In this section, then, we define terms that are common throughout the book. The most important of them, of course, is *gene*. A gene is a segment of a molecule of deoxyribonucleic acid (DNA) that is involved in *polypeptide* synthesis and found at a specific location on a chromosome. In other words, it is the smallest unit of development. A polypeptide is a chain of amino acids leading to the development of proteins. The term *genetic*, then, refers to that which is determined by genes—it is not synonymous with *congenital*, which means only that the trait is present at birth for any reason (including inheritance). The *genome* is the full complement of DNA, that is, the total genetic information stored in the chromosomes of an organism. We read much press about the human genome project, a project begun in 1990 and to be completed by 2005, to identify and locate (i.e., map) all the genes. Genes are carried on the *chromosomes* that are found in every cell of the body that has a nucleus. In humans, there are 23 pairs of chromosomes (= 46, the *diploid* number); each member of the pair is said to be *haploid*. In humans, one of these pairs is the sex chromosomes, X and Y; all the other chromosomes are called *autosomes*. It is the Y chromosome that makes males male. Chromosomes that correspond in structure, position, and origin are said to be *homologous*. A *homozygote* is an individual who has identical genes at a given position on the chromosome. A *heterozygote*, then, is one who has different genes at a given locus.

It isn't necessary that all the genes in our genome appear in our offspring (Mendel's third law). If a genetic trait—say, blue eyes—passes from either or both parents to a child, we speak of *penetrance* to say that the trait penetrated in order to be expressed. The extent to which a trait penetrates is called *expressivity* (or expression). For example, it is possible for deaf parents to produce no deaf children, or all of their children could be deaf, or only some of their children might be deaf; this is penetrance. It is also possible, though, for some of those hearing-impaired children to have poorer hearing than their siblings; this is expressivity. We followed a family in which both parents and both children were deaf. Their mother had a recessive form of deafness (Pendred syndrome), but the children did not. Their father had a dominant gene for deafness that penetrated to both children. However, one of the children had poorer hearing than the other: expressivity.

What, then, is meant by recessive and dominant? A *recessive* trait appears only in children whose parents are homozygous, that is, carrying the same gene. *Dominant* inheritance occurs in children of heterozygotes; in other words, only one parent needs to pass the gene. The probability that a recessive trait would appear is 25% because both parents must carry the gene and each parent also has another *allele* (any alternative form of a gene) at the same locus. Genes found at the same site on the chromosome are said to be linked. Two or more traits could be transmitted across generations because they are determined by linked genes (Thompson, 1986). So the child could receive both genes for that trait from the parents, or could receive neither gene for that trait from the parents, or could receive one of each allele (Figure 1.1). Only if both genes were passed would the trait appear. There are five to ten different gene locations for deafness (Carrel, 1977). Given that only one parent needs to carry the gene for a heterozygous trait,

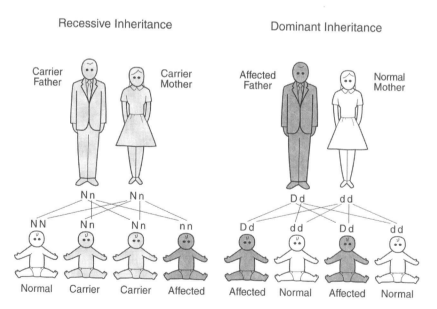

FIGURE 1.1   Recessive and dominant inheritance. Reprinted with permission from Lubs (1983).

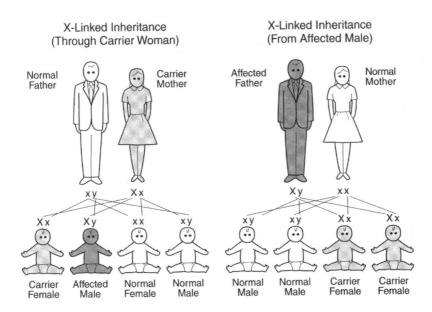

X-Linked Inheritance
(Through Carrier Woman)

X-Linked Inheritance
(From Affected Male)

Normal
Father

Carrier
Mother

Affected
Father

Normal
Mother

x y   X x   X y   x x

X x   X y   x x   x y   x y   x y   X x   X x

Carrier   Affected   Normal   Normal   Normal   Normal   Carrier   Carrier
Female   Male   Female   Male   Male   Male   Female   Female

FIGURE 1.2   X-linked inheritance. Reprinted with permission from Lubs (1983).

the odds are 50% that it would appear in the descendants. It is important to recall, though, that these odds recur with each pregnancy.

There are also some few disorders that are said to be X linked, that is, they are carried on the X chromosome and not on any autosome. Since males have only one X chromosome, these disorders are always passed from mother to son; they never express in daughters, but the daughters can be carriers (Figure 1.2). It is only the mother's allele on the X chromosome that matters. There are no known Y linked disorders.

Two more things are important. First is the *phenotype*. Phenotype is the total nature of a person in terms of anatomy, physiology, and biochemistry—and possibly behavior. It is the total of detectable characteristics produced by the interaction of the genotype and the environment. Your phenotype is who you are (biologically speaking), and any given phenotype is created both by your genes and by effects of the environment. For example, prenatal viral disease is well known to lead to congenital deafness, that is, a deaf phenotype. That has nothing to do with genes. On the other hand, your *genotype* is the full complement of your genes whether or not expressed. It is apparent, therefore, that phenotype can be changed with no change of genotype. The patient who expresses the sequelae of prenatal disease probably has had no change of genotype and has no increased probability of passing on that trait.

Can the genotype be changed? Indeed; and that is what is called a *mutation*, a permanent heritable change. Mutations are not necessarily either good or bad; they are only changes of genotype. It is probably a good guess to claim that virtually all changes of the human phenotype over the history of our species have been mutations. Batshaw (1997) observed that the incidence at which a mutation occurs in the population depends on the difference between the rate of mutation production and the rate of mutation removal, that is, although mutations may appear at some rate over some time in a given population, some mutations are lethal and therefore disappear from the population. He said further that some mutations are actually helpful in the normal process of evolution.

IV. SOME INFORMATION

This book is not limited to biological and clinical concerns. What follows in the succeeding chapters are the biological, clinical, and ethical consequences of our knowledge. We cover first the biological matters and then turn our attention to clinical concerns. But, what is meant by ethical consequences? What might ethical consequences be? What is the role of the genetic counselor? The possibility exists for genetic discrimination. Suppose that a certain person has a family history of a genetic disease. This person doesn't have the disease and may never have the disease, yet can be discriminated against because of the possibility of the disease arising. Who does the discrimination? It is possible that employers, prospective employers, and insurers could do it. This is a most serious matter that merits our attention.

We need also to consider the ethical consequences of gene therapy. Are we proposing to create a super human or to correct a genetic defect? If the latter, how? Who decides which patients do and which do not get such treatments? These are intriguing, and even frightening, questions; we must ask them. We must also consider the ethical principles underlying genetic counseling. No ethical genetic counselor would ever tell a family that they should or should not reproduce. They need to be told only what the odds are for a trait to penetrate. It is the prospective parents' decision, but it should be an informed decision based on known risk probabilities.

These kinds of questions have given rise to a program called ELSI (ethical, legal, and social implications of the human genome project). ELSI has four major priorities: (1) issues about informed consent, privacy, commercialization, and the possibility of patenting genes; (2) the clinical integration of new genetic techniques; (3) privacy and fairness in the use of genetic information; and (4) education about genetics for the general public as well as health professionals and other professionals.

Communicative disorders are indeed heritable. Many of them, probably most, really are inherited. Our ability to understand and to treat our patients and their families hinges on our appreciation of genetics.

REFERENCES

Baker, O. (1999). Faulty control gene underlies retardation. *Science News*, *156*, 214.

Barrett, S., Beck, J. C., Bernier, R., *et al.* (1999). An autosomal genomic screen for autism. *American Journal of Medical Genetics*, *88*, 609–615.

Batshaw, M. L. (1997). Heredity. In M. L. Batshaw (Ed.), *Children with disabilities* (pp. 17–33). Baltimore: Brookes.

Brancal, B., & Ferrer, M. (1998). Análisis perceptual de las características del habla en personas afectas de ataxias hereditarias. *Revista Logopedia, Foniatría, y Audiología*, *18*, 213–224.

Carrel, R. E. (1977). Epidemiology of hearing loss. In S. E. Gerber (Ed.), *Audiometry in infancy* (pp. 3–16). New York: Grune & Stratton.

Felsenfeld, S., McGue, M., & Broen, P. A. (1995). Familial aggregation of phonological disorders: Results from a 28-year follow up. *Journal of Speech and Hearing Research*, *38*, 1091–1107.

Ganetzky, B. (2000). Tracking down a cheating gene. *American Scientist*, *88*, 128–135.

Gates, G. A., Couropmitree, N. N., & Myers, R. H. (1999). Genetic associations in age-related hearing thresholds. *Archives of Otolaryngology—Head and Neck Surgery*, *125*, 654–659.

Gerber, S. E. (1990). Review of a high risk register for congenital or early-onset deafness. *British Journal of Audiology*, *24*, 347–356.

Gerber, S. E. (1998). *Etiology and prevention of communicative disorders*. San Diego: Singular.

Godai, U., Tatarelli, R., & Bonnani, G. (1976). Stuttering and tics in twins. *Acta Genetica Medicae et Gomellologiae*, *25*, 369–375.

Grobstein, C. (1988). *Science and the unborn*. New York: Basic Books.

Hallahan, D. P., & Kauffman, J. M. (1997). *Exceptional learners* (7th ed.). Boston: Allyn & Bacon.

Hallahan, D. P., Kauffman, J. M., & Lloyd, J. W. (1996). *Introduction to learning disabilities*. Boston: Allyn & Bacon.

Ingham, R. J. (1987). Stuttering: Recent trends in research and therapy. In H. Winitz (Ed.), *Human communication and its disorders* (pp. 1–63). Norwood, NJ: Ablex.

Jung, J. H. (1989). *Genetic syndromes in communication disorders*. Boston: College-Hill.

Kapur, Y. P. (1996). Epidemiology of childhood hearing loss. In S. E. Gerber (Ed.), *The handbook of pediatric audiology* (pp. 3–14). Washington, DC: Gallaudet University Press.

Kelly, T. E. (1986). *Clinical genetics and genetic counseling* (2nd ed.). Chicago: Year Book Medical.

Konigsmark, B. W. (1971). Hereditary congenital severe deafness syndromes. *Annals of Otology, Rhinology, & Laryngology*, *80*, 269–288.

Lahey, M., & Edwards, J. (1995). Specific language impairment: Preliminary investigation of factors associated with family history and with patterns of language. *Journal of Speech and Hearing Research*, *38*, 643–657.

Lubs, M.-L. (1983). In M. J. Krajicek & A. I. Tearney (Eds.), *Detection of developmental disorders in children* (2nd ed.). Austin: ProEd.

McGuirt, W. T., & Smith, R. J. H. (1999). Connexin 26 as a cause of hereditary hearing loss. *American Journal of Audiology*, *8*, 93–100.

Mendel, G. (1865). *Versuche über Pflantzenhybriden*. Brünn: Verhandlungen des Naturvorschenden Vereins.

Nelson, S. E. (1939). The role of heredity in stuttering. *Journal of Pediatrics*, *14*, 642–654.

Nelson, S. E., Hunter, N., & Walter, M. (1945). Stuttering in twin types. *Journal of Speech Disorders, 10,* 335–343.

Nuland, S. B. (2000). The misty crystal ball. *American Scholar, 69*(2), 129–132.

Peterson-Falzone, S. J. (1989). Basic concepts in congenital craniofacial defects. In K. R. Bzoch (Ed.), *Communicative disorders related to cleft lip and palate* (3rd ed.) (pp. 37–46). Boston: College-Hill.

Regehr, S. M., & Kaplan, B. J. (1988). Reading disability with motor problems may be an inherited subtype. *Pediatrics, 82,* 204–210.

Rice, M. L. (1996). Of language, phenotypes, and genetics: Building a cross-disciplinary platform for inquiry. In M. L. Rice (Ed.), *Toward a genetics of language* (pp. xi–xxv). Mahwah, NJ: Erlbaum.

Shprintzen, R. J. (1997). *Genetics, syndromes, and communication disorders.* San Diego: Singular.

Sparks, S. N. (1982). *Birth defects and speech–language disorders.* San Diego: College-Hill.

Spitz, R. V., Tallal, P., Flax, J., & Benasich, A. A. (1997). Look who's talking: A prospective study of familial transmission of language impairments. *Journal of Speech, Language, & Hearing Research, 40,* 990–1001.

Thompson, M. W. (1986). *Genetics in medicine* (4th ed.). Philadelphia: Saunders.

Tomblin, J. B., & Buckwalter, P. R. (1998). Heritability of poor language achievement among twins. *Journal of Speech, Language, & Hearing Research, 41,* 188–199.

Willig, S., Moss, S., & Lapham, E. V. (2000, March 14). The new genetics: What does it mean to us? *ASHA Leader, 4–5,* 10.

Wolff, P. H., Melngailis, I., Obregon, M., & Bedrosian, M. (1995). Family patterns of developmental dyslexia, Part II: Behavioral phenotypes. *American Journal of Genetics, 60,* 494–505.

Wolff, P. H., Melngailis, I., & Kotwica, K. (1996). Family patterns of developmental dyslexia. Part III: Spelling errors as a behavioral phenotype. *American Journal of Medical Genetics, 67,* 378–386.

Zoll, B. (1999, September). Zur Genetik der Sprachentwicklungsstörungen. *Sprach-Stimme-Gehör,* 127–180.

2

DELINEATION OF GENETIC COMPONENTS OF COMMUNICATIVE DISORDERS

GLENN E. GREEN

*Departments of Surgery, Pediatrics,
and Speech & Hearing Sciences
University of Arizona
Tucson, Arizona*

RICHARD J. H. SMITH

*Molecular Otolaryngology Research Laboratory
University of Iowa
Iowa City, Iowa*

I. Historical Aspects
    A. Common Environmental Exposures
    B. Common *in utero* Exposures
    C. Common Cultural Experiences
    D. Stochastic Variation
II. Genetic Inheritance Patterns
    A. Mendelian Inheritance
    B. Non-Mendelian Inheritance
    C. Penetrance and Expressivity
    D. Chromosomal Inheritance
    E. Multifactorial Inheritance
III. Identification of Genetic Components
    A. Twin Study
    B. Family Study
    C. Segregation Analysis

IV. Identification of Loci and Genes
    A. Protein Approaches
    B. Candidate Gene Approaches
    C. Positional Approaches
    D. Association Studies
    E. Animal Models
    F. Verification of Findings
V. Medical Significance
    A. Diagnostics
    B. Genetic Counseling
    C. Prognostics
    D. Therapeutics

I. HISTORICAL ASPECTS

Despite a frequently poor understanding of the development of most communicative disorders, strong evidence supports the existence of underlying genetic components. First appreciated even before the work of Gregor Mendel, the importance of hereditary factors in the development of various types of communicative disorders is suggested by the presence of multiple affected individuals within a single family. One hopes that, by delineating these genetic components, the etiology and pathogenesis will be more greatly understood and will lead to more accurate diagnoses, genetic counseling, prognoses, and treatment.

Since prehistoric times, characteristics have been known to pass from parents to their children. However, it was not until the nineteenth century that discoveries by Mendel established genes as the basis for inheritance. Deoxyribonucleic acid (DNA) was identified subsequently as the physical material by which information passes from parental cell to progeny cell (see, e.g., Watson, 1953). It was with the appreciation that genes were composed of DNA that the anatomic basis for Gregor Mendel's work was understood. The DNA of a single cell, packaged into bundles as chromosomes, holds enough information for the complete development of an adult. Through the human genome project, the human DNA sequence along with a complete list of its genes will offer unprecedented opportunities to decipher how this information leads to differences among individuals in disease and health (Stausberg *et al.*, 1999).

The central concept of genetics is the relation between *genotype* and *phenotype*. The phenotype is the physical appearance of an individual along with any manifestation of disease. The genotype is the complete genetic make-up (DNA) of an individual. To various degrees, phenotype is determined by genotype. However, a number of factors, including education and environmental exposures, also impact on the phenotype. The terms "nature" and "nurture" have been used to describe the effect of genetic and environmental influences on a trait. Both types of influences are usually present, affecting the outcome for an individual. For example, a deaf child raised in medieval times would be illiterate and unable to communicate, largely because of the environment in which he was raised. In contradistinction, a deaf child with Renier syndrome—microcephaly, mental retardation, spastic diplegia, and severe sensorineural hearing loss—raised today would be similarly illiterate and unable to communicate, largely because of the genetic basis of his deafness (Gustavson *et al.*, 1993). Identifying the genetic component of a disease is often difficult. This chapter reviews various ways that genes can impact on a genetic disorder and ways of delineating that risk.

The presence of a genetic component of a disease can be difficult to identify. Evidence supporting a genetic component includes familial clustering of cases, increased incidence in consanguineous matings (i.e., matings between closely related individuals), increased incidence within genetically segregated communities, increased risk to the children or siblings of affected individuals, and concurrence of identical twins for the disorder.

When more than one member in a family is affected by the same rare condition, it is tempting to speculate that there is a genetic contribution to the etiology. Indeed, before the laws of genetics were known, some communicative disorders were known to have a hereditary component often thought of as atavistic, from the Latin *atavus*, meaning "grandparent's great-grandfather." Traits were known to spread from generation to generation, recurring several times in a family.

However, it should be realized that there are several nongenetic reasons why a disease phenotype, causally unrelated to a genetic predisposition, can be seen recurrently in the same family. These nongenetic familial etiologies should be explicitly remembered when postulating a genetic contribution to a particular disorder. Heritability studies, as discussed below (see Section III), use statistical techniques to separate the genetic and environmental influences.

A. COMMON ENVIRONMENTAL EXPOSURES

Members of a family are frequently exposed to the same environmental insults. This may lead to recurrence. A poor or rich educational environment will usually have a marked effect on language outcomes. For example, the child of a mother with a cleft palate may develop hypernasal speech from mimicry, which, if not treated early in life, may be recalcitrant to treatment later. The combined effects of such factors as age, sex, education, parental education, early intervention, and household income may be appreciable, obscuring the effects of genetic factors.

B. COMMON *IN UTERO* EXPOSURES

A shared *in utero* exposure can lead to familial aggregations of problems. Fetal exposure to rubella can result in concurrence of deafness in identical twins. The hoarseness from juvenile-onset recurrent respiratory tract polyposis is caused by the human papilloma virus, which may spread from mother to child. Medical conditions—such as diabetes, lupus, and phenylketonuria—can all result in sequelae that can give the appearance of a genetic relationship.

C. COMMON CULTURAL EXPERIENCES

Shared religious and cultural values and exposures may lead to apparent familial segregation. One example is the language used in the home. Dialects and language-related difficulties, despite recurrence in a family, may be due to a shared cultural (rather than genetic) etiology. Differences in dietary habits, abuse of illicit drugs, and parental expectation may all result in a phenotype that can be misconstrued as being of genetic origin. Fetal alcohol syndrome—a constellation of features that may include a characteristic facial appearance, cleft lip and palate, and hearing loss—is one of many examples.

Association studies, where a trait is matched to a chromosomal pattern (as discussed below, Section IV.D), are particularly laden with problems due to shared environmental exposures. Any genetic characteristic found more frequently in a subpopulation will show positive association with environmental characteristics of that group. For example, genetic marker HLA-A1 (human leukocyte antigen, an antigen important for cell-mediated immunotoxicity) is associated with the ability to speak Mandarin, not because the ability to speak Mandarin has a genetic origin, but rather because Chinese are more likely to have the marker HLA-A1 and are more likely to speak Mandarin.

D. STOCHASTIC VARIATION

By chance, two members of a family may develop the same condition with no underlying genetic or environmental predisposition. Also, some members of a family may acquire a condition for reasons completely unrelated to other members of the family. A *phenocopy* is an individual with a phenotype similar to other members of a family but with a different etiology. An example would be an individual with noise-induced hearing loss who has brothers with nonsyndromal genetic hearing loss. However, some stochastic events may be influenced to some degree by a genetic predisposition (Kurnit *et al.*, 1987).

II. GENETIC INHERITANCE PATTERNS

Gregor Mendel first delineated the methods by which genetic factors are transmitted. Although most communicative disorders appear to have a complex inheritance pattern, a select group of communicative disorders has inheritance patterns that directly parallel those observed by Mendel in pea plants.

The simplest interaction between gene and phenotype is when a mutation within a single gene results in a clearly defined phenotype. Many genes have DNA sequences that vary from individual to individual. These different forms of a gene are each termed *alleles*. Most of this DNA variation is of no appreciable consequence and is ascribed as *benign polymorphism*. However, sometimes the change in DNA structure does result in a recognizable difference in phenotype.

Each person generally has two copies of each gene, one copy on the maternally inherited chromosome and one copy on the paternally inherited chromosome. The broadest exceptions are the genes found on the sex chromosomes: the X and Y chromosomes. (The other 22 chromosomes are called *autosomes*.) For the X chromosome, males usually have only one copy, while females usually have two copies. Thus, most people can have, or carry, two alleles for each gene. If the two alleles for a gene are identical, the person is *homozygous* for the gene. If the two alleles differ, the person is *heterozygous*. The most common allele is usually called the *wild-type* (i.e., the type usually found in nature). When a person carries two non-wild-type alleles, the person is *compound heterozygous*.

Gregor Mendel was the first individual to identify the law of segregation (see Chapter 1). Succinctly, the law of segregation states that the alleles inherited from our parents remain discrete entities rather than merging. For each gene, only one of two alleles is passed on to an individual's child. Whether the parent's phenotype is also passed on to a child is dependent on several additional factors, discussed below in this section.

A. MENDELIAN INHERITANCE

Gregor Mendel first discovered the basis of heredity in his studies of pea plants. He developed the concepts of dominant and recessive genes. In a heterozygous state, the dominant phenotype will be expressed and the recessive phenotype will be camouflaged. Each of these Mendelian patterns is known to account for the inheritance pattern of several communicative disorders.

Many disease-causing alleles cause a phenotypic change in the heterozygous state. These alleles are termed *dominant*. In an autosomal dominant disorder, individuals inheriting a mutant gene develop the disease phenotype. From the law of segregation, on average, half of the children of an affected individual will likewise inherit the disease-causing allele.

In contradistinction, for a *recessive* disorder to occur, both alleles must be affected. An individual with only one mutant allele will not develop the phenotype and is called a carrier. From the law of segregation, by chance, one in four children born to two carriers will be affected, having inherited both the maternal and paternal mutant alleles. Two out of four children will inherit exactly one copy of the mutant allele (either the maternal or the paternal copy) and will be unaffected carriers. One in four will inherit both the maternal and paternal wild-type alleles and be a noncarrier. Carriers and noncarriers are indistinguishable from a phenotypic standpoint. Thus, an average of two of three phenotypically normal children of two carriers will be carriers, and one of three will be a noncarrier.

In an *X-linked* disorder, the gene is passed on the X-chromosome. Nearly all X-linked disorders are recessive. For X-linked recessive disorders, a woman who has the mutant allele will not have the phenotype. By chance, half of a carrier's sons will inherit the mutant X-allele, and will be affected because they have no normal copy of the gene. This is known as *hemizygosity*. The other half will inherit the wild-type allele. All of the daughters of an affected man will be carriers of the mutant allele, but none of his sons will inherit his X-chromosome.

B. NON-MENDELIAN INHERITANCE

Outside of the typical Mendelian inheritance patterns, there are several other means by which a mutant allele can be made manifest. Although markedly dissimilar in mechanism, these atypical inheritance patterns are grouped as non-Mendelian inheritance (Austin & Hall, 1992).

In rare cases, both alleles of a gene are inherited from the same parent. An individual may inherit a double copy of an allele from one parent and no alleles from the other parent (*uniparental disomy*). In this case, despite only one parent being a carrier for a recessive disease, a child still may be homozygous for this mutation and develop the disease phenotype.

Much more frequently, there is a variation between the use of the genes inherited from one's mother and the genes inherited from one's father. Genes that are expressed exclusively from the maternally inherited allele or the paternally inherited allele are *imprinted*. For genes with imprinting, only one allele is activated. In this case, a mutant allele will cause phenotype changes only if it is inherited from the mother (maternal imprinting) or the father (paternal imprinting). Angelman syndrome—a disorder characterized by mental deficiency, inappropriate laughter, a characteristic facial appearance, and the absence of speech development—is due exclusively to maternally derived deletions in the 15q11.2–q13 region and imprinting (Williams *et al.*, 1990).

In unusual cases, the effects of a mutation may become worse in succeeding generations, a process called *anticipation*. This is related usually to progressive expansion of a repeated stretch of DNA. Myotonic dystrophy—a muscular dystrophy with early involvement of head and neck musculature resulting in characteristic speech and swallowing difficulties—is caused by progressive amplification of a trinucleotide repeat in the noncoding portion of a serine–threonine kinase gene such that succeeding generations have increasingly virulent manifestations (Sabouri *et al.*, 1993).

In addition to 23 pairs of nuclear chromosomes, cells will usually contain several mitochondrial chromosomes. Mitochondria are organelles that contain DNA, ribosomes, and enzymes. The mitochondrial DNA may differ in sequence among the mitochondria found within a single cell. In the process of egg formation, most of the mitochondria become a single type (*homoplasmy*), although some mitochondria may continue to be different (*heteroplasmy*). Because an egg contains many more mitochondria than a spermatozoan, mitochondrial DNA is inherited nearly exclusively from one's mother. *Mitochondrial inheritance*, also called cytoplasmic inheritance, is marked by both sons and daughters of an affected woman (but not an affected man) having the mutant phenotype. Due to homoplasmy, children are often more severely affected than their mother. Deafness is associated with many syndromic and nonsyndromic mitochondrial mutations, and may be a preeminent cause of deafness in some populations (Estivill *et al.*, 1998).

Other factors can result in apparently complex inheritance patterns. Some genes have a very high spontaneous mutation rate. These *de novo* mutations result in a dominant disease appearing in a family with no previous history of the disorder. These *de novo* mutations rarely occur only in the germline cells. In this case, a parent can sire many children with a dominant disease despite not having the disease. *De novo* mutations can also affect exclusively non-germline cells. These somatic mutations result in the affected person having the disease, but that person is at no risk to pass on the disease to their children.

Illegitimacy, mislabeled specimens, adoption, and incorrectly constructed pedigrees may all result in an unusual appearance to the pedigree and should be specifically excluded.

C. PENETRANCE AND EXPRESSIVITY

In classic Mendelian genetics, phenotypic identity occurs among individuals with the same genotype. However, many individuals have widely different phenotypes despite inheriting identical alleles. When an individual inherits a disease-causing gene, yet does not develop the disease phenotype, the gene is nonpenetrant. By definition, nonpenetrant individuals cannot be distinguished phenotypically from their siblings who do not have mutant genes. The *penetrance* of a disease is the proportion of individuals showing the expected phenotype. Decreased penetrance markedly hampers efforts to identify disease-causing genes.

The *expressivity* is the degree to which the phenotype is manifested in penetrant individuals. When the phenotype is not the same among all individuals with a mutation, a gene is said to have variable expressivity. Expression may vary both within a family and among families. Diseases with marked intrafamilial variation that nonetheless have a consistent phenotype within any particular family usually have distinct mutations. Other factors such as the background genotype may also have an effect. Branchio-oto-renal syndrome—deafness, renal abnormalities, and branchial cleft cysts—may have marked differences in phenotype, with various degrees of renal abnormalities from complete kidney failure to normal kidney function (Smith & Schwartz, 1998).

Penetrance and expressivity may vary by sex. In *sex-limited inheritance*, only one sex exhibits the trait; in the other sex it is nonpenetrant. In *sex-influenced inheritance*, the expression of the phenotype varies between the sexes or the penetrance varies between the sexes. For most communicative disorders, sex-influenced inheritance, rather than X-linked inheritance, is the more likely explanation for a high proportion of affected males.

D. CHROMOSOMAL INHERITANCE

In many disorders, the causative defect involves much more than a discrete portion of a single gene. Deletion of a small portion of a chromosome may result in a distinct phenotypic constellation or syndrome. Velocardiofacial syndrome—a relatively common cause of cleft palate or submucous cleft palate associated with hypernasal speech and subtle facial anomalies, specific learning difficulties, cardiac abnormalities, and aberrant internal carotid arteries—is characterized by deletions in a specific portion of the long arm of chromosome 22 (Ryan *et al.*, 1997). Delineation of this region has led to the use of FISH (fluorescent *in situ* hybridization) with a labeled DNA probe as the primary means of diagnosis of this syndrome at present.

As the area of deletion or duplication becomes larger, progressively more genes become affected. This leads to a *contiguous gene syndrome* with altered function of a series of chromosomally adjacent genes. Individuals with contiguous gene syndromes and microdeletions of chromosomes are often the most valuable patients for direct identification of a gene's location in that the locus can be inferred directly from the location of the chromosomal abnormality.

Other chromosomal abnormalities involve large portions of chromosomes or entire chromosomes. Trisomy 21—the most common form of Down syndrome—for example, consists of an entire extra chromosome 21. Monosomy is loss of a chromosome and is exemplified by the single X chromosome seen in individuals with Turner syndrome—characteristic facial and body appearance, gonadal abnormalities, cardiac defects, and frequent hearing loss. Most monosomies and trisomies are not compatible with life.

Chromosomal abnormalities are usually inherited in a dominant fashion. Usually, a strong family history is absent since most chromosomal abnormalities occur *de novo*. Certain specific chromosomal rearrangements—such as a Robertsonian translocation (i.e., one formed from two acrocentric chromosomes and containing the long arms of both and the centromere of one)—can predispose to recurrence despite a normal phenotypic appearance of the carrier.

E. MULTIFACTORIAL INHERITANCE

Most communicative disorders do not have a single, clearly defined genetic etiology. A phenotype that does not exhibit classic Mendelian inheritance pattern is said to have a *complex inheritance pattern* (Lander & Schork, 1994). Complex inheritance patterns occur in most *heterogeneous* diseases that have multiple different phenotypically indistinguishable etiologies. These are especially seen in deaf marriages, where multiple different mutant Mendelian genes may be present in each spouse, including genes unrelated to the cause of deafness for a particular individual. Complexity also occurs when a genotype does not yield a consistent phenotype, whether because of penetrance, expressivity, environmental influences, or chance.

For many communicative disorders, it appears that several genes combine to determine phenotype. A single gene that controls the phenotypic effect of another locus is said to exhibit *epistasis*. This modifier locus determines the phenotypic expression of the second locus. For example, DFNB26—recessive deafness occurring in a large Pakistani family—has been found to have a limited penetrance. This penetrance appears to be modulated by a single additional locus (Riazuddin *et al.*, 1999). More commonly, several genes may interact to produce the phenotype, a process called *polygenic inheritance*. Polygenic inheritance is most easily demonstrated in laboratory animals, where the effect of strain background on gene expression may be clearly seen. However, this process may also play a role in human communicative disorders such as DFNB15—recessive deafness in a consanguineous Indian family—which has been shown to have two chromosomal locations shared among all affected members (Chen *et al.*, 1997).

To differentiate among heterogeneity, epistatic effect, and polygenic inheritance, the inheritance patterns of several genomes within a family or segregation analysis is usually required (as discussed below, Section III.C). Environmental factors may also have a prominent role in some diseases. For example, the mitochondrial mutation 1555A>G results in deafness much more frequently in individuals exposed to aminoglycoside antibiotics (Estivill *et al.*, 1998).

III. IDENTIFICATION OF GENETIC COMPONENTS

The goal of genetic studies is to identify the role of genes in determination of phenotype. Determining whether a trait has a genetic component is often not straightforward. A study that determines the amount of genetic contribution to a trait is called a heritability study. *Heritability* is an expression of the degree to which total phenotypic variation is due to genetic variation.

The basis behind all heritability studies is a comparison in the phenotypes between persons who share much genetic material with those who share little genetic material. If individuals sharing much genetic material are more likely to have the disease than those sharing less, then genetic factors are deduced to play a significant role in the phenotype. On the other hand, a lack of difference in the likelihood of disease appearance implies that genetic factors do not play a significant role. Heritability (H), by definition, is the ratio of genetic variance (V_G) to phenotypic variance (V_T). Phenotypic variance is the sum of genetic variance and environmental variance (V_E):

$$H = V_G/(V_G+V_E)$$

To properly determine the heritability of traits, an analysis of environmental effects must be included. Also, it should be noted that heritability is dependent on the environment being studied. For example, deafness in an impoverished area with high rates of infection-related deafness will have a lower heritability than deafness in an affluent area.

A. TWIN STUDY

In a twin study, the concordance of a phenotype in identical twins is compared to the concordance in fraternal twins. Identical twins share 100% of their genetic material, while fraternal twins share approximately only 50% of their genetic material. If identical twins are more likely than nonidentical twins to share a phenotype, a genetic component can be deduced. If identical twins are several times more likely to share a phenotype, the existence of multiple interacting genes is likely. Theoretically, heritability equals two times the difference in variability between fraternal and identical twins divided by the total variance. In most twin studies, the existence of subtle environmental differences between fraternal and identical twin environments must be accounted for (Guo, 1999).

Twin studies have been valuable in identifying genetic predisposition to many complex communicative disorders. Even in the general population, differences in verbal aptitude and phonological decoding ability are highly heritable (Light *et al.*, 1998). In other words, much of the difference in verbal aptitudes and phonologic decoding ability among individuals is genetically, rather than environmentally, related in the United States.

Especially valuable twin studies evaluate twins who were adopted by different families and raised separately. In this unique setting, the role of shared environmental factors is particularly reduced, enabling stronger deduction of genetic components.

B. FAMILY STUDY

With the exception of *de novo* mutations, if having one child with a disease does not increase the probability of having a second child with the disease, there is no hereditary component. Risch (1990) developed the use of R, representing the relative risk, in identification of loci. For example, the relative risk of a sib (R_s) for dyslexia equals the ratio of the probability of a sib of someone with dyslexia having dyslexia divided by the random chance for someone to have dyslexia. The relative risks of extended family members are especially helpful in identifying genetic components of a communicative disorder. A comparison of risk ratios by relationship enables estimation of the number of genes involved in a trait and mode of inheritance, despite phenocopies and decreased penetrance. For quantitative rather than qualitative traits, heritability is the equivalent of relative risk, which can be solved using various algorithms (de Andrade *et al.*, 1999).

C. SEGREGATION ANALYSIS

Segregation analysis examines statistically the clustering of diseases within families and can be applied only to relatively common disorders. The expected ratios of affected individuals of various relation to the index are compared under different models of inheritance. Through statistical analysis of large numbers of individuals, the probabilities of different inheritance patterns for the disease are compared. Segregation studies also allow estimates of allele frequencies, penetrance, and the proportion of diseases due to hereditary and nonhereditary components. Because individuals with affected sibs are usually more likely to be counted in a segregation analysis, it is imperative to correct for ascertainment bias (Shute & Ewens, 1988).

IV. IDENTIFICATION OF LOCI AND GENES

Genetic contributions to a disease can be identified through three basic approaches: the traditional genetics approach, the candidate gene approach, and the positional approach. In traditional genetics, the aberrant protein is first identified; and, from knowledge of the amino acid composition of the protein, the encoding gene is determined. In the candidate gene approach, the pathophysiology of the disease suggests a gene to examine for mutations. In positional genetics, formerly called reverse genetics, the chromosomal location for the disease is determined and the gene is identified within this chromosomal location (see Section IV.C). The vast majority of disease-causing loci have been identified through positional or combination positional–candidate approaches.

A. PROTEIN APPROACHES

Sometimes, through enzymatic studies or other direct techniques, the aberrant protein underlying a disease process can be identified directly. For example, the inner ear protein Connexin 26 forms part of the ability to maintain normal auditory function. Mutations in the *GJB2* gene, which codes for Connexin 26, have been identified as the cause of as many as half of the incidents of nonsyndromic, severe to profound, sensorineural deafness (McGuirt & Smith, 1999).

Previously, protein sequencing followed by the use of molecular probes based on the genetic code would be used to probe a genetic library to find the encoding gene. Alternatively, antibodies prepared to the protein can be used to screen genes that have been cloned in such a way that they are expressed by the bacteria. Then the identified gene is screened for mutations. This approach was used to determine many of the first-identified hereditary diseases, such as sickle cell anemia and the thalassemias. It has also been used to identify the prototypes of many families of functionally related proteins, such as the calcium channel subunits. This approach has also been used to identify the cochlear protein Organ of Corti Protein II (OCP2), which is not known to be associated with any hearing disorder. This approach, however, is inapplicable to nearly all communicative disorders (Brown *et al.*, 1996).

B. CANDIDATE GENE APPROACHES

Sometimes a specific constellation of symptoms is highly suggestive of an etiologic basis for a condition. In the candidate gene approach, a protein that is putatively related to the disease is examined for mutations in affected individuals. This approach has proven most helpful in various types of syndromic disorders, where the constellation of symptoms can suggest a possible protein. For example, the constellation of deafness in association with prolongation of the cardiac QT interval (Jervell and Lange–Nielsen syndrome) suggested a mutation in a cardio–cochlear potassium channel gene (Green *et al.*, 1994). Subsequent examination of cardio–cochlear potassium channel genes identified etiologic mutations (Neyroud *et al.*, 1997; Tyson *et al.*, 1997).

If a gene is localized to a specific chromosomal area, as discussed below, the genes in that area can be examined. One of these genes may suggest a pathogenic process and become a candidate gene. This positional–candidate approach is often able to identify the cause of a disease.

C. POSITIONAL APPROACHES

The recent explosion in disease loci identification has occurred through positional approaches to identifying genes. In positional approaches, no knowledge of the disease process is needed. In fact, many of the genes identified have yielded novel understanding of pathogenic mechanisms. The first step in the positional approach is to identify the chromosomal location, or *locus*, of the gene. Subsequently, fine mapping and mutation analysis are used to identify the involved genes.

1. Identifying the Loci

Based on Mendel's law of independent assortment, genes on different chromosomes are inherited independently of one another; if a paternal copy of one gene is passed to a child, it is equally likely that the maternal or paternal copy of a gene will be passed on to a child. The situation is different when two genes are on the same chromosome: if a man's paternally inherited copy of one gene is passed to a child, it is more likely that the man's paternally inherited copy (as opposed to the maternally inherited copy) of the second gene will be passed also. The closer two genes are on a chromosome of a child, the more likely both copies originated from the same grandparent. This phenomenon is called *linkage*. When there is complete identity between the origin of two loci, the loci are completely linked. The chromosomal location of a disease-related allele is determined by identifying complete linkage between a disease and marker loci, loci of known location. These marker loci can be used to verify or disprove linkage if they are polymorphic. The large and successful effort to identify hundreds of highly polymorphic markers enables the identification of disease-linked locations for families of adequate size and clear inheritance pattern (Murray *et al.*, 1994). Under proper conditions, and with enough patients, these markers can be used to identify a locus with only affected pairs of relatives based on the increased sharing of the disease-causing chromosomal location (Guo & Elston, 1999)

If an unpositioned locus is linked to a gene of known chromosomal location, the location of the unpositioned locus can be inferred (Lander & Schork, 1994). During meiosis, the maternal and paternal alleles can be partially mixed in a *crossover* or *recombination*. The presence of crossovers limits the amount of the chromosome that is completely linked. The initial steps of a positional approach are to establish linkage between a phenotype and a previously positioned locus and then to delineate the area of complete linkage or nonrecombination.

By chance, alleles on different chromosomes can be inherited from the same parent, a false linkage. To avoid incorrectly positioning a genetic locus, much stricter p-values are maintained in genetics in comparison to other scientific fields. The p-values are usually expressed as an LOD score, the logarithm of the odds of an event occurring by chance to the odds of an event occurring if there is linkage. By convention, linkage is established between a phenotype and a locus when the LOD score is greater than or equal to 3 ($p < 0.001$) and refuted when the LOD score is less than or equal to -2 ($p < 0.01$).

If a disease has a genetic component, the most straightforward means to identify the related gene is to study large families where the inheritance is Mendelian. For a dominant disease, a locus can potentially be identified with DNA from 12 affected members. For a fully penetrant disease, unaffected sibs of affected individuals can be substituted.

For a recessive disease, approximately six affected members of a single family would be required. Outside of segregated communities, it is very difficult to identify this many patients. Consanguineous families, commonly found in some cultures, provide a stronger ability to identify recessive loci. The power of consanguineous marriages stems from the fact that both of the mutant alleles usually come from a single progenitor. The identification of this area of homozygosity by descent increases the power of this method. In an uncle–niece marriage, five affected members are needed to identify a locus. Even fewer affected children are needed to identify a locus from a first-cousin marriage (four affected children) or a second-cousin marriage (only three affected children).

Computer analysis is prerequisite for confirmation of locus identification. Programs such as the widely used LINKAGE program can include parameters for phenocopies and decreased penetrance. Consanguineous families, which contain the same ancestors on both sides of the family tree, a loop, pose additional computing problems that have been solved (Becker et al., 1998). Alternative methods have been designed to identify concurrently multiple interacting genes involved in complex multigenic disorders (Bhat et al., 1999).

Complex traits become much more solvable when subcomponents with a Mendelian inheritance can be culled out. Methods used to do this include carefully delineating the clinical phenotype, especially with identification of subtle syndromic stigmata; identifying patients with specific time periods of onset (e.g., congenital deafness or delayed loss of speech ability); limiting study to families with a clearly delineated phenotype; examination of specific ethnic groups; and identification of families who are likely to have a common genetic etiology and that are large enough for a linkage study. For the many communicative disorders that are quantitative, rather than qualitative, different methods are required to delineate hereditary loci (de Andrade et al., 1999).

2. Fine-Mapping

After a locus is linked, the interval in which the gene is located is narrowed. Polymorphisms are examined near the linkage site until the interval is precisely defined in which there is complete concordance between the inherited chromosomal segment and the phenotype. Genes in this chromosomal segment historically would be determined through laboratory methods. Currently, the results of extensive mapping and gene identification enable electronic databases to be searched to identify the genes in the interval. Raw DNA sequence can also be examined for genes using established, but still imprecise, algorithms. Completion of the human genome project will enable direct knowledge of the genes within the interval.

3. Identifying the Mutation

After the genes within the narrowly defined region are demarcated, they are sequentially examined for disease-causing mutation. Knowledge of the function of the gene may suggest more likely candidates within this interval. To examine a gene for mutations, the boundaries of each splice-site are determined. The entire portion of the gene encoding the protein is screened. To identify the causative mutation, splicing-related noncoding sequence and regulatory domains may need to be examined as well. There are several well-developed methods for mutation identification (Forrest *et al.*, 1995).

D. ASSOCIATION STUDIES

In contrast to positional studies that identify consistent chromosomal concurrence with a phenotype, association studies identify consistent allelic concurrence with a phenotype. The classic association studies were between disease phenotype and HLA alleles.

Association studies may be positive for three reasons. First, the allele may be causing disease. Second, the allele may be chromosomally adjacent to the true locus. In such a case, as the chromosomal segment with the disease is passed to subsequent generations, the alleles near that locus are also consistently passed through the population. When the true locus and adjacent alleles match more frequently than would be expected by random assortment, the marker allele is said to be in *linkage disequilibrium*. Third, positive associations can arise due to subpopulations that are more likely to have a gene and more likely to have a particular allele, a process known as *population admixture*.

To reduce the chance of spurious association, it is important to try to obtain a homogeneous population and to select a control group of equivalent ethnicity in looking at marker alleles. A test to verify the findings of a heritability study is a transmission disequilibrium test. In this test, a second sample from the same population is used to determine whether parents who are heterozygous for the associated allele more frequently pass that allele to affected individuals than to unaffected individuals.

E. ANIMAL MODELS

Animal models can be used to complement many of the techniques described. The particular value of the mouse model for hereditary hearing loss has been reviewed by Probst and Camper (1999). Because animals can be specifically bred with one another and because specific strains exist, it is often very easy to rapidly determine the chromosomal location of Mendelian loci. More complex inheritance patterns, especially multifactorial inheritance patterns, are particularly amenable to a mouse model.

To a large extent, the chromosomal order and location of genes are conserved among mammals, a relation called *synteny*. Thus, if the genetic location in the mouse is known, often the homologous location in the human genome can be determined from the location of adjacent genes. Also, if a mouse gene is known, the homologous human gene can be examined for mutations. Due to the great similarity between mouse and human genes, homologous human genes can be identified through the polymerase chain reaction with degenerate primers or by library screening or by computative examination of electronic databases.

Other methods of gene identification are suitable exclusively to examination of an animal model. In the phenotype rescue approach, various genes are inserted into the mouse genome to identify a mouse with a normal phenotype. The etiologic gene can be inferred from the gene that restored or rescued the wild-type phenotype, as for DFNB3—a form of recessive nonsyndromal deafness (Wang *et al.*, 1998).

Happenstance insertions in transgenic knockout mice may disrupt a gene leading to a phenotype of interest as was seen by Alagramam *et al.* (1999). The disrupted gene can often readily be determined using knowledge of the transgenic insert.

F. VERIFICATION OF FINDINGS

Regardless of the technique employed, identification of a mutation within a gene does not establish the gene as the etiology. Additional corroboration is needed. To verify that a mutation is not a benign polymorphism, several control individuals from the same ethnic group as the affected individuals should be screened for a similar mutation. The identification of similar mutations in unrelated families and the identification of *de novo* mutations in individuals without a family history is strongly supportive of correct gene identification. The gold standard at present is the generation of an animal model with a homologous mutation; the concurrence of phenotype establishes the mutation as the cause of the disorder. Unfortunately, animal equivalents of many communicative disorders may not be as clearly identifiable as morphologic disorders.

V. MEDICAL SIGNIFICANCE

Identification of the etiology of a disorder in a particular patient carries valuable medical information. Broadly, benefits may accrue in diagnostics, genetic counseling, prognostics, or treatment.

A. DIAGNOSTICS

Direct molecular diagnostic tests are the first benefit accrued from the identification of pathogenic genes. The unrivaled precision of genetic tests allows for more accurate comparison of treatment modalities and outcomes, improving the caliber of research for therapeutic intervention. Genetic tests enable diagnoses to be made prenatally and well before the onset of any overt symptoms or in the presence of only subtle manifestations. The ability to make early, accurate diagnoses enables early intervention to be implemented and studied (see Chapter 11).

A molecular diagnosis may also eliminate the need for a medical diagnostic work-up. The medical diagnostic work-up for different communicative disorders is avoided, possibly including such non-benign diagnostic tools as lumbar punctures, tissue biopsies, and general anesthetics for imaging studies.

Molecular diagnostic tests may also identify individuals at high risk through broad-based screening procedures. However, decreased penetrance and variable expressivity may limit more widespread clinical implementation.

B. GENETIC COUNSELING

The second benefit of a molecular diagnosis is genetic counseling. Often, precise Mendelian recurrence risks can be assigned after a molecular diagnosis. Even when a molecular diagnosis cannot be made, exclusion of certain genetic etiologies may improve counseling. For example, in nonfamilial deafness, genetic testing for *GJB2* mutations—highly prevalent mutations (3% carrier rate in the Midwestern United States) that cause much of hereditary deafness, especially in families with no history of deafness—separates two groups, one having a Mendelian recurrence chance of 25% and the other having a recurrence chance of 14% (Green *et al.*, 1999).

C. PROGNOSTICS

Medical prognostic ability may improve with molecular diagnosis. By precisely defining separate groups, the response of those groups to different therapeutic interventions can be compared. The risk of rare complications may also be identified and appropriate screening procedures instituted. For example, the identification of *GJB2* mutations in deafness identifies a group with excellent response to cochlear implantation and a group at low risk for deafness comorbidities such as mental retardation or vision loss.

D. THERAPEUTICS

Rarely, after determining the cause of a disorder, a previously unsuspected intervention becomes obvious. Also, specific avoidance measures may be suggested to avoid complications. For example, in Jervell and Lange–Nielsen syndrome—deafness accompanied by a heart repolarization abnormality—specific drugs should be avoided that otherwise may precipitate sudden death. Since a molecular diagnosis can be made even prenatally, known medical and educational interventions can be begun prior to the development of any overt symptoms, probably improving outcomes. The identification of the molecular basis of a disorder enables further studies on the pathophysiology of disease. Homologous animal models may be generated to study different therapeutic interventions more rigorously than is possible with humans.

Determining whether these types of interventions or direct genetic manipulation can alleviate the problems of communicative disorders remains one of the exciting endeavors of our time.

REFERENCES

Alagramam, K. N., Kwon, H. Y., Cacheiro, N. L., Stubbs, L., Wright, C. G., Erway, L. C., & Woychik, R. P. (1999). A new mouse insertional mutation that causes sensorineural deafness and vestibular defects. *Genetics, 152,* 1691–1699.

Austin, K. D., & Hall, J. G. (1992). Nontraditional inheritance. *Pediatric Clinics of North America, 39,* 335–348.

Becker, A., Geiger, D., & Schaffer, A. A. (1998). Automatic selection of loop breakers for genetic linkage analysis. *Human Heredity, 48,* 49–60.

Bhat, A., Heath, S. C., & Ott, J. (1999). Heterogeneity for multiple disease loci in linkage analysis. *Human Heredity, 49,* 229–231.

Brown, K. A., Leek, J. P., Lench, N. J., Moynihan, L. M., Markham, A. F., & Mueller, R. F. (1996). Human sequences homologous to the gene for the cochlear protein OCP-II do not map to currently known non-syndromic hearing loss loci. *Annals of Human Genetics, 60,* 385–389.

Chen, A., Wayne, S., Bell, A., Ramesh, A., Srisailapathy, C. R., Scott, D. A., Sheffield, V. C., Van Hauwe, P., Zbar, R. I., Ashley, J., Lovett, M., Van Camp, G., & Smith, R. J. (1997). New gene for autosomal recessive non-syndromic hearing loss maps to either chromosome 3q or 19p. *American Journal of Medical Genetics, 71,* 467–471.

de Andrade, M., Amos, C. I., & Thiele, T. J. (1999). Methods to estimate genetic components of variance for quantitative traits in family studies. *Genetic Epidemiology, 17,* 64–76.

Estivill, X., Govea, N., Barcelo, E., Badenas, C., Romero, E., Moral, L., Scozzri, R., D'Urbano, L., Zeviani, M., & Torroni, A. (1998). Familial progressive sensorineural deafness is mainly due to the mtDNA A1555G mutation and is enhanced by treatment of aminoglycosides. *American Journal of Human Genetics, 62,* 27–35.

Forrest, S., Cotton, R., Landegren, U., & Southern, E. (1995). How to find all those mutations. *Nature Genetics, 10,* 375–376.

Green, G. E., Drescher D. G., & Beisel, K. W. (1994). Identification of a cardiac-type potassium channel expressed in the mouse cochlea. *Abstracts of the Association for Research in Otolaryngology, 17,* 320.

Green, G. E., Scott, D. A., McDonald, J. M., Woodworth, G. G., Sheffield, V. C., & Smith, R. J. (1999). Carrier rates in the midwestern United States for *GJB2* mutations causing inherited deafness. *Journal of the American Medical Association, 281*, 2211–2216.

Guo, S. (1999). The behaviors of some heritability estimators in the complete absence of genetic factors. *Human Heredity, 49*, 215–228.

Guo, X., & Elston, R. C. (1999). Linkage information content of polymorphic genetic markers. *Human Heredity, 49*, 112–118.

Gustavson, K. H., Anneren, G., Malmgren, H., Dahl, N., Ljunggren, C. G., & Backman, H. (1993). New X-linked syndrome with severe mental retardation, severely impaired vision, severe hearing defect, epileptic seizures, spasticity, restricted joint mobility, and early death. *American Journal of Medical Genetics, 45*, 654–658.

Kurnit, D. M., Layton, W. M., & Matthysse, S. (1987). Genetics, chance, and morphogenesis. *American Journal of Human Genetics, 41*, 979–995.

Lander, E. S., & Schork, N. J. (1994). Genetic dissection of complex traits. *Science, 266*, 2037–2048.

Light, J. G., DeFries, J. C., & Olson, R. K. (1998). Multivariate behavioral genetic analysis of achievement and cognitive measures in reading-disabled and control twin pairs. *Human Biology, 70*, 215–237.

McGuirt, W. T., & Smith, R. J. H. (1999). Connexin 26 as a cause of hereditary hearing loss. *American Journal of Audiology, 8*, 93–100.

Murray, J. C., Buetow, K. H., Weber, J. L., Ludwigsen, S., Scherpbier-Heddema, T., Manion, F., Quillen, J., Sheffield, V. C., Sunden, S., Duyk, G. M., Weissenbach, J., Gyapay, G., Dib, C., Morrissette, J., Lathrop, G. M., Vignal, A., White, R., Matsunami, N., Gerken, S., Melis, R., Albertsen, H., Plaetke, R., Odelberg, S., Ward, D., Dausset, J., Cohen, D., & Cann, H. (1994). A comprehensive human linkage map with centimorgan density. *Cooperative Human Linkage Center (CHLC). Science, 265*, 2049–2054.

Neyroud, N., Tesson, F., Denjoy, I., Leibovici, M., Donger, C., Barhanin, J., Faure, S., Gary, F., Coumel, P., Petit, C., Schwartz, K., & Guicheney, P. (1997). A novel mutation in the potassium channel gene KVLQT1 causes the Jervell and Lange–Nielsen cardioauditory syndrome. *Nature Genetics, 15*, 186–189.

Probst, F. J., & Camper, S. A. (1999). The role of mouse mutants in the identification of human hereditary hearing loss genes. *Hearing Research, 130*, 1–6.

Riazuddin, S., Castelein, C. M., Friedman, T. B., Lalwani, A. K., Liburd, N., Naz, S., Smith, T. N., Riazuddin, S., & Wilcox, E. R. (1999). A novel nonsyndromic recessive form of deafness maps to 4q28 and demonstrates incomplete penetrance. *American Journal of Human Genetics, 65*, A101.

Risch, N. (1990). Linkage strategies for genetically complex traits, I: Multilocus models. *American Journal of Human Genetics, 46*, 222–228.

Ryan, A. K., Goodship, J. A., Wilson, D. I., Philip, N., Levy, A., Seidel, H., Schuffenhauer, S., Oechsler, H., Belohradsky, B., Prieur, M., Aurias, A., Raymond, F. L., Clayton-Smith, J., Hatchwell, E., McKeown, C., Beemer, F. A., Dallapiccola, B., Novelli, G., Hurst, J. A., Ignatius, J., Green, A. J., Winter, R. M., Brueton, L., Brondum-Nielsen, K., Scambler, P. J., et al. (1997). Spectrum of clinical features associated with interstitial chromosome 22q11 deletions: A European collaborative study. *Medical Genetics, 34*, 798–804.

Sabouri, L. A., Mahadevan, M. S., Narang, M., Lee, D. S., Surh, L. C., & Korneluk, R. G. (1993). Effect of the myotonic dystrophy (DM) mutation on mRNA levels of the DM gene. *Nature Genetics, 4*, 233–238.

Shute, N. C., & Ewens, W. J. (1988). A resolution of the ascertainment sampling problem. III: Pedigrees. *American Journal of Human Genetics, 43*, 387–395.

Smith, R. J. H., & Schwartz, C. (1998) Branchio-oto-renal syndrome. *Journal of Communication Disorders, 31*, 411–421.

Stausberg, R. L., Feingold, E. A., Klausner, R. D., & Collins, F. S. (1999). The mammalian gene collection. *Science, 286*, 455–457.

Tyson, J., Tranebjaerg, L., Bellman, S., Wren, C., Taylor, J. F., Bathen, J., Aslaksen, B., Sorland, S. J., Lund, O., Malcolm, S., Pembrey, M., Bhattacharya, S., & Bitner-Glindzicz, M. (1997). IsK and KvLQT1: Mutation in either of the two subunits of the slow component of the delayed rectifier potassium channel can cause Jervell and Lange–Nielsen syndrome. *Human Molecular Genetics*, *6*, 2179–2185.

Wang, A., Liang, Y., Fridell, R. A., Probst, F. J., Wilcox, E. R., Touchman, J. W., Morton, C. C., Morell, R. J., Noben-Trauth, K., Camper, S. A., & Friedman, T. B. (1998). Association of unconventional myosin MYO15 mutations with human nonsyndromic deafness DFNB3. *Science*, *280*, 1447–1451.

Watson, J. D. (1953). Molecular structure of nucleic acids. *Nature*, *171*, 371.

Williams, C. A., Zori, R. T., Stone, J. W., Gray, B. A., Cantu, E. S., & Ostrer, H. (1990). Maternal origin of 15q11-13 deletions in Angelman syndrome suggests a role for genomic imprinting. *American Journal of Medical Genetics*, *35*, 350–353.

3

PRENATAL AND POSTNATAL CRANIOFACIAL DEVELOPMENT

SYLVAN E. STOOL

Department of Otolaryngology
The Children's Hospital of Denver
Denver, Colorado

I. PHYLOGENETIC ASPECTS AND EMBRYOLOGY

It is appropriate that an early chapter of a text on communicative disorders be devoted to the broad subject of the development of the craniofacial complex. This is the major region involved in diseases and disorders of the ears, nose, and throat and serves as the entryway to the air and food passages. The more we know about the embryology, growth, and development of the face and about the various factors involved in normal variations and anomalies of this region, the better will be our understanding of the many communicative disorders that may affect infants and children, as well as adults.

The first region that the clinician and, indeed, the layperson inspects on encountering another person is the face. An impression of the face and an evaluation of the facial type and facial expression are usually made instantly. After this, the general body type and posture are noted, and the degree of interpersonal communication is ascertained. DeMeyer (1975) stated

> One glance at the patient's face may settle the diagnostic issue, an Augenblick, or eyeblink diagnosis, in which the clinician immediately knows what syndrome the patient has. I am neither describing nor advocating the hasty careless snap judgment. I am merely pointing out that the clinician, utilizing the pattern recognition attributes of his own brain, sometimes can diagnose abnormal faces with the speed and certainty with which he distinguishes the faces of family and friends.

On the basis of certain facial features, the clinician may decide that a recognizable syndrome identifies the patient with a group of similar patients more than it does with the individual's own family. Therefore, the face and the cranial configuration contribute immeasurably to the total, or gestalt, diagnosis. Any observer can appreciate that there is great variation in the appearance of the normal face. In addition, there are certain characteristics that we associate with facial types almost on an instinctive basis. These variations and expectations in facial types can be appreciated by examining Figure 3.1, which is a sketch of a group of white children from the same grammar school class. The variations in facial configuration are obvious: there are round, oval, and triangular faces. Individual characteristics of the eyes and the nose also show tremendous variation. A diagnosis of an abnormality that is based on facial configuration may be difficult to make unless the observer knows the hereditary background of the individual. However, some abnormalities, such as Down syndrome, are expressed by similar facial features regardless of the child's origin. Thus, although we recognize great variations in facial type as being normal, we also instinctively recognize other features as being abnormal in a particular individual on the basis of our ability to assess facial patterns in the context of age, race, and hereditary background.

The human craniofacial complex is the result of at least 500 million years of progressive development. These structures, which developed in the anterior portion of an ancestral organism, were designed to obtain and maintain first contact with the environment. The pattern that developed in the invertebrates was continued in the vertebrates; and, according to Krogman (1974), there can be no doubt that the craniofacial complex from its beginning was a multistructured, highly integrated, diversely systemized center for almost every life need of the organism. In the development of the craniofacial complex in the human embryo and the fetus, the form and functions that have evolved for many millions of years take shape in fantastically rapid sequence. Those structures that required many millions of years of natural selection to evolve may form in minutes or hours in a human. This is especially true in the embryonic stages of development and is the reason

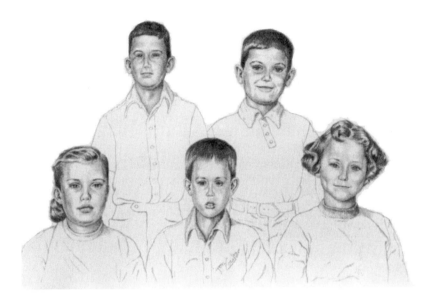

FIGURE 3.1   Children from a sixth-grade class. Note the variation of facial types, even though all are the same age and race. Reprinted with permission from Stool (1996).

that any interference with these processes in the early embryonic stages may have catastrophic consequences in the developing human. The embryogenesis of the craniofacial complex is indeed an amazing phenomenon, as form and function must relate to one another with an almost unbelievable precision and at exactly the right time. To appreciate the structures and the physiologic processes that those of us interested in disorders and diseases of the ears, nose, and throat so frequently see go awry, we begin this chapter with an abbreviated review of the normal human head. Therefore, this section is concerned primarily with the cranium, the base of the skull, the face, and the eyes, and concentrates on the broad concepts involved in the development of these structures.

Since many of the advances in embryology of interest to those involved with craniofacial anomalies have occurred because of a better understanding of subcellular events, these events are presented. A general overview of the structure of the human face is presented first, followed by a discussion of the cellular and molecular events that lead to the facial configuration. This method of presentation parallels the way in which the clinician usually views patients with anomalies of this region.

A. PLAN OF THE HUMAN FACE

In humans, the assumption of an upright posture has been associated with a number of anatomic developments, as can be appreciated from an examination of

Figure 3.2A,B. With the enlargements of the brain, especially of the frontal region, and the concomitant rotation of the eyes to the midline, there has been a relative decrease in the intraorbital distance in humans compared with that in lower mammals. This has resulted in a smaller region at the root of the nose and a shortening of the muzzle, or snout. Thus, humans have close-set eyes and a short narrow snout, narrow noses that do not interfere with binocular vision.

The growth of the frontal lobes and other evolutionary changes have resulted in flexure of the cranial base, as illustrated in Figure 3.2C, making the face appear to hang from the base of the skull. Other less obvious changes have occurred, such as rotation of the olfactory bulbs and nerves, so that the nasal region in humans has a vertical orientation and most of its important functional components are housed within the face. This placement of the face within the flexure of the cranial base may be of some clinical significance; any condition that affects the cranial base may have some secondary effects on the airway and, ultimately, on the speech mechanisms.

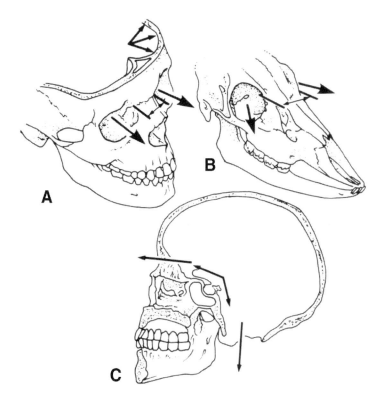

FIGURE 3.2   (A) Plan of the human face demonstrating an enlargement of the frontal lobes in the human and rotation of the orbit, resulting in a narrow nasal root, in contrast to a lower animal (B). (C) Flexure of the cranial base results in an alteration of facial alteration. Reprinted with permission from Stool (1996).

Prenatal Development of the Face

The development of the face from midembryonic through midfetal life is illustrated in Figure 3.3. The embryo at about 3 to 4 weeks of age is illustrated in Figure 3.3A. At this stage, the embryo does not have a face; the head is composed of a brain covered with a membrane, and the anterior neuropore is still present.

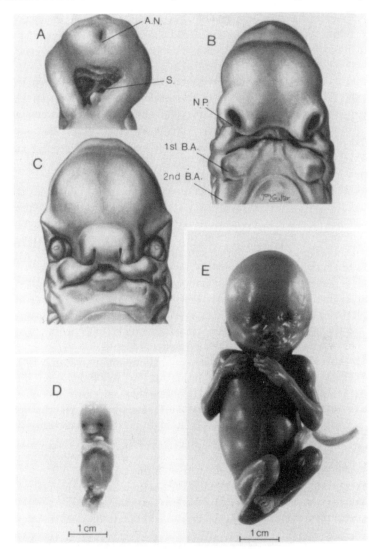

FIGURE 3.3   Prenatal facial development. (**A**) An embryo of 3 to 4 weeks. AN = anterior neuropore; S = stomodeum. (**B**) An embryo of 5 to 6 weeks. NP = nasal pit; 1st BA = first branchial arch; 2nd BA = second branchial arch. (**C**) An embryo of 7 to 8 weeks. (**D**) A fetus of 8 to 9 weeks. (**E**) A fetus of 3 to 4 months. Fetal specimens are from the Krause Collection, the Cleft Palate Center, University of Pittsburgh. Reprinted with permission from Stool (1996).

The eyes, which are represented by optic vesicles, are the lateral aspects of the head, as in fish, and the future mouth is represented by a stomodeum. It is only in the latter part of this period of embryonic growth that nasal pits develop. At the embryonic age of 5 to 6 weeks, as illustrated in Figure 3.3B, the general shape of the face has begun to develop. The frontonasal process is prominent; the nasal pits are forming laterally; and, with the increase in size of the first and second branchial arches, there is a suggestion of a mouth. In the subsequent weeks of embryonic life, as illustrated in Figure 3.3C, the structures that we associate with the human face—jaws, nose, eyes, ears, and mouth—will take on human configurations.

During this period of rapid growth and expansion, there is also tremendous differential growth (i.e., growth rates are not uniform for all tissues). Thus, the development of a human baby is not merely the enlargement or rearrangement of a previous form but, by differential growth, the development of a new configuration. This is a concept that has been difficult for students to comprehend, perhaps because of the tendency for different stages of embryonic development to be illustrated with drawings of equal size.

The embryonic period ends at about 8 weeks, when the embryo has achieved sufficient size and form so that facial characteristics can be recognized and photographed at actual size, as shown in Figure 3.3D. At this stage of late embryonic or early fetal development, the facial features are characterized by the appearance of hypertelorism; during subsequent growth, it will appear as though the eyes are moving closer together. This is not happening, however; the eyes continue to move farther apart, but the remainder of the face is growing at a much more rapid rate, and thus it appears that the eyes are moving closer together; hypertelorism is actually decreasing as a result of differential development. These observations may be of importance in understanding some of the craniofacial syndromes in which hypertelorism is a prominent feature.

The continued rapid growth and change in configuration, not only of the face but also of the extremities and body during the next few months, are illustrated in Figure 3.3E. The fetus has facial features that are easily recognized and associated with the human. The ears, nasal alae, and lips are well developed, and the head constitutes a large portion of the body mass—a relationship that will exist at birth and gradually change during extrauterine life.

The concept of differential growth is vital to the comprehension of both prenatal and postnatal development. Although this concept is difficult to grasp when the student must view development of structures of different ages magnified to the same size and when illustrations are in two dimensions, it is important to visualize the process in three dimensions, in addition to the fourth dimension—time.

B. FORMATION OF THE CRANIOFACIAL COMPLEX

The structures and the factors that form the craniofacial complex have been the subject of investigation by embryologists for many years, and their study has involved use of a number of sophisticated, time-consuming techniques. Among the most interesting studies has been the research of Johnston (1975) into the development and migration of cells in the neural crest. These cells are initially composed of ectoderm found at the junction of the neural plate and surface ectoderm. Figure 3.4A shows the neural crest cells forming around the anterior neuropore. It has been shown that the face of the amphibian, as well as that of

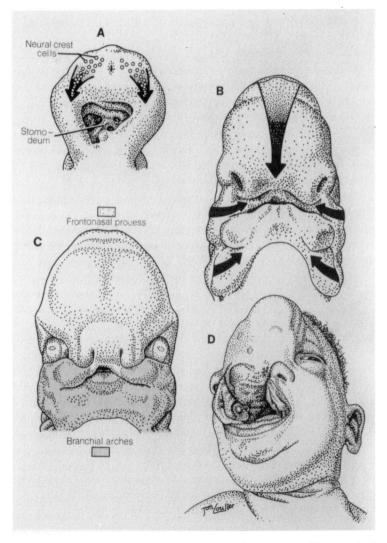

FIGURE 3.4   Formation of the craniofacial complex. (A) An embryo of 3 to 4 weeks showing development and beginning migration of neural crest cells. (B) Migration of neural crest cells in the forebrain and the branchial arches. (C) Contributions to the face of the frontonasal process and branchial arches. (D) Malformation caused by failure of neural crest migration. Reprinted with permission from Stool (1996).

mammals, develops as a consequence of massive cell migrations and the interactions of loosely organized embryonic tissue. In most of the body, this embryonic tissue is derived from mesoderm; however, in the craniofacial complex, neural crest cells give rise to a large variety of connective and nervous tissues of the skull, face, and branchial arches. Therefore, this ectodermal tissue constitutes the majority of the pluripotential tissue of the face. The sequence of events after the initial formation of neural crest cells is illustrated in Figure 3.4B. The differentiation, proliferation, and migration of those cells are critical in the formation of the face.

Migration occurs at different rates. For instance, the cells that form the frontonasal process are derived from the forebrain fold, and their migration is relatively short as they pass into the nasal region. However, the cells that form the mesenchyme of the maxillary processes have a considerably longer distance to migrate, since they must move into the branchial arches, where they surround the core-like mesodermal muscle plates. In Figure 3.4C, the ultimate distribution of neural crest cells from the frontonasal process and from the branchial arches is illustrated. Since this mesenchymal tissue contributes the majority of the soft tissues and bone to the face, future proliferation or migration may be responsible for a number of abnormalities, such as orofacial clefts. An illustration of a severe facial abnormality due to failure of migration is illustrated in Figure 3.4D. Less severe clefts of the lip, the palate, or both may also develop. In some cases, such as with severe holoprosencephaly, not only are mesodermal tissues involved, but there are central nervous system abnormalities as well.

C. DIVISIONS OF THE HUMAN FACE

From the foregoing, it can be seen that the human face may be divided embryologically, as illustrated in Figure 3.4C. The median facial structures arise from the frontonasal process, and the lateral structures arise from the branchial arches. This dual embryonic origin provides a basis for dividing the face into three vertical segments. The central segment, primarily the frontonasal process, includes the nose and the central portion of the upper lip. The two lateral segments that arise from the branchial arches may be called the otomaxillomandibular segments. For convenience of description, the face can also be divided into three almost equal horizontal planes. The upper, or frontal, horizontal segment derives solely from the frontonasal process. The middle or maxillary segment derives from the maxillary process of the first branchial arch, and the prolabium comes from the frontonasal process. The third horizontal segment, the lower or mandibular segment, comes from the mandibular process of the first branchial arch.

Prenatal Craniofacial Skeletal Components

The craniofacial skeleton provides support and protection for the human's most vital functions. Conceptually, it is a region with two divisions: one that is involved with the central nervous system, the *neurocranium*; and one that is involved with respiration and mastication, the *visceral cranium*. The craniofacial skeleton consists of four components: cranial base, cranial vault, nasomaxillary complex, and mandible.

The skeletal structures originate spontaneously from two types of bone. One type of bone is first formed in cartilage, and the other is derived from membrane. In general, the bones of the skull that represent the earliest phylogenetic structures are first formed as cartilage, which subsequently ossifies; the more recently developed craniofacial structures are derived from membranous bone.

The components and structures of the fetal craniofacial complex are illustrated in Figures 3.5 through 3.8. Figure 3.5 is a parasagittal section through the cranial base and the facial structures. The cranial base is cartilaginous and provides a floor for the calvaria and a roof for the face. The nasal space and nasopharynx are part of the airway system. Although the airway is not functional in the fetus, alterations of the cranial base during fetal life may affect its subsequent development. Figure 3.6 shows the cartilaginous continuity of the cranial base and nasal septum, as well as the arrangement of the fetal facial bones and teeth around the cartilaginous nasal capsule. The nasal septum is attached to the cranial base and the palate and, thus, constitutes a large portion of the skeletal structure in the fetal midface. Although there is much difference of opinion on this subject, growth of craniofacial cartilage is considered by some to be of prime importance in facial development.

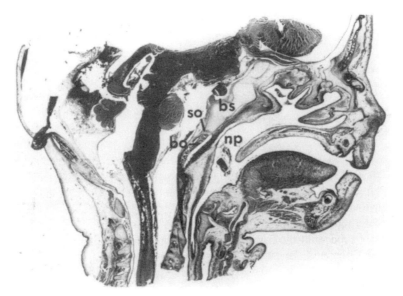

FIGURE 3.5   Photomicrograph of a parasagittal section of a 15-week-old fetal head: bo = basiocciput; bs = basisphenoid cartilage; np = nasopharynx; so = sphenooccipital synchondrosis. From the Krause Collection, the Cleft Palate Center, University of Pittsburgh. Reprinted with permission from Stool (1996).

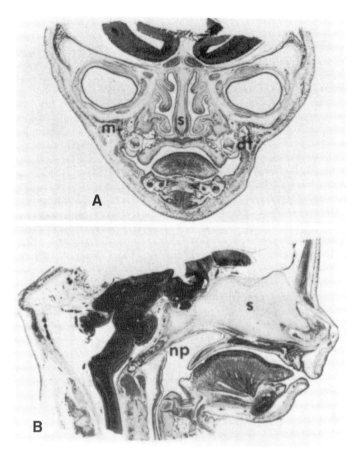

FIGURE 3.6 (A) Coronal section of a 15-week-old fetal head. (B) Sagittal section of a 15-week-old fetal head. dt = deciduous tooth germ; m = maxillary bone center; np = nasopharynx; s = nasal septum. Reprinted with permission from Stool (1996).

As mentioned, the craniofacial skeletal complex is composed of bones of different embryonic origins. Figure 3.7 shows the bones of cartilaginous origin (dark stipple) and those of membranous origin (light stipple); cartilage that is of branchial arch origin is indicated by solid black. In general, the base of the skull and the sphenoid, petrosal, and ethmoid bones are of cartilaginous origin. The growth of the cartilage of the cranial base will be primarily at the cartilaginous synchondroses until the cartilage is replaced by bone; thereafter, growth will be at the periosteal margins. Most of the cranial and facial bones are membranous, and growth takes place primarily at the margins of these bones. The major facial bones are formed from multiple ossification centers, which subsequently produce single bones in later fetal life. The importance of understanding the dual embryonic origin of the skeleton is that many diseases that affect the craniofacial

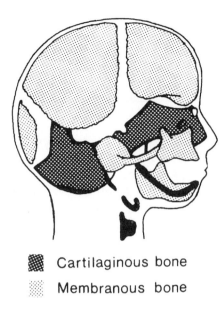

■ Cartilaginous bone

▒ Membranous bone

FIGURE 3.7   Schematic illustration of the components of the fetal craniofacial complex of membranous origin (light stipple) and cartilaginous origin (dark stipple). The cartilage of branchial arch origin is indicated in black. Redrawn with permission from Stewart and Prescott (1976). Reprinted with permission from Stool (1996).

complex may be manifested because of their influence on particular types of bone; for example, achondroplasia, which affects bones of cartilaginous origin, usually results in a characteristic alteration of facial configuration.

The sequential development of the fetal skeleton has been studied extensively by radiographic methods. However, it is anticipated that developments such as magnetic resonance imaging will provide better visualization of the relationship of the various tissues and improve our understanding of craniofacial morphogenesis. Figure 3.8 illustrates the definition of the structures that may be obtained by this technique. In addition, ultrasonography is a method of *in-vivo* study that has achieved wide clinical use. This technique permits prenatal study not only of structure but also of function. Figure 3.9 illustrates some of the information that may be obtained. These studies confirm many of the observations made by Hooker (1939) and Humphrey (1970) (Figure 3.10).

D. DEVELOPMENT OF CRANIOFACIAL ARTERIES, MUSCLES, AND NERVES

Figure 3.11 illustrates the development of the cranium, arteries, nerves, and muscles during embryonic and early fetal life. The characteristics of these struc-

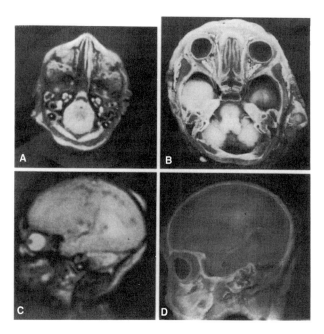

FIGURE 3.8   (A) Transverse magnetic resonance image (T-weighted) of a 24-week-old aborted fetus at the level of the orbital floors and inner and middle cars. (B) Transverse section through the fetal head at the level of the orbits at 28 weeks gestation. (C) Sagittal magnetic resonance image of the fetal head (T-weighted). (D) Sagittal section of the fetal head at 24 weeks gestation. Reprinted with permission from Stool (1996).

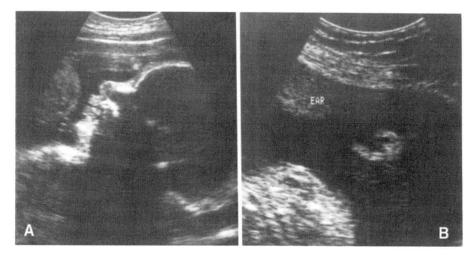

FIGURE 3.9   Ultrasound demonstration of the profile of a fetal face and a fetal car at 31 to 32 weeks of gestation. Reprinted courtesy of Landon M. Hall, MD, Pittsburgh, PA. Reprinted with permission from Stool (1996).

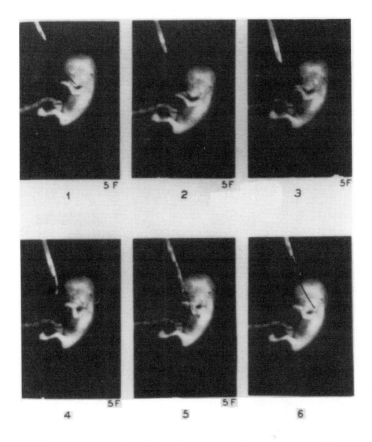

RESPONSE TO ARM TENDON STRETCHING

PROBABLE MENSTRUAL AGE — 9.5 WEEKS

FIGURE 3.10   Photograph of the original work of Davenport Hooker showing fetal response to tactile stimulation. Reprinted with permission from Stool (1996).

tures are discussed in their respective sections because their growth and development are interrelated.

1. Arteries

Figure 3.11A shows that the early arterial supply to the head consists primarily of the dorsal aorta and an arch with a small branch coming from it, which is the primitive internal carotid artery. Figure 3.11B shows an embryo of about 6 weeks, when the first and second aortic arches and their arteries have formed. As the face continues to develop, these vessels will ultimately disappear. The internal carotid

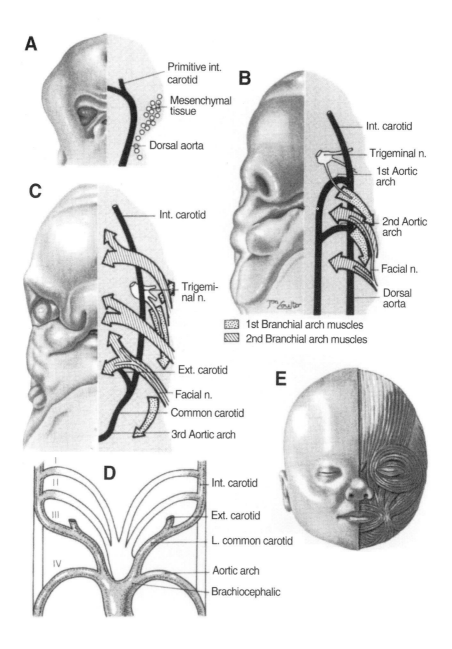

FIGURE 3.11   Development of the craniofacial arteries, muscles, and nerves. (**A**) A 3- to 4-week-old embryo. (**B**) A 5- to 6-week-old embryo. (**C**) A 7- to 8-week-old embryo. (**D**) The fate of the aortic arches (shaded vessels persist). After Avery (1990). (**E**) Distribution of the facial musculature in the 15-week-old fetus. After Gasser (1967). Reprinted with permission from Stool (1996).

artery at this stage has increased in size, and the facial muscles are beginning to develop in a laminar fashion. One group of muscles develops a lamina that grows posteriorly, and the other group of muscles comes from a lamina that extends anteriorly.

The nerves are beginning to develop as outgrowths of the central nervous system. The skull base forms, and foramina exist where bone forms around any preexisting soft tissue (blood vessels or nerves). The fifth cranial nerve (trigeminal), which will ultimately supply sensation to the face, is really a combination of three nerves with ophthalmic, mandibular, and maxillary divisions and a division to the muscles of mastication. The seventh cranial nerve, which is the nerve supply to the second branchial arch, has also begun its development. By the time the embryo has facial characteristics that appear more human (Figure 3.11C), the blood supply to the face and cranium has developed the pattern that will persist into fetal and postnatal life. Figure 3.11D illustrates the formation of the arterial supply.

2. Muscles

By the end of embryonic life, the facial musculature has become well developed and has migrated extensively superiorly into the craniofacial region. Figure 3.11E shows the muscles contributed by the various laminae. The first branchial arch contributes the muscles that lie beneath the musculature of the second branchial arch and, in general, have a different orientation. These muscles include the temporal, masseter, pterygoid, mylohyoid, and anterior belly of the digastricus as well as the tensor muscle of the velum palatinum and the tensor muscle of the tympanum.

3. Nerves

The nerve supply to the muscles of the face has been described by Gasser (1967) and is discussed in detail by him in May's (1986) book on the facial nerve. These cranial nerves are mixed nerves, having autonomic, sensory, and motor components. By the time the fetus has reached 37-mm crown–rump length, all of the peripheral branches of the facial nerve are identifiable.

E. MOLECULAR CONTROL OF CRANIOFACIAL DEVELOPMENT

The subject of embryology is a complex one, running the gamut from descriptive chronology of events that transpire during prenatal life to details of genetic types and mutations and how they affect the individual proteins and nucleic acids that are part of the molecular biology of the embryo. The transformation of a fertilized egg into a baby is a remarkable orchestration of cell migration, cell differentiation, programmed cell death, and differential growth. The information that controls this incredibly complex process is encoded in the DNA. Since each cell in the body contains the entire genome, the control of the expression of the different genes in the DNA is crucial to differentiation of the developing organism. Thus, an understanding of the control of DNA is central to the understanding of morphogenesis (see Chapter 2).

Molecular Biology and Morphogenesis

The plan that determines the major regions of the body is established early in the developing embryo. A critical determination that must be made is axis deline-ation or polarity. Mechanisms that determine the anterior–posterior axis, the dorsal–ventral axis, and left–right symmetry operate early in embryonic develop-ment and have been the subject of intense investigation.

The transmission and control of patterning data are complex, and the signal transduction system is modulated at all points. Establishment of the three layers (ectoderm, mesoderm, and endoderm) and the subsequent subdivision of the layers and tissue differentiation are under genetic and epigenetic control. Developmental control genes, peptide growth factors, and cytoskeletal elements are important in this process of establishing and coordinating sequential boundary formation. The regulatory mechanisms may act in cascading fashion, such that a homeobox gene product (see below) regulates a peptide growth factor in the mesoderm, which in turn activates another homeobox gene in the neural ectoderm. Concentration gradients also control development in that different concentrations of the signaling molecule produce differing cell fates. The state of the responding cell is also important; receptor expression patterns and ligand affinities vary at different times throughout embryogenesis.

While neural crest cell migration has long been appreciated, other classes of cells are being identified. Neural plate cells, mytoblasts, angioblasts, and placode-derived cells also migrate, either independently or in concert with other cells. Advances in immunocytochemistry, *in-situ* hybridization transgenic reporter genes, explanation experiments, and molecular probes are all providing insights into the way by which genetic information is transformed into specific tissues and organs.

F. CONCLUSION

Progress in identifying the mechanisms of control of human facial development has been accelerated by advances in molecular genetics. Identification of the genes responsible is a crucial step toward an ultimate understanding of the development of the face. Mapping and identification of the genes associated with craniofacial abnormalities will eventually elucidate the biochemical, cytochemical, and mo-lecular mechanisms that control the development of the human face. Elucidation of the molecular mechanisms of human craniofacial anomalies may suggest approaches for their amelioration, correction, and ultimate prevention (see Chap-ter 7).

II. POSTNATAL CRANIOFACIAL GROWTH
AND DEVELOPMENT

Growth implies an increase in dimension and mass, whereas development implies a progression to more adult characteristics. Here, we first describe the appearance of the soft tissues of the human head and then examine the underlying skeletal components in order to relate the development of these components to some of the basic principles and concepts of cartilage and bone growth. The infant face rarely projects an image of the adult configuration. Conversely, it is usually impossible to attempt to identify an adult by examination of his or her "baby pictures." The face of an infant or child is not a miniature of an adult face but has definite proportions different from those of the adult. The changes that take place during maturation are part of a differential growth process. In general, newborns, regardless of their ethnic backgrounds, resemble each other more than each one does his or her parents. The different proportions of infant and adult faces have been studied extensively by artists and anthropologists and are appreciated almost instinctively by laypersons. These changes in facial configuration and proportions are illustrated in Figure 3.12. The infant has a very prominent forehead because of the early development of the cerebral hemisphere in relation to the face. About 90% of the child's facial height are achieved by 5 years of age, whereas 90% of facial width are attained by 2 years. Thus, the young child's head appears round.

The face of the infant is diminutive compared with the calvaria. As seen in Figure 3.12, the proportion of facial mass to cranial mass, viewed laterally, is 1 to 3. Subsequent growth in childhood alters this proportion so that the ratio becomes about 1 to 2½, whereas in adolescents and adults the proportion becomes 1 to 2. However, if this proportion does not change as described, the adult is frequently referred to as having a "baby face." In addition, because the soft tissues of the face include fat, the external appearance does not necessarily reflect the underlying musculoskeletal structure of the face. Thus, the underlying proportions may change, but the general outline of the adult face may still appear childlike. The infant face has a "flat" configuration, which changes during adolescence when sharper angles develop as a result of orbital, mandibular, and nasal growth. The maxilla and mandible grow to accommodate the primary dentition (20 teeth), followed by the permanent dentition (32 teeth). The chin of the infant is almost nonexistent but is usually a prominent structure in adults as a result of mandibular growth and development. The cheekbones are notable in adults because of loss of baby fat and rotation of the skeletal components. The ears of the infant appear to be very low-set, because the head in general is more ovoid than elongated; the ears appear to "rise" with growth because of the increase in the vertical dimension of the lower facial height. The configuration of the ear remains the same throughout life, although its mass increases.

The most prominent facial features, the relationship of which has become characteristic of human faces, are the nose and eyes. The nose of the infant has a

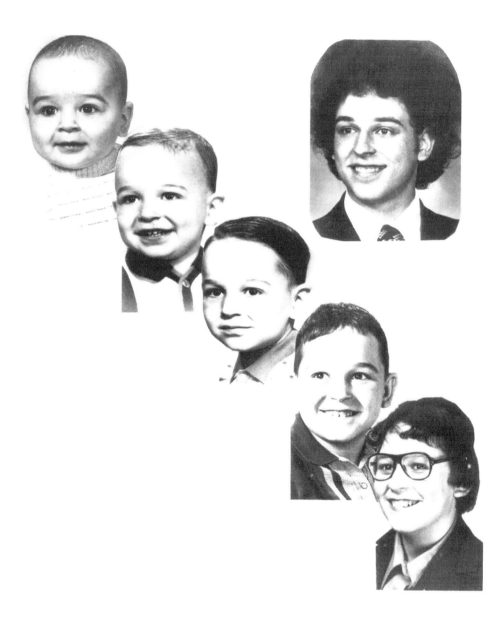

FIGURE 3.12 Postnatal growth of a Caucasian boy. The diagonal from above downward shows the boy at ages 6 months, 2 years, 4 years, 8 years, and 12 years; the photograph in the upper right corner is the same child at 18 years. In the infant, the proportion of face mass to cranial mass is 1 to 3; during childhood, it gradually changes to 1 face mass to 2½ cranial mass. From adolescence through adult life, it is 1 face mass to 2 cranial mass. Reprinted with permission from Stool (1996).

distinctive "pug" appearance. It is diminutive and remains so throughout most of childhood. During adolescence and later, especially in males, there is an increase in length, breadth, and protrusion of the nose, which is related to the increase in airway. The growth of the face can be explained more easily if a subordinate position is given to the craniofacial skeleton, while a leading role is designated to the soft tissues and the functional components that play a part in the activities of the face. In these, the maintenance of the airway is predominant. Humans are the only animals with a truly external nose, and this particularly human trait is subject to many variations, depending in part on ethnic background.

The relationship between vertical dentofacial morphology and respiration in adolescents has been studied by Fields and colleagues (1991), who compared normal and long-face subjects aged 11 to 17 years. Both morphologic and contemporary respirometric techniques were used for the two groups and resulted in no significant differences being found in airway impairment, although different oronasal breathing modes were present.

The eyes of infants appear to be wide-set, with a very prominent inner canthal fold, giving an appearance of hypertelorism because of the lack of vertical dimension of the face. If the infant's face is bisected horizontally, the eyes are located in the inferior half of the face. During childhood, the eyes appear to move upward, but in fact the lower half of the face grows more than the upper half, so the maxilla and mandible become more prominent. In older children, the eyes are placed midway in the face. In adolescence, with further growth and development of the lower half of the face relative to the upper half, the eyes finally appear to be just above the dividing line. This adult configuration is the result of differential growth of facial components. The same principle may be used to explain why in adults the eyes are less prominent than they appear to be in children; with growth of the supraorbital rim during adolescence, less of the eye is exposed.

Even though somatic growth is measured by height and weight recordings during childhood and adolescence, there is no reason to assume that it terminates at adulthood. A study conducted by Behrents (1985), as an extension of the Bolton–Brush longitudinal growth studies, revealed continuing growth of the craniofacial complex throughout all age levels, similar in direction to adolescent alterations but of lesser magnitude and rate.

A. GROWTH CONCEPTS

Parallel evaluation of the cranium and of other parts of the skeleton is the basis for the clinical distinction of generalized skeletal disorders from cranial abnormalities (Pierce *et al.*, 1977). Therefore, to understand the normal morphologic changes that occur with growth, as well as craniofacial abnormalities, it is important to describe some basic concepts of skeletal growth: bone formation, remodeling, and displacement.

1. Bone Formation

Humans possess an endoskeleton that is fabricated from specialized connective tissue: cartilage and bone. Cartilage is a special, tough, pliable tissue that has the capacity to form in regions that experience direct pressure; it does not always calcify and does not necessarily have a surface membrane. Its most important feature in the craniofacial complex is its ability to function as a precursor or model for bone. The characteristics of bone are hardness and rigidity and the possession of a surface membrane, or periosteum. It is a complex substance that is viewed by the chemist as a compound of protein, polysaccharide, mineral, and cellular constituents. To the histologist, it is a tissue composed of osteogenic cells and intracellular matrix. To the gross anatomist, it is an organ with vascular and nerve supplies.

The cells of cartilage and bone are derived from fetal mesenchymal tissue, which has a fairly uniform and undifferentiated appearance. These cells differentiate into chondroblasts and osteoblasts. Osteoblasts secrete a matrix that mineralizes and surrounds and encases them; they mature into osteocytes. Multinucleated giant cells called osteoclasts, which are known to destroy mineralized bone, also develop. They do not act on uncalcified bone—a fact of some importance in certain dysplasias—but they play an important role in the process of destruction and deposition of these cells.

Bone always forms in preexisting connective tissue. When this tissue is cartilage, the process is called endochondral ossification; when it is noncartilaginous, it is called intramembrane ossification. The sequence of events is illustrated in Figure 3.13. Membranous bone in the skull forms as a layer of mesenchyme with foci of condensation. These areas of condensation begin to ossify, and the process extends until the areas meet to form suture lines. Craniosynostosis (see Chapter 7) will result if premature closure of sutures in the cranium occurs.

Endochondral ossification is a more complex process that is easier to visualize in the tubular bones. The mesenchyme condenses and then undergoes chondrification. This forms a precise model for future bone surrounded by a limiting membrane. Formation of a periosteal collar is followed by development of a primitive marrow cavity and an ossification center, which forms at the end of the bone. It is possible to identify four distinct segments in the tubular bone. The epiphysis is covered by an articulator cartilage in tubular bones and includes the ossification center. The physis, or growth plate, is a very narrow but highly active region that consists of four zones, all related to chondrogenesis. The metaphysis is a zone where the transformation, or change of growing cartilage, into bone takes place. Growth in length is achieved primarily through the activities of the cells in the metaphysis. This is also an important region in the remodeling process. Eventually, when growth ceases, the physis will undergo ossification and disappear. The diaphysis is the shaft of the bone.

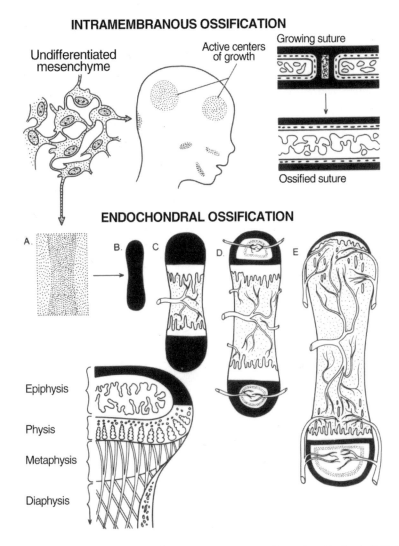

FIGURE 3.13 Mechanism of formation of the two types of bone found in the skull. Undifferentiated mesenchyme is the presence of both. Intramembranous ossification mesenchyme condenses to form centers of growth, which enlarge until they meet to form a suture. Growth proceeds at these sutures and remains active until the stimulus is removed and the suture ossifies. *Endochondral ossification*: (**A**) endochondral bone formation also begins with condensation; (**B**) cartilage anlage is formed; (**C**) vascular mesenchyme forms a primary marrow and periosteal collar forms; (**D**) ossification centers develop at the extremities, resulting in the four segments illustrated in the lower left; (**E**) eventually, the bone is completely ossified and the segmental differences disappear. The segments of a typical long bone are shown in the lower left. *Epiphysis*: a secondary ossification center covered with cartilage. *Physis*: the cartilage growth plate. *Metaphysis*: the segment in which cartilage is transformed into bone by endochondral bone formation. *Diaphysis*: the shaft separating the growing ends. Redrawn with permission and in part from Rubin (1964) and Williams and Wendell-Smith (1969). Reprinted with permission from Stool (1996).

2. Remodeling and Displacement

In the craniofacial complex, growth and development depend on two separate but interrelated processes: displacement, which involves motion between bones, and remodeling, which involves a change in the configuration of the bone while displacement is occurring. Bone grows by a continuous process of deposition and resorption. This is not a uniform process throughout the entire bone but is a differential growth process. If this were not so, the adult skeleton would be the same as the fetal configuration. The mechanism by which these two different but complementary functions are achieved is influenced by a number of factors, such as surface stress and various nutritional, hormonal, and genetic influences. The biodynamics have been studied for years and are still undergoing conceptual changes.

In the simplest terms, bone growth occurs when bone is both deposited by osteoblastic activity and resorbed during osteoclastic activity. At any time during the growth process, entire regions of a bone may be found to be undergoing localized deposition or resorption. These areas undergoing change are known as growth fields, and the entire surface of a growing bone may be composed of such localized fields, the cumulative effects of which provide for increase in bone size and change in shape.

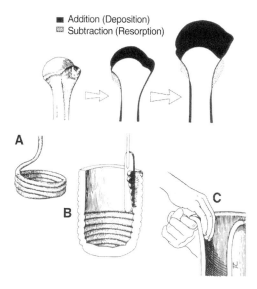

FIGURE 3.14   The concept of remodeling is illustrated. To prevent distortion of growing bone, there is osteoclastic cutback at the metaphysis. An example is this tubular bone, in which there is addition (deposition) at the epiphysis and subtraction (resorption) at the metaphysis. The concepts involved in skeletal growth and development are illustrated using the analogy of the ancient coil technique of clay construction: (**A**) the initial step is formation by deposition (addition); during this process, there is concomitant removal, resorption (subtraction), resulting in differential growth; (**B**) the final configuration is achieved by these two processes as well as an additional one, displacement (**C**). Reprinted with permission from Stool (1996).

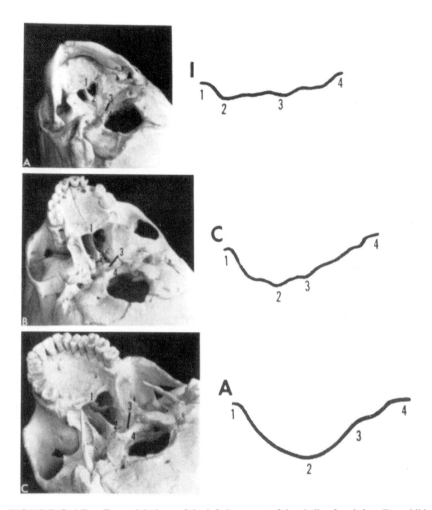

FIGURE 3.15   Tangential views of the inferior aspect of the skulls of an infant (I), a child (C), and an adult (A). All illustrate the change in configuration of the nasopharynx. The anatomic landmarks are: 1 = the posterior nasal spine; 2 = the junction of the vomer with the base of the skull; 3 = the sphenooccipital synchondrosis; and 4 = the edge of the foramen magnum. The change in size and configuration of the posterior choanae and nasal airway can be appreciated. Reprinted with permission from Stool (1996).

In long bones, this concept is fairly easy to visualize. Growth of long bones is best described by the "V principle." Growth at the metaphysis (Figure 3.14) involves endochondral bone formation, which effectively separates or displaces the epiphysis from the metaphysis. The pattern of growth can then be described as an expanding V, as shown in Figure 3.15. Anything that interferes with this process will result in an abnormal configuration. In the tubular bones, this concept is fairly easy to visualize. For a bone to increase in length and retain its normal shape, it is necessary to add and subtract bone. This is illustrated in Figure 3.14.

The craniofacial region is a much more complex area, and perhaps the process of bone growth in this region can best be visualized by describing the technique by which an artist working with clay might construct a bowl using coils. A basic hollow form is constructed, to which clay is added superficially. The edges may be smoothed to achieve a pleasing configuration. To keep the wall thickness uniform, it may be necessary to remove (subtract) some clay from the inner surface of the bowl (resorption). If a change in configuration is desirable, it can be accomplished by applying pressure to the inner surface (displacement) and modeling the outer surface. Although this simple explanation is of some help in understanding the mechanics of bone formation, it does not explain why these events occur in humans.

For the clinician, it is important to realize that bone formation begins in the fetus and undergoes constant changes throughout life. This twofold process is important not only in the formation of craniofacial structures but also in the growth of other bones. In a series of investigations utilizing both cross-sectional and longitudinal material, Israel (1968) came to the conclusion that, with aging, the cranial skeleton and vertebrae basically gain in all dimensions studied.

The effects of abnormal bone formation can well be illustrated in human skull growth (Figure 3.16). In achondroplasia, all bone forming from cartilage (having a cartilaginous precursor) is abnormal, including the chondrocranium. This results in a shortened skull base, a flattened palate, a sunken bridge of the nose, and a general reduction in the development and size of the facial region (Figure 3.16B).

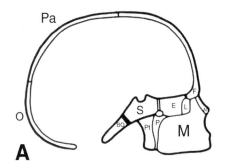 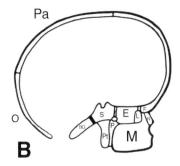

FIGURE 3.16   (A) Normal skull. The bones of the calvaria, cranial base, and upper face. The position of the sphenooccipital synchondrosis is shown in black. M = maxilla; N = nasal bone; F = frontal bone; L = lacrimal bone; E = ethmoid; P = vertical plate of the palatine bone; S = body of the sphenoid; Pt = pterygoid plate; O = occipital; BO = basioccipital. (B) Achondroplastic skull. Note the foreshortened skull base, sunken bridge of the nose, and general reduction in the development and size of the facial region. Reprinted with permission from Stool (1996).

The growth of the calvaria, which does not rely on ossification of cartilage for growth, is unhindered.

A certain group of disorders is affected by alterations in membranous bone formation. For instance, a craniometaphyseal abnormality involves alterations of the remodeling process, which are best understood by examination of the extremities. Some systemic diseases, such as hemolytic and iron deficiency anemias, may first be recognized in the cranium. Obviously, complete diagnosis of some cranial abnormalities necessitates evaluation of the remainder of skeleton.

3. Postnatal Skeletal Growth

The external features and some of the basic concepts of growth of the craniofacial complex have been discovered. We now examine the changes that occur in the skeleton. Skeletal growth is more readily assessed and easily documented than soft tissue growth as it is subject to graphic examination and physical measurements. The methods yield good estimates of skeletal proportions. Because of the availability of these tools, skeletal growth parameters have come to be widely used as indices for growth evaluation. Skeletal age is one of the "magic ages" used to ascertain the normality of growth and development. Usually, this is evaluated not only with cephalometric radiography but also by examination of the extremities, most commonly the wrist.

The skull is a complex structure formed from many component bones that articulate along an intricate network of sutures. The final location of each bone is determined by a composite of many different localized growth processes as well as regional changes. Figure 3.17A presents frontal views of the skulls of a newborn, a child, and an adult; 3.17B shows three-quarter views; 3.17C shows these same skulls with the infant and the child enlarged to the same size as the adult so that the vertical dimensions are equal. This provides a graphic means of illustrating changes in proportion.

Growth and development of the craniofacial complex are discussed as involving the cranium, mandible, and nasomaxillary complex. The bones that compose the cranium must be considered in two parts, the calvaria (roof) and the basicranium (floor), because distinctly different circumstances and modes of growth are involved for each.

B. CRANIUM

1. Calvaria

The calvaria is constructed from the frontal and parietal bones and portions of the temporal, occipital, and sphenoid bones. At birth, the bones are separated by six fontanelles bridged by fibrous tissue. The anterior fontanelle is the last to close, at about 18 months. As seen in Figure 3.17C, the skull of an infant is almost round. Sullivan (1986) made the following comparison: the curvature of the surface of

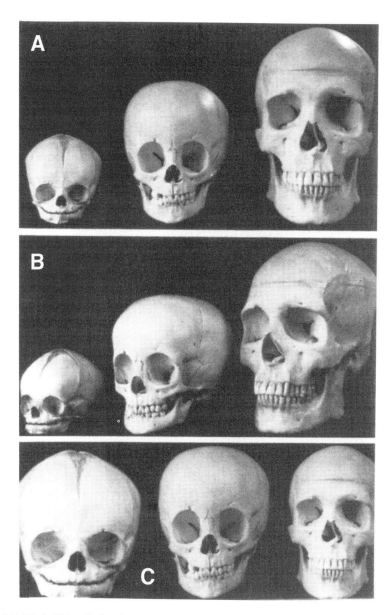

FIGURE 3.17   Skulls of a newborn, a child, and an adult illustrate skeletal changes during growth and development. (**A**) Frontal view. (**B**) Three-quarter view. (**C**) The newborn and the child skulls have been enlarged to the same size as the adult skull to demonstrate the changes in proportion with growth. The outward displacement of the bones of the calvaria is accompanied by changes in their regional curvatures. Ectocranial and endocranial periosteal surfaces are predominantly depository and I endosteal surfaces are resorptive. However, localized changes in surface contours are produced by opposite combinations, particularly in areas near sutural junctions. Adapted from Enlow (1990). Reprinted with permission from Stool (1996).

a large sphere is less than that of a small sphere. The adult calvaria is larger than the infant's and shows a corresponding reduction in curvature (Figure 3.17C).

2. Basicranium

The basicranium is a particularly fascinating region that has been the subject of much investigation. Phylogenetically, it is the oldest skeletal component; anatomically, it has been considered the cornerstone of craniofacial growth. The basicranium is formed from the basal part of the occipital, the sphenoid, the petrous part of the temporal, and the ethmoid bones. It is composed primarily of bones formed by the ossification of cartilage precursors. Synchondroses, in addition to sutures, are present in the cranial base. They represent regional adaptation to the pressure-located areas of the growing cranium. In the case of the sphenooccipital synchondrosis, ossification takes place on both the sphenoidal and the occipital faces of the cartilage. (This is in contrast to ossification in the epiphyseal cartilage of a long bone, which occurs on only one surface.)

Investigators do not agree on the exact role of cartilage in craniofacial development. The sphenooccipital synchondrosis has been presumed to represent the primary growth site of the basicranium. This assumption has been the subject of much controversy, and whether the synchondrosis acts as a primary growth center or not, it must not be regarded as the only mechanism participating in cranial base growth, although it continues active growth until 18 to 20 years of age. The anterior cranial base stabilizes in early childhood with the closure of the sphenoethmoidal synostosis. This provides a convenient area of superimposition for comparing longitudinal cephalometric records of craniofacial growth. Additionally, future growth of the maxillary complex will be affected by early closure of the sphenoethmoidal synchondrosis, as occurs in the craniosynostoses. This results in various degrees of sagittal and vertical maxillary deficiency.

It is difficult to visualize the basicranium from the anterior view. Figure 3.18, which is a tangential view of the inferior aspect of the skull, reveals that the nasomaxillary complex covers the anterior portion, beneath the anterior cranial fossa. The posterior portion of the cranial base provides the roof of the nasopharynx. In the infant, this line is relatively flat, but with growth and development it assumes a more curved appearance in the child. This is due not only to increased depth, which results from remodeling of the palate, but also to the flexure of the basicranium. These changes provide an enlarged nasal airway to meet the requirements of gas exchange and speech resonance in the adult.

For the otolaryngologist, this region is important for several reasons. Many bone dysplasias affecting the skeleton may also affect the cranial base. As major nerves and vessels passing through foramina in the basicranium become involved, classic symptoms result. One such example is osteopetrosis with facial palsy. Also, the size of the nasopharyngeal airway is determined in part by the configuration of the basicranium, and this has an effect on respiration and middle-ear function

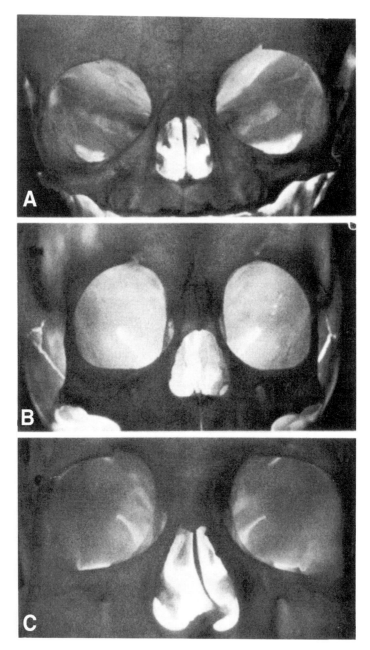

FIGURE 3.18   Skulls of a newborn (**A**), a child (**B**), and an adult (**C**) that have been transilluminated to emphasize the change in the relationship of the floor of the orbit to the floor of the nose. In the newborn and the child, there is little separation; however, in the adult the distance increases because of downward growth and displacement of the floor of the nose and upward growth of the floor of the orbit. Reprinted with permission from Stool (1996).

because of the dynamics of airflow. Finally, the ear may also be affected as the osseous Eustachian tube passes through the cranial base, and the muscles that control the cartilaginous portion of the tube originate from it.

C. MANDIBLE

The human mandible is a membrane bone that forms in close association with Meckel's cartilage, the first branchial arch cartilage. At birth, the bone is in two parts joined in the midline by the symphysis mandibularis, which closes by the end of the first year of life. The mandible is unusual in having a secondary growth cartilage under the surface of the articular condyle.

In studying craniofacial growth, it is often helpful to recognize that the bones of the face grow in a pattern balanced among its parts. Growth (increase in size or change in location) of one bone or portion of bone must be met with a congruent change in other bony parts of the face if an imbalance in the overall pattern of growth is to be avoided. Enlow (1990) identified particular areas of the facial skeleton that fit into this unique part–counterpart pattern. For example, the anterior cranial fossa, the palate, and the corpus of the mandible are considered to be counterparts of the bony maxillary arch. Growth changes occurring in any one of these parts must be accompanied by congruent changes in each of the others if the existing relationships are to be preserved. As the maxillary dental arch lengthens, so must the corpus of the mandible for the normal relationship between them to be preserved. The mandibular ramus and the middle cranial fossa are also considered to be counterparts. Growth of the middle cranial fossa must be matched by changes in the ramus, which again serves to maintain a balanced pattern of facial growth.

The condyle grows in whatever direction and to whatever extent it must to provide a functional occlusal position for the dental arch. Although controversy still exists, many investigators currently hold that the condylar cartilage may not perform an actual primary role in mandibular growth and development, but rather that it is an important adaptive site of growth. In a study regarding shape change in the mandible during adolescence, Dibbets *et al.* (1987) found further support for the theories that postulate local control factors for mandibular growth. They noted that the growth process of the mandible does not always proceed at a uniform rate for corpus and ramus, concluding that the growing mandible may favor either at any specific time.

Nasomaxillary Complex

The nasomaxillary complex consists of the nasal, lacrimal, maxillary, zygomatic, palatine, and pterygoid bones and the vomer. It can be seen (see Figure 3.4A) that this regional complex is closely related to the anterior segment of the cranium formed by the frontal, ethmoid, and sphenoid bones. Any relative forward growth of the anterior cranial base will carry the "upper facial region" with it into a more anterior position. Development of the nasomaxillary complex has been the subject of extensive investigation. Although long ago it was observed that growth of these structures occurs downward and forward, the mechanism of such growth has been the subject of debate. The problem has been that it is difficult to design studies in which the variables are effectively controlled. In addition, this is a complex anatomic region that is difficult to visualize from one perspective. Growth in this region occurs in both the horizontal and the vertical planes, and different segments grow at various rates. This can be appreciated by examining Figure 3.18, which shows the change in configuration and relationship of the orbits and the nasal apertures with age in the skulls of a newborn, a child, and an adult. All have been transilluminated so that the changes in density of the bone and the outline of the nasal apertures are more apparent.

The remodeling changes in the orbit are very complex, as many bones are involved, each of which undergoes different amounts of growth and displacement. One of the most marked changes is the difference in the relationship of the floor of the nose to the floor of the orbit. In newborns they are almost level; in children there is some separation. However, in adults there is a marked change due to the downward displacement of the entire maxilla. This change is more complex, as the floor of the orbit is displaced superiorly and the floor of the nose is displaced inferiorly. The change in the bony septum with age is rather dramatic. In the newborn, the septum appears straight, and in the adult skull shown in Figure 3.18C, there is marked septal deviation, a common finding. It is interesting that the breadth of the nasal bridge does not increase noticeably from early childhood to adulthood, although the shape of the nasal aperture changes from almost circular to pear shaped—a characteristic that shows marked racial variation.

The biomechanical force for displacement of the nasomaxillary complex is the subject of much controversy. It may be due to the expansion of the nasal septum; however, Latham (1970) believed that it is due to traction on the septopremaxillary ligaments. Early principles noted by van der Klaauw were strengthened and advanced by Moss (1962) as the functional matrix theory, which proposes that the genetic determinants of skeletal growth do not reside within the actual bony part itself. That is, the pacemakers of the displacement and the bony remodeling processes occur in the surrounding soft tissue parts. It is important to understand that the functional matrix concept describes essentially what happens during displacement and remodeling but is not intended to explain how this growth happens or what the regulating processes actually are at the tissue and cellular levels.

Another factor that influences the nasomaxillary complex is dentition. There is little evidence in the newborn's jaw of the dental structures that will develop. However, Figure 3.19, which shows the maxilla and mandible of a child, reveals a palisade of multi-tiered primary and permanent teeth in many stages of development. The growth and development of teeth and related dental architecture have been studied extensively. Early surgical intervention necessitates care in placing

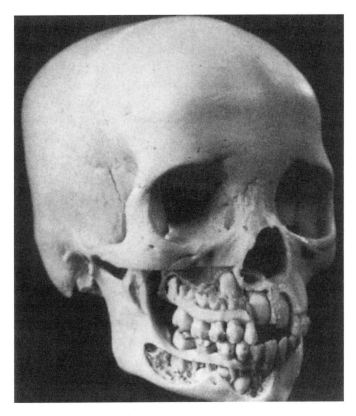

FIGURE 3.19   Skull of a child demonstrates mixed dentition. The multi-tiered battery of teeth is partially responsible for the increase in the vertical and horizontal dimension of the jaws with increasing age. Reprinted with permission from Stool (1996).

the osteotomy cuts to avoid interrupting the developing succedaneous teeth, as the distances between the orbit and the alveolar ridge are shallow.

The development of the craniofacial skeleton has been investigated widely by means of standardized cephalometric radiographs, employing this technique to explore relationships between upper airway obstruction and craniofacial growth. Cephalometric studies have also been undertaken to examine sexual dimorphism in the craniofacial complex. Ingerslev and Solow (1975) found that the cranium was, on the average, smaller in the female than in the male group except as regards the nasal bone, the foramen magnum, and the interorbital distance. The female group showed a more prominent frontal bone and a less prominent nasal bone than the male group. Bibby (1979) noted that the patterns of craniofacial morphology in males and females appear to be identical except in posterior facial height. In addition, the male skulls were 8.5% larger than the female skulls.

Many factors have been shown to affect craniofacial growth and development. A detailed description of each is not given here, but Figure 3.20 provides an overall view of both the general growth factors and the local factors postulated to influence craniofacial growth. In strong contrast to the many factors known to influence general growth, little information is available concerning the local control mechanisms that guide the growth of the bones and the development of the craniofacial skeleton. Much is known of what happens, but little is known about *how* it happens.

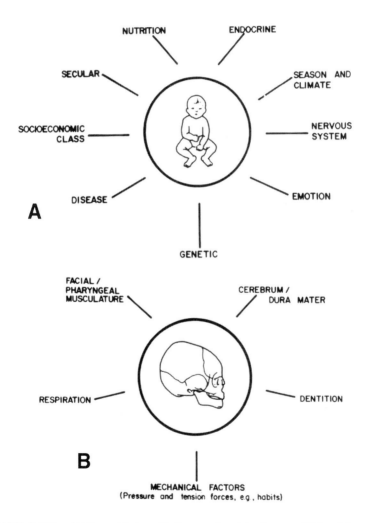

FIGURE 3.20 (**A**) General factors affecting growth and development. (**B**) Local factors postulated to affect craniofacial growth. Reprinted with permission from Stool (1996).

III. FUNCTIONS OF THE HUMAN CRANIOFACIAL COMPLEX

In this chapter, we have discussed prenatal and postnatal development and have alluded to some of the many functions of the craniofacial complex: respiration, olfaction, speech, digestion, hearing, balance, vision, and neural integration. The tissue components of this complex can be classified as skeletal tissue, soft tissue, and functional spaces (nasopharyngeal and oropharyngeal). Space permits only a brief discussion of these functions; but, since the musculature is intimately related to skeletal development, it is discussed in more detail.

A. EYE

One of the most salient elements of human evolution has been the development of vision as a dominant sense. It was this sense that enabled primitive humans to survive as a species and to develop our present state of technology. The development of binocular vision enabled humans to evolve a system of eye–hand coordination that their increased cerebral function can utilize.

B. EAR

The ear has the dual functions of hearing and balance. The balance mechanism is of earlier phylogenetic development and is represented by paired organs that are connected to the brain. Hearing is a person's most important contact with the environment, for without adequate hearing, speech and oral communication will not develop (see Chapters 5 and 6).

C. NOSE

The sense of smell, which is of such importance in the lower animals, is one of the less important basic functions in humans. However, the conditioning of inhaled air and the provision of a nasal airway are two important functions of the nose in respiration.

D. MOUTH

As the initial portion of the digestive tract, the mouth has a vital function, and although it may be temporarily bypassed by artificial means, the ultimate growth and development of the organism will be affected if the anatomy of this area is altered. Speech, which utilizes both the air and food passages, is a relatively recent phylogenetic function. However, for humans, speech is one of the major achievements and represents the most important means of communication and expression. The neuromuscular functions of the craniofacial complex are concerned with both the aesthetic and the expressive functions of the face. The human face covers a highly complicated skeletal framework with extremely flexible and expressive soft tissue. It is capable of an amazing number of motions and has the ability to convey emotion. Since the face is not covered, even slight facial malformations and deformities may be difficult to conceal and can seriously affect the appearance, and thus the interpersonal relationships, of a child. This was expressed beautifully by Charles Bell in 1833:

> The human countenance performs many functions—in it are combined the organs of mastication, of breathing, of natural voice and speech, and of expression. These motions are performed directly by the will; here also are seen signs of emotions, over which we have but a very limited or imperfect control; the face serves for the lowest animal enjoyment, and partakes of the highest and most refined emotions.

The distribution of the facial musculature is illustrated in Figure 3.21, which demonstrates the relationship of the various facial muscle masses. Facial movements that occur during fetal life were described by Hooker (1939) and discussed in detail by Humphrey (1970). At birth, the infant's musculature is involved primarily with the functions of suckling and swallowing. The airway is maintained, and there are primitive facial reflexes that provide some expression. Experiments have shown that there are responses to taste such as sweet and sour. Early postnatal facial expressions are largely imitations, but most of the facial muscles are used for mandibular stabilization and airway functions. During subsequent postnatal growth and development, there will be tremendous changes in the facial neuromusculature. According to Enlow (1990), more study has been given to the growth of the craniofacial skeleton than to that of the neuromusculature. One reason for this is that it is much more difficult to study the neuromusculature of the face than it is to study its bone structures; consequently, we know less about the facial and jaw muscles (and are less certain of what we do know) than we do about bones and teeth.

During the early periods of embryonic growth, an intimate functional relationship exists between the muscles and the bones to which they are attached. Obviously, when the bones grow, the muscles also must change their size and shape. As a consequence, the muscles occupy different positions, and there is constant adjustment in the attachments of muscles to the skeleton. For instance, changes in the vertical dimensions of the skull will result in a reorientation of the angles at the musculo–osseous junctions.

The influence of the facial musculature on skeletal growth depends on the region involved. Since the most powerful of the facial muscles are involved with mastication, the influence of musculature on the dentition and especially on the mandible will be considerable. Muscles of the airway and food passages compete for influence with the tongue, one of the most powerful muscles of the head.

As a final comment on postnatal craniofacial growth and development, just as the embryo begins as an undifferentiated cell mass, so the newborn appears as an undifferentiated craniofacial complex. Because of differential growth, highly developed individual characteristics will appear as the newborn matures. In the

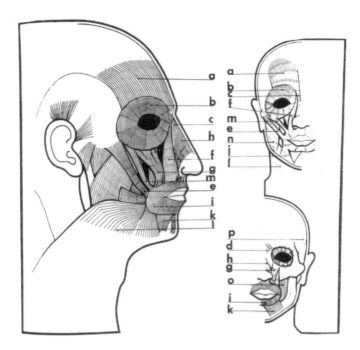

FIGURE 3.21   The distribution of the facial muscles and the complexity of this musculature are illustrated. The muscles originate in laminar form and segment into specific muscles: a = frontalis; b = orbicularis oculi; c = procerus; d = corrugator; e = zygomaticus major; f = levator labii superioris at alae nasi; g = levator labii; h = compressor naris; i = orbicularis oris; j = depressor anguli oris; k = depressor labii inferioris; l = platysma; m = zygomaticus minor; n = masseter nonexpressive; o = buccinator nonexpressive; and p = temporal nonexpressive. After Gasser (1967). Reprinted with permission from Stool (1996).

skeleton, osteoblastic and osteoclastic activity leads to bone deposition, resorption, and displacement. The stimuli for alterations in skeletal development are both genetic and environmental, and it is a balance of these two factors that is responsible for the ultimate craniofacial configuration. Research in craniofacial growth has led to the realization that the mechanisms controlling the growth processes in the face are complex, interrelated, and interdependent. Models of facial growth have evolved from those based on strict genetic predetermination to new paradigms that view the craniofacial complex as highly adaptive and under both local and epigenetic control mechanisms. Growth of the mandible alone is seen to be modulated by a highly complex cybernetic system involving both local and peripheral feedback mechanisms and hormonal and central nervous system influences. The functions of the craniofacial complex, the most characteristic of which in humans are binocular vision (so important in eye–hand coordination), speech, and an infinite variety of facial expressions, have evolved over millions of years. It is understandable that we should desire to know more about this very important area of development, but it is also obvious why study of the craniofacial complex involves deep concentration and unusual effort to yield results. There are numerous theories regarding facial growth, ranging from intrinsic genetic factors controlling the mechanisms of growth to functional or environmental determinants. Gene concepts or paradigms have shifted with new knowledge and changing frameworks of reference, so that currently a combination of genetic and environmental or functional determinants predominates our understanding of an epigenetic paradigm.

REFERENCES

Avery, T. (1990). *Developmental anatomy* (7th ed.). Philadelphia: Saunders.

Behrents, R. G. (1985). *Growth in the aging craniofacial skeleton* (Monograph No. 17). Craniofacial Growth Series. Ann Arbor: Center for Human Growth and Development, University of Michigan.

Bell, C. (1833). *The nervous system of the human body*. Papers presented to the Royal Society on the Subject of Nerves. Stereotyped by Duff Green for the Register and Library of Medical and Chirurgical Science.

Bibby, R. E. (1979). A cephalometric study of sexual dimorphism. *American Journal of Orthodontia, 76,* 256–259.

DeMeyer, W. (1975). Median facial malformations and their implications for brain malformations. In D. Bergsma (Ed.), *Morphogenesis and malformation of face and brain* (pp. 155–181). New York: Liss.

Dibbets, J. M., deBruin, R., & Van der Weele, L. (1987). *Shape change in the mandible during adolescence* (Monograph No. 20). Craniofacial Growth Series. Ann Arbor: Center for Human Growth and Development, University of Michigan.

Enlow, D. H. (1973). Growth and the problem of the local antral mechanism. *American Journal of Anatomy, 178,* 2.

Enlow, D. H. (1990). *Handbook of craniofacial growth*. Philadelphia: Saunders.

Fields, H. W., Warren, D. W., Black, K., & Phillips, C. H. (1991). Relationship between vertical dentofacial morphology and respiration in adolescents. *American Journal of Orthodontia and Dentofacial Orthopedics, 99,* 147–154.

Gasser, R. (1967). The development of the facial nerve in man. *Annals of Otology, Rhinology, and Laryngology, 76,* 37–56.

Hooker, D. (1939). Fetal behavior. *Association for Research in Nervous and Mental Disease, XIX: Interrelationships of mind and body* (pp. 237–243). Baltimore: Williams & Wilkins.

Humphrey, T. (1970). Reflex activity in the oral and facial area of the human fetus. In J. Bosma (Ed.), *Second symposium on oral sensation and perception* (pp. 195–233). Springfield, IL: Thomas.

Ingerslev, C. H., & Solow, B. (1975). Sex differences in craniofacial morphology. *Acta Odontologica Scandinavica, 33,* 85–94.

Isaacson, G., & Mintz, M. C. (1986a). Magnetic resonance image of the fetal temporal bone. *Laryngoscope 96,* 1343–1346.

Isaacson, G., & Mintz, M. C. (1986b). Prenatal visualization of the inner ear. *Journal of Ultrasound in Medicine, 5,* 409–410.

Isaacson, G., Mintz, M. C., & Crelin, E. S. (1986). *Atlas of fetal sectional anatomy*. New York: Springer-Verlag.

Israel, H. (1968). Continuing growth in the human cranial skeleton. *Archives of Oral Biology, 13,* 133–137.

Johnston, M. C. (1975). The neural crest in abnormalities of the face and brain. *Birth Defects Original Articles Series, 11,* 1–18

Krogman, W. (1974). Craniofacial growth and development: An appraisal. *Yearbook of Physical Anthropology, 18,* 31–64.

Latham, R. A. (1970). Maxillary development and growth: The septomaxillary ligament. *Journal of Anatomy, 107,* 471–478.

May, M. (1986). *The facial nerve.* New York: Thieme.

Moss, M. L. (1962). The functional matrix. In B. S. Kraus & R. A. Riedel (Eds.), *Vistas in orthodontics* (pp. 85–97). Philadelphia: Lea & Febiger.

Pierce, R. H., Mainen, M. W., & Bosma, J. F. (1977). *The cranium of the newborn infant.* DHEW Publication No. (NIH) 76-788. Bethesda, MD: U.S. Department of Health, Education, & Welfare.

Rubin, P. (1964). *The dynamic classification of bone dysplasias.* Chicago: Year Book.

Stewart, R., and Prescott, G. (Eds.) (1976). *Oral facial genetics.* St. Louis: Mosby.

Stool, S. (1996). Phylogenetic aspects and embryology. In C. D. Bluestone, S. E. Stool, and M. Kenna (Eds.), *Pediatric Otolaryngology* (pp. 1–18). Philadelphia: Saunders.

Sullivan, P. G. (1986). Skull, jaw, and teeth growth patterns. In F. Falkner & J. M. Tanner (Eds.), *Human growth,* Vol. 2: *Postnatal growth* (pp. 381–412). New York: Plenum.

Williams, P., and Wendell-Smith, C. (1969). *Basic human embryology* (2nd ed.). Philadelphia: Lippincott.

4

MORPHOGENESIS AND GENETICS OF INNER EAR DEVELOPMENT AND MALFORMATION

DOROTHY A. FRENZ

Department of Otolaryngology
Department of Anatomy and Structural Biology
Albert Einstein College of Medicine
Yeshiva University
New York, New York

JUAN REPRESA

Department of Otolaryngology
University of Valladolid
Valladolid, Spain

THOMAS R. VAN DE WATER

Department of Otolaryngology
Department of Neuroscience
Albert Einstein College of Medicine
Yeshiva University
New York, New York

69

I. INTRODUCTION

The membranous labyrinth of the inner ear is comprised of a complex array of fluid-filled cavities and is derived from an epibranchial placode of surface ectoderm (Van De Water, 1988). The sequential expression of patterning genes in the anlagen of the inner ear establishes regional molecular differences that initiate distinct programs of cell proliferation, cell migration, cell differentiation, and cell death. As a result, histogenic domains are created and the otic anlagen becomes transformed into a three-dimensional arrangement of epithelial cells. These ultimately form a vestibular portion (three semicircular ducts with cristae and utricle and saccule with their maculae) and an auditory portion of the inner ear (a coiled cochlear duct with its organ of Corti). Surrounding the membranous labyrinth of the inner ear is the protective bony labyrinth, which is derived from condensed mesodermal mesenchyme in the periotic region. This chapter reviews the morphogenesis of the membranous and bony labyrinths of the inner ear and the gene expression that regulates the cellular and molecular processes responsible for transformation of the otic anlagen into a fully functional inner ear.

II. MORPHOGENESIS OF THE INNER EAR

A. MEMBRANOUS LABYRINTH

The inner ear develops from cephalic surface ectoderm that forms the otic placode. Each otic placode thickens, then invaginates to form the otic vesicle (otocyst), the epithelial primordia from which the vestibular and cochlear regions of the membranous labyrinth develop. The otocyst elongates dorsoventrally to form the pars superior (dorsal vestibular) and pars inferior (ventral cochlear) portions, with the intermediate region giving rise to the utricle and saccule (Lewis & Li, 1967). The anlagen of the endolymphatic duct, one of the first recognizable structures to develop, appears as a finger-like projection from the dorsomedial surface of the otocyst. The duct extends from the developing otocyst and ends in a pouch that will eventually develop into the endolymphatic sac. While during the early stages of fetal development the duct and pouch extend straight out from the inner ear, during later stages of fetal development and early postnatal development the duct curves, achieving a downward angle of 30 to 60°. At 5 weeks of fetal development in the human, the pars superior portion of the otocyst produces two ridge-like structures that, over the next 2 weeks, form the semicircular ducts. A developmental series of photomicrographs illustrating this series of morphogenetic events in the mouse is shown in Figure 4.1.

Coincident with the onset of vestibular morphogenesis (i.e., 5 weeks), cochlear morphogenesis begins when the pars inferior portion of the otocyst starts to elongate and curl in on itself. By 8 weeks of fetal development, the cochlear duct has coiled one full revolution; by 10 weeks, two revolutions. At approximately 25 weeks, the duct has completed 2.5 revolutions and has achieved adult size and shape. The ductus reuniens (i.e., the proximal narrowing of the cochlear duct where it communicates with the saccule) becomes progressively more attenuated during this period of cochlear development (Anson et al., 1960).

The statoacoustic ganglion develops as an aggregation of cells medial and rostral to the developing otocyst. Neurons that arise from this placodally derived tissue originate primarily from a portion of the medial aspect of the otocyst that will later form the macula utriculus (Van De Water, 1986). Two different portions of cells comprise this cluster of neurons: a lateral portion comprised of large cells that exhibit alkaline phosphatase reactivity and a medial portion comprised of smaller cells that do not demonstrate alkaline phosphatase reactivity. The large cells from the lateral portion eventually migrate and form both the *partes magnocellulares* of the vestibular ganglion and the spiral ganglion (Bretos, 1980). The smaller cells form the medial portion from the *partes parvocellulares* of the vestibular ganglion. Neural crest cells invade the statoacoustic ganglion at an early stage of development, extending along the branches of the VIIIth cranial nerve to the crista ampullares and macula utriculus as prospective Schwann cells (D'Amico-Martel & Noden, 1983). Small clusters of neural crest-derived neurons may contribute to the vestibular afferent network of the statoacoustic ganglion. A schematic of the placodal origins of the auditory and vestibular neurons that comprise the VIIIth nerve ganglion in the chick embryo is seen in Figure 4.2.

The sensory structures of the inner ear are derived from the same neuroectoderm that gives rise to the statoacoustic ganglion and the nonsensory regions of the membranous labyrinth. The macula utriculus develops from the inner epithelial lining beginning in the 7th to 8th week of development. Two basic cell types form within the developing macula: supporting cells, which produce a gelatinous substance that forms the otolithic membrane, and sensory cells, which develop into type I and II vestibular hair cells. Type I cells produce one long kinocilium and very tall stereocilia that extend up through the otoconial layer in hair cell bodies enveloped by calyx-type afferent nerve endings. Type II sensory cells produce only short sensory hairs and hair cell soma that are contacted by button-type afferent nerve endings. Type I cells, which are localized mostly in the central zone, are innervated primarily by thick fibers and are static receptors (displacement of the cupula) with a regular discharge pattern. Type II cells, found mostly in the peripheral zone, are innervated by small fibers and are dynamic receptors (endolymph movement) with an irregular discharge pattern.

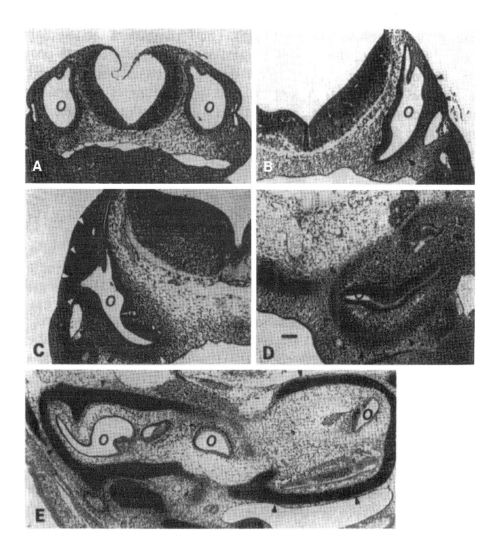

FIGURE 4.1   Photomicrographs of a cross-section of the head of a mouse embryo at 11 days (**A**), 12 days (**B**), 13 days (**C**), 14 days (**D**), and 16 days (**E**) of gestation. The developing otocyst (O) undergoes a series of complex morphogenetic stages as the periotic mesenchyme first condenses (arrows in **B** and **C**) and later chondrified (arrows in **D** and **E**). Note the close contouring of the cartilaginous capsule around the otocyst in **E**, particularly around the semicircular duct on the left-hand side. Ossification begins shortly after 16 days, using the cartilaginous capsule as a template.

By the 14th to 16th week of human development, the superficial appearance of the maculae resembles that seen in the adult. The differentiation of these sensory cell types does not appear to be under the influence of ingrowing nerve fibers

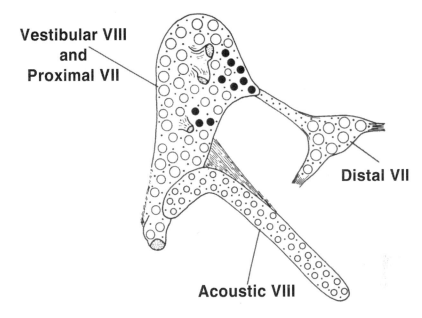

FIGURE 4.2   A diagrammatic reconstruction of the right VIIth and VIIIth cranial nerve ganglion complex of a 12-day-old chick embryo, indicating the tissue origins of the neurons, satellite cells, an Schwann sheath cells. These results are based on orthotopic transplantation of neural crest cells from quail embryos to chick embryo host. ◯ = placodal neurons; ● = neural crest neurons; small black dots = neural crest satellite cells and Schwann cells. Reprinted with permission from D'Amico-Martel and Noden (1983).

since synaptic contacts do not occur until approximately 24 hours after differentiation is evident (Tanaka *et al.*, 1975). Additional evidence of the independence of hair cell differentiation from neuronal influences has been demonstrated by the progression of both electrophysiologic and morphologic differentiation in denervated vestibular explants (Rusch *et al.*, 1998). Although much of the innervation and differentiation is completed during fetal development, both the crista and macula utriculus undergo continued postnatal development. In the rat, the utricle undergoes major morphological changes as late as postnatal day 32, while the cristae postnatally change their shape and size, and demonstrate evidence of ciliogenesis (Killackey & Belford, 1979).

At about 8 weeks gestation, the cristae ampullaris first appear in the human embryo as localized thickenings of the sensory epithelium. The cells forming the crista differentiate into two basic types: supporting and sensory. The development and function of the sensory cells are similar to those observed in the maculae. Each of the sensory cells eventually becomes connected to a dendrite of one of the ampullary branches of the vestibular nerve.

The cupula first appears during mouse vestibular development as a thin amorphous membrane that later becomes compact and fibrous (Ma *et al.*, 1997). Well-developed cupular canals, which resemble those observed in the cupula of the human, are present in the cupullary membrane by 6 days of postnatal development. While in the central zone of the crista, tall stereociliary bundles are in contact with a part of the cupular canal, in the subcupular space the stereociliary bundles are short and freestanding. In the periphery of the crista, the cupular canals are smaller, and disappear at the extreme periphery. As a result, only the tall stereociliary bundles are in direct contact with the cupula. Both the supporting cells of the sensory epithelium and the transitional cells of the crista ampullaris secrete cupular material (Lim & Anniko, 1985). As late as 7 weeks gestation in the human embryo, only poorly formed hair cell stereociliary bundles have been observed (Dechesne *et al.*, 1985). Sensory receptors begin to appear in both the utricular macula and cristae between the 7th and 8th weeks of development. By 23 weeks of gestation (human), the cristae have attained adult form (Lim & Anniko, 1985).

The sensory receptor of the cochlear duct forms from placodal ectoderm. The posterolateral wall of the developing cochlear duct begins to differentiate during the 8th week of human development as concurrently the scala vestibuli and scala tympani begin to form. Fusion of the anterior wall of the scala media with the scala vestibuli results in the formation of Reissner's membrane; fusion of the posterior wall of the scala media with the scala tympani forms the basilar membrane.

Differentiation of the organ of Corti parallels the development of the cochlea. In the embryonic mouse, the hair cells and supporting cells of the organ of Corti have their greatest number of terminal mitoses from gestation age 14–18 days (Ruben, 1967), the equivalent of 6–12 weeks in the developing human. Terminal mitoses of future hair cells occur first at the apex of the mouse cochlear duct and last at the base, while the pattern of cytodifferentiation is from base to apex. In contrast, the pattern of cytodifferentiation in the chick basilar papilla follows the opposite orientation (i.e., from apex to base), with stereocilia bundles appearing first in the distal portion of the papilla and later in the proximal portion.

At approximately 11 weeks of human development, the organ of Corti consists of a thickened pseudostratified epithelium with an extracellular matrix on its luminal surface that will eventually form a tectorial membrane. Studies in the mouse embryo have revealed that the tectorial membrane develops in two parts: the major tectorial membrane, which originates as an amorphous covering of the medial surface of the greater epithelial ridge (Lim & Anniko, 1985), and the minor tectorial membrane, which is derived from primordial supporting cells of the lesser epithelial ridge. The inner and outer hair cells of the cochlea are initially not covered by the tectorial membrane. However, by gestation day 18 in the mouse, the inner hair cells in all turns of the cochlea are covered by the major tectorial membrane (Rueda *et al.*, 1996). By day 19, the minor tectorial membrane covers the outer hair cells in the basal turn. Whereas the stereocilia of the inner hair cells become detached from the tectorial membrane after postnatal day 14, the stereocilia of the outer hair cells remain attached. A transient attachment of the tectorial membrane to the organ of Corti is provided by the marginal pillar cells (Lenoir *et al.*, 1987; Rueda *et al.*, 1996).

The inner and outer hair cells originate from the greater and lesser epithelial ridges of Kolliker's organ, respectively. In the embryonic mouse, inner and outer hair cells in the basal turn of the cochlea can be recognized by gestation age 15 days (Lim & Anniko, 1985), while in the developing human the tunnel of Corti and hair cells appear at the basal turn by the 16th week of gestation. By 25 weeks of gestation (human), the organ of Corti has attained an adult-like configuration (Anson & Donaldson, 1981). The numerous short, thin stereocilia that initially cover the apical hair cell surface are reduced in number as the sensory cells mature. However, the remaining stereocilia grow progressively taller. Typical of most mammalian systems, the mouse auditory hair cells have kinocilia only during development. Even though the organ of Corti is morphologically mature in the 14-day-old mouse neonate, a single kinocilia remains on the apical surface of each auditory hair cell (Lim & Anniko, 1985). By day 21 in the postnatal mouse, no kinocilia are present on the apical auditory hair cell surface, suggesting that full sensory maturation is delayed in the mouse until at least 21 days gestation.

The stria vascularis can be first identified as a protrusion of strial marginal cells on the luminal surface of the scala media. This protrusion disappears as the marginal cells mature. At about 6 days postnatally, the characteristic flat hexagonal cell surface and numerous microvilli of the mature strial marginal cell become defined. In the gerbil stria vascularis, adult vasculature is not achieved until postnatal days 8 to 10 (Axelsson *et al.*, 1986). During this period, the rapid development of the stria vascularis precedes the development of cochlear function. This pattern suggests that full development of the stria vascularis may be associated with the ionic composition of the endolymph and the onset of auditory function.

Morphogenesis of cochlear ganglion cell peripheral processes begins at 3 to 5 days of incubation in the developing chick (Cotanche & Sulik, 1984). Fibers that emerge from the ganglion grow in a uniform fashion toward the yet undifferentiated receptor neuroepithelium. Hair cells become distinguishable from the surrounding epithelium at 8 to 9 days *in ovo*. By 11 to 13 days *in ovo*, nerve fibers develop large, bulbous preterminal swellings located near the bases of the target hair cells. These preterminal swellings disappear by 14 to 17 days (*in ovo*), and the endings transform into mature foot-shaped extensions at the base of each of the hair cells. The synchrony between hair cell differentiation and synaptogenesis is suggested to reflect a nerve–target cell recognition and interaction (Dechesne & Pujol, 1986; Van De Water & Ruben, 1983; Whitehead & Morest, 1985).

B. BONY LABYRINTH (OTIC CAPSULE)

The otic capsule appears initially at 6 weeks of human embryonic development as a condensation of mesodermal (periotic) mesenchyme around the developing otocyst. By 8 weeks of gestation, the condensed mesenchyme has formed a fully chondrified otic capsule that serves as a template for the subsequent formation of the endochondral bony labyrinth. The developing otocyst plays an integral role in the induction and subsequent morphogenesis of the otic capsule. Experiments in embryonic mice demonstrate that chondrogenic differentiation of the otic capsule, and its eventual shape, are both dependent on the presence and normal development of the neuroectodermal otocyst (McPhee & Van De Water, 1986). More recently, studies in high-density culture of mouse inner ear mesenchyme and epithelium have confirmed the control of otic capsule chondrogenesis by otic epithelial–periotic mesenchymal tissue interactions (Frenz & Van De Water, 1991). At early stages of otic capsule development, otic epithelium is required for the induction of chondrogenic differentiation. Consequently, factors that are endogenous to the otocyst epithelium have a significant influence on otic capsule chondrogenesis. These factors include members of the transforming growth factor ($TGF\alpha$), bone morphogenetic protein (BMP), and fibroblast growth factor (FGF) families (Frenz et al., 1992, 1994, 1996 1998; Frenz & Liu, 1998).

In developing humans, the cartilaginous otic capsule persists until the 15th to 16th week of fetal development, at which time ossification centers begin to develop, first in the region at the base of the cochlea and utriculus, and later in the distal portion of the cochlea. By week 19, ossification is nearly complete, except in the region overlying the posterior and horizontal semicircular canals. The posterolateral portion of the posterior semicircular canal ossifies at 20–21 weeks of development, with final ossification of the otic capsule occurring in the area of the ante fenestrum at 22–23 weeks.

The fully developed otic capsule is a trilaminar structure, consisting of three distinct layers of bone: an outer periosteal layer of lamellar compact bone that blends peripherally with the rest of the petrous portion of the temporal bone; an internal periosteal layer of lamellar compact bone that provides attachment to the membranous structures of the labyrinth; and a middle layer of endochondral bone that never fully ossifies and is thus histologically unique (Jahn, 1988). This middle, endochondral layer maintains islands of cartilage surrounded by processes of bone. The reason for the persistence of these islands of cartilage, referred to as *globuli interossei*, may be due to a lack of mechanical stress (Jahn, 1988). Alternatively, it has been speculated that the cartilage rests may serve to cushion the cochlea or to permit vibration of the cochlea for bone conduction (Jahn, 1988; Pedziwiatr, 1971). The combination of intrachondral and endochondral bone is unique to the bony labyrinth (Anson et al., 1960) and may be associated with the localized formation of otosclerotic lesions in this tissue and that of the incompletely ossified structures surrounding the stapedial footplate.

III. GENETIC PATTERNING OF INNER EAR DEVELOPMENT

Analyses of inner ear development in mice with targeted single and/or multiple gene inactivations (null mutations) are beginning to reveal insights into the way patterning genes function to establish the regionalization of inner ear development (Bermingham et al., 1999; Morsli et al., 1999). As a result, new genes with expression domains restricted to particular anatomic sectors of the developing otocyst and/or to specific cell phenotypes have been described (Torres & Giraldez, 1998). Genes expressed during inner ear development can encode for transcription factors, membrane receptors, growth factors, or cell adhesion molecules (Torres & Giraldez, 1998). Transfection of the inner ear with a viral vector that contains a marker gene is also a powerful tool to establish mechanisms of cell phenotype selection that participates in the formation of the unique patterns of tissues that compose the sensory receptors of the adult inner ear (Fekete et al., 1998).

A. REGIONAL SPECIFICATION: PATTERNING OF COCHLEA VERSUS VESTIBULE

The sequential expression of patterning genes (e.g., Hmx3, Pax2) is thought to be the mechanism that underlies how the different tissues of the developing otic anlagen are correctly assembled into their appropriate three-dimensional morphology within the inner ear (Fekete, 1996). It is also known that both the chorda mesoderm and the hindbrain contribute to the induction of the developing otic primordium that is needed for otic placode specification and invagination (Van De Water & Represa, 1991). In-vitro fate mapping of the developing mouse otocyst indicates that, by the time of its formation (i.e., E11), this otic anlagen has become a mosaic for the development of inner ear sensory structures with respect to the dorsoventral, anteroposterior, and lateromedial axes (see Figure 4.3) (Li et al., 1978). Basically, the dorsal portion (pars superior) of the otocyst is committed by this stage to produce vestibular sensory receptors—for example, the semicircular ducts with their associated ampullae with cristae—and the ventral portion (pars inferior) is programmed to differentiate into the cochlear duct with its organ of Corti sensory receptor epithelium. Fate mapping of the mouse otocyst is summarized into eight anatomic sectors in Figure 4.3. The anterior semicircular duct and its associated crista develop from the dorsoanterior portion of the otocyst. The lateral semicircular duct originates from the dorsolateral wall of the otocyst and its associated crista from the dorsolateral anterior section. The posterior semicircular duct and its associated crista develop from the dorsoposterior portion of the otocyst. The utricle and utricular macula are derived from the upper middle third of the medial and lateral walls of the otocyst. The saccule and saccular macula are derived from the lower middle third of the medial wall of the otocyst.

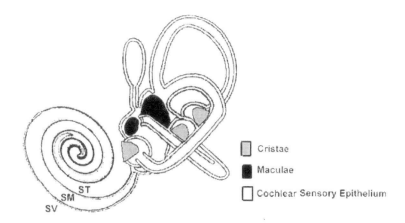

DORSO-MEDIAL ANTERIOR
2 Ducts (Anterior,Lateral)
1Crista (Anterior)
Utriculo-Saccular spaces (Utricle, Saccule)
2 Maculae (Utricular, Saccular)

DORSO-LATERAL ANTERIOR
1 Duct (Anterior)
1Crista (Anterior)
Utriculo-Saccular spaces (Utricle, Saccule)

DORSO-MEDIAL POSTERIOR
1 Duct (Posterior)
1Crista (Posterior)
Utriculo-Saccular space (Utricle)

DORSO-LATERAL POSTERIOR
2 Ducts (Posterior, Lateral)
1Cristae (Posterior)
Utriculo-Saccular space (Utricle)

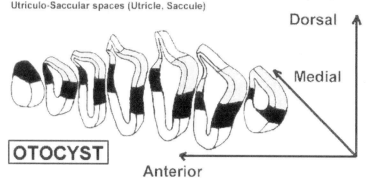

VENTRO-MEDIAL ANTERIOR
Cochlear Duct
Cochlear Sensory Epithelium
Utriculo-Saccular spaces (Utricle, Saccule)
2 Maculae (Utricular, Saccular)

VENTRO- LATERAL ANTERIOR
Cochlear Duct
Cochlear Sensory Epithelium
Utriculo-Saccular spaces (Utricle, Saccule)
2 Maculae (Utricular, Saccular)

VENTRO-MEDIAL POSTERIOR
Cochlear Duct
Cochlear Sensory Epithelium
Utriculo-Saccular space (Utricle)

VENTRO- LATERAL POSTERIOR
Cochlear Duct
Cochlear Sensory Epithelium
Utriculo-Saccular space (Utricle)

FIGURE 4.3   Fate map of inner ear sensory receptors represented as originating from eight different anatomical sectors of the mouse otocyst. Reprinted with permission from Represa *et al.* (2000).

The cochlea, with its sensory and secretory epithelium, develops from both the anterior and posterior regions of pars inferior.

Patterning of the inner ear into prospective vestibular and auditory sensory areas is associated with restriction of gene expression domains during the early stages of otic development (i.e., placode to vesicle stages). Dorsolateral areas that form vestibular epithelium express *Hmx2, Hmx3, dlx3, mshC, mshD, Sox9, p75, lmx1, gbx3, sek1, BMP7,* and *igf1* genes. In contrast, the ventromedial areas, where the putative auditory receptor forms, express *Pax2, dlx4, fgf2, fgf3, BMP4, notch,* and *Ncam.* Figure 4.4 summarizes this anatomic pattern of expressed genes in the otic vesicle in the dorsolateral and ventromedial areas.

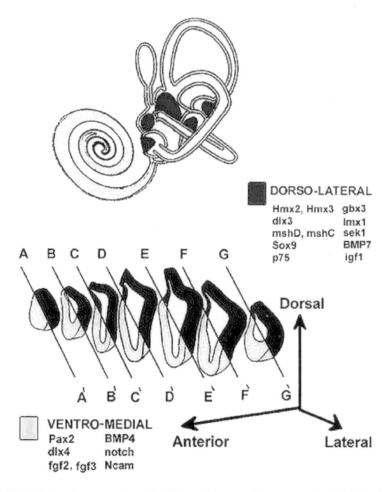

FIGURE 4.4   Representation of the differential pattern of gene expression in the dorsolateral and ventromedial segments of the mouse otocyst. Reprinted with permission from Represa *et al.* (2000).

One model of cell fate specification proposes intersecting loci of the patterns of gene expression in an attempt to explain the regionalization of sensory receptor development (Fekete, 1996). An example of the consequences of a loss of expression of a single patterning gene is the effect of knocking out (null mutation) a single ventral patterning gene, that is, paired-box gene 2 (*Pax 2*) on the formation of the cochlea (Torres *et al.*, 1996). *Pax 2* transcripts are expressed in the ventromedial region of the otocyst, and the membranous labyrinth of the *Pax2* null mutant mouse shows agenesis of the cochlea contrasted to the normal development of vestibular sensory receptors. However, such a dramatic effect in response to the loss of a single gene is unusual, with the more typical effect being a much less dramatic phenotype, reflecting redundancy in the expression domains and action of the patterning genes during otic anlagen development. This concept of gene redundancy in the development of the inner ear is exemplified by the overlapping pattern of expression of two closely related homeobox-containing genes (*Hmx2* and *Hmx3*) in the dorsolateral region of the otocyst (Hadrys *et al.*, 1998; Wang *et al.*, 1998). *Hmx2* and *Hmx3* genes are expressed in overlapping patterns early in the developing mouse otocyst. However, null mutation of the *Hmx3* patterning gene produces only a limited vestibular defect (i.e., utriculo–saccular fusion and lack of a horizontal crista ampullaris), with a complete agenesis of only one of the vestibular receptors (Wang *et al.*, 1998). Future analyses of the inner ear structure of *Hmx2* knockout and *Hmx2/Hmx3* double knockout mutants will determine the extent of redundancy between the *Hmx2* and *Hmx3* patterning genes. Figure 4.5A,B shows examples of mediolateral patterning of the inner ear reflected by the differential and complementary expression patterns of the *Pax2* (Figure 4.5A) and *Hmx3* genes (Figure 4.5B) in the early development of the mouse otocyst.

B. PATTERNING OF TISSUE AND CELL FATE SPECIFICATION

During inner ear development, a series of fate decisions have to be made, for example, neuronal versus nonneuronal, sensory versus nonsensory, and hair cell versus support cell.

One of the earliest morphogenetic events is the thickening of the ventral wall of the otic vesicle, followed by a delamination and then emigration of neuroblasts from the neurogenic regions of the otocyst into the underlying mesenchyme to form the statoacoustic (VIIIth nerve) ganglion (Van De Water, 1988). Grafting experiments in chick and quail embryos (Van De Water, 1988), as well as viral microinjection techniques, have revealed that the potential to generate neurons in the chicken embryo is determined between the placodal and vesicle stages of inner ear development (Represa, unpublished results). Therefore, the selection for the neuroblast cell phenotype of the cochlear and vestibular ganglia occurs after irreversible determination of the otic cup and marks the starting point of the cell-fate specification period within the otic anlagen. Neuroblasts can be observed delaminating from the anteroventral region in the otic cup. Figures 4.5C and 4.5D

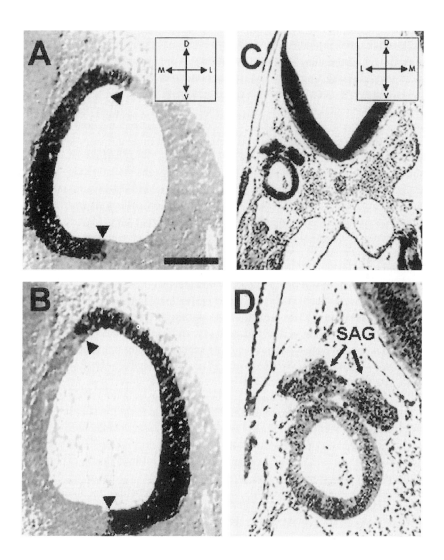

FIGURE 4.5   Examples of gene patterning and establishment of polarity in the developing inner ear. (**A,B**) E9.5, mouse otocyst, *in-situ* hybridization. (**A**) Distribution of *Pax-2* transcripts in the E9.5 otocyst (arrowheads). (**B**) Distribution of *Hmx3* transcripts in the E9.5 otocyst (arrowheads). (**C,D**) A hematoxylin- and eosin-stained transverse section through a chicken embryo otocyst that was rotated 180° at the otic cup stage and then incubated for 2 days *in ovo*. The statoacoustic ganglion (SAG; VIIIth nerve ganglion) in the rotated otic anlagen has established itself in an aberrant position dorsal to the otocyst. The normal position for the SAG is ventromedial and anterior to the otocyst. Rotation of the otic cup shows that the dorsoventral polarity with respect to gangliogenesis is already established by this stage of inner ear development in the chicken embryo. Scale bar equal to 50 μm in **A** and **B**, 250 μm in **C**, and 100 μm in **D**. Reprinted with permission from Represa *et al.* (2000).

show an example of specification of the region of neurogenesis revealed by anomalous position (i.e., dorsal orientation) of the statoacoustic (VIIIth nerve) ganglion in a chicken embryo where the otic cup has been rotated 180° after the establishment of the dorsoventral axis (Represa, unpublished results). In Figure 4.6 the injection of a single otic pit neuroepithelium cell with a retroviral vector shows that several neuroblasts have originated from this single labeled neuroectoderm precursor cell (Represa, unpublished results). Several vertebrate homologues (e.g., *notch, delta, serrate*) of insect lateral inhibition genes have been described to be present in the chick otic anlagen at the time of lineage segregation of neuroblasts (Adam *et al.*, 1998). Concurrent with the specification of neurogenic areas in the chick otic cup, *BMP4* (bone morphogenic protein 4) is expressed in two patches that flank the neurogenic areas (Oh *et al.*, 1996). Functional studies are needed to clarify the relevance of this expression pattern of *BMP4* during neurogenesis in the developing otic anlagen. The *neurogenin-1* (*ngn-1*) gene has been shown to be essential for neuroblast determination in the murine otic anlagen, because the inner ears of *ngn-1* null mutants lack both a vestibular (Scarpa's) and an auditory (spiral) ganglion (Ma *et al.*, 1998).

Another critical developmental decision is the specification of sensory versus nonsensory groups of cells in the otic anlagen. As development progresses, groups of different patterning genes are expressed parallel to the generation of sensory and nonsensory patches within the auditory and vestibular sensory receptors. Several classes of genes are expressed: (a) genes encoding transcription factors, such as *dlx3, dlx4, GH6, SOHO-1, otxl otx2, mshC, mshD, Hmx2, Hmx3*, and *Pax-2*; (b) genes encoding secreted factors, for example, *fgf-2, fgf-3, wnt-3, Xwnt-4, BMP-4*, and *BMP-5*; and (c) genes encoding receptor tyrosine kinases, for example, *ret* and *sek-I*. Some of these genes are specific for putative sensory epithelium—for example, *dlx2, dlx4, mshC, mshD, Ghox7, mlx1, msal, BMP4, sek1, p75, Ncam*, and *GCR*—while other genes, such as *BMP7* and *Lcam* are expressed in nonsensory areas. One gene has been described that is expressed in both sensory and nonsensory areas of the otocyst, *Hmx3*.

BMP4 is a very early marker of putative sensory epithelium in the developing inner ear (Morsli *et al.*, 1998; Wu & Oh, 1996). The gene expression pattern of *BMP5* (similar to that of *BMP4*) is transient and disappears by the otic vesicle stage of development (Oh *et al.*, 1996). In contrast, expression of the *BMP7* gene is extensive and begins at the otic placode stage of development. By E5 in the chicken embryo, the expression patterns of *BMP4* and *BMP7* differ among both the vestibular and auditory sensory receptors. In the vestibule, *BMP7* gene expression becomes segregated from the main sensory tissue areas at the onset of the differentiation of the sensory receptor epithelium, whereas *BMP4* expression was found to become restricted to the area of the differentiating supporting cells. In contrast, the expression pattern of *BMP7* in the cochlea becomes restricted to the sensory tissue and, as development proceeds, localizes to the area of the supporting cells, whereas *BMP4* gene expression becomes localized to the areas of the differentiating putative hair cells. In addition to *BMP4, Msx-1* and *P75*

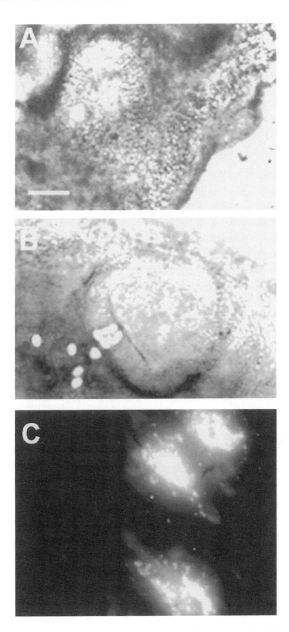

FIGURE 4.6   Lineage tracing using microinjection of single neuroepithelial cells with a retroviral vector expressing a marker protein suggests that segregation of neuroblasts occurs from single neuroectoderm precursor cells. Both neuronal and nonneuronal cell lineages arise from a common progenitor cell within the otic ectoderm. (A–C) Expression of retroviral vector marker protein. (A) Labeling of the otic cup. (B) Labeling of the otic vesicle wall and neuroblasts that have emigrated during the process of gangliogenesis of the statoacoustic ganglion. (C) Individually labeled neuroblasts of the statoacoustic ganglion. Reprinted with permission from Represa *et al.* (2000).

(low-affinity pan-neurotrophin receptor) are markers for the sites of the develop-ing cristae of the semicircular ducts. Based on the expression patterns of these three genes (*BMP4*, *Msx-1*, and *P75*), the temporal pattern of commitment and differentiation of sensory organs has been defined in chick embryos (Wu & Oh, 1996). The anterior and posterior cristae appear first, followed sequentially by the macula of the saccule, the lateral crista, the basilar papilla and lagena, the macula of the utricle, and the macula neglecta.

A series of recent experiments in chicken embryos (Chang *et al.*, 1999; Gerlach *et al.*, 2000) has shown that ectopic expression of a gene, *noggin*, that antagonized the action of the *BMP4* gene product, disrupts both the formation of the semicir-cular ducts (nonsensory) and their cristae (sensory). In the developing mouse inner ear, a similar pattern of the origins of sensory receptors can be defined by the sequential expression pattern of the *BMP4*, *lunatic fringe* (*Fng*), and *Brn 3.1* genes (Morsli *et al.*, 1998). One other gene product was also found to affect the forma-tion of the semicircular ducts in the mouse, and that is the cell guidance molecule netrin. The inner ears of null mutants for the *netrin* gene all displayed malforma-tion of their semicircular ducts, implicating this gene as an essential gene for the proper morphogenesis of the semicircular ducts (Salminen *et al.*, 2000). The *otx1* and *otx2* genes (murine orthologues of *Drosophila aorthodenticle Otd* gene) are expressed in the area fated to form both vestibular and auditory sensory receptors (Morsli *et al.*, 1999). Null mutation of the *otx1* gene affects both auditory and vestibular structures, and the development of these inner ear sensory receptors was more profoundly affected in the inner ears of *otx1* null mutants that are heterozygous (+/–) for the *otx2* gene (Morsli *et al.*, 1999). Null mutation of *otx2* results in early death of affected embryos prior to otic morphogenesis. However, if the *otx2* gene is knocked out and the resultant homozygotic embryos rescued by knocking in an *otx1* gene under the control of the promoter of the *otx2* gene, then the *otx2* null mutants have a more severe disruption of inner ear development (Van De Water, unpublished data). These results suggest that both *otx1* and *otx2* represent boundary genes that affect the development of both the vestibule and the cochlea. There is a suggestion from these *otx1* knockout and *otx2* knockout and *otx1* knock-in experiments that these patterning genes also influence the three-dimensional morphologic relationship between the cochlea and the vesti-bule.

Once the specification of sensory organs has been established, the specification of hair cell versus supporting cell occurs next. Mouse *Brn3.1*, a *Pou*-domain transcription factor gene, is expressed in all the sensory areas of the otocyst (Erkman *et al.*, 1996; Xiang *et al.*, 1998). Targeted mutation of this factor results in the loss of all inner ear hair cells, showing that the expression of *Brn 3.1* constitutes, in both auditory and vestibular receptor epithelium, an absolute re-quirement to insure the survival of the newly generated hair cells (Erkman *et al.*, 1996; Xiang *et al.*, 1998). Maturation of the supporting cells also appears to be impaired in the inner ears of these *Brn 3.1* null mutants, suggesting that active hair cell-supporting cell interactions are required to support the survival of the supporting cell lineage (Erkman *et al.*, 1996; Xiang *et al.*, 1998). Lineage tracing using retroviral transfection suggests that hair cell and supporting cell lineages arise from a common population of progenitor cells and do not segregate until very late in inner ear development (Fekete *et al.*, 1998). The molecular mechanisms that allow for differentiation of the two phenotypes from a single pool of progenitor cells are just beginning to be understood. Recent analyses of the inner ears of two new null mutants, *Jagged-1* and *Math1*, have implicated the *Notch-Delta* signaling pathway (Lanford *et al.*, 1999) and *Math1* (Bermingham *et al.*, 1999) in the selection of a developmental choice between hair cell and supporting cell phenotypes in the developing mouse inner ear.

A final consideration in the genetic patterning of the inner ear is the role of the sequential expression of growth factor genes and their role in specifying the development of both the otic capsule and the perilymphatic spaces, which act to protect and nourish the membranous labyrinth. The bony labyrinth of the inner ear is formed as a result of the initial process of endochondral bone formation that forms the cartilaginous otic capsule. The formation of the cartilaginous otic capsule involves reciprocal tissue interactions between the epithelium of the otocyst and its surrounding periotic mesenchyme. Hence, aside from regulating the cellular and molecular processes that establish patterning of the membranous labyrinth, patterning genes in the otic anlagen also affect the differentiation and morphogenesis of the periotic mesenchyme to produce an endochondral bony labyrinth. These genes encode for secreted factors, including members of the *TGFβ*, *FGF*, and *BMP* families of growth factors (Frenz *et al.*, 1992; Frenz & Liu, 1998). In response to induction by FGFs (FGF2, FGF3), chondrogenic differentiation of the periotic mesenchyme begins with the formation of cellular condensations within the surrounding mesenchyme (Frenz *et al.*, 1994; Frenz & Liu, 1998). As these regions of condensed mesenchyme differentiate into cartilage, they are acted on by secreted factors that include *TGFβ* and *BMP2* (Frenz *et al.*, 1992, 1996), ultimately forming a fully chondrified otic capsule, with its perilymphatic spaces, that serves as the template for subsequent formation of the bony labyrinth, scala vestibuli, and scala tympani of the adult inner ear and temporal bone.

ACKNOWLEDGMENTS

This work was supported by The Hearing Research Fund of the Communication Disorders Institute of Montefiore Medical Center

REFERENCES

Adam, J., Myat, A., LeRoux, I., Eddison, M., Henrique, D., Ish-Horowicz, D., & Lewis, J. (1998). Cell fate choices and the expression of Notch, Delta and Serrate homologues in the chick inner ear: Parallels with drosophila sense-organ development. *Development, 125*, 4645–4654.

Anson, B. J., & Donaldson, J. A. (1981). *Surgical anatomy of the temporal bone.* Philadelphia: Saunders.

Anson, B. J., Hanson, J. S., & Richany, S. F. (1960). Early embryology of the auditory ossicles and associated structures in relation to certain anomalies observed clinically. *Annals of Otology, Rhinology, & Laryngology, 69*, 427–447.

Axelsson, A., Ryan, A., & Woolf, N. (1986). The early postnatal development of the cochlear vasculature in the gerbil. *Acta Otolaryngologica, 101*, 75–86.

Bermingham, N. A., Hassan, B. A., Price, S. D., Vollrath, M. A., Ben-Arie, N., Eatock, R. A., Bellen, H. J., Lysakowski, A., & Zoghbi, H. Y. (1999). Math1: An essential gene for the generation of inner ear hair cells. *Science, 284*, 1837–1841.

Bretos, M. (1980). La morphogenese primordial du ganglion stato-acoustique et de l'oreille interne chez l'embryon de souris, II: Etude de l'evolution des ebauches chez l'embryons de 101/2 à 12 jours. *Archiv Belgique, 91*, 77–113.

Chang, W., Nunes, F. D., De Jesus-Escobar, J. M., Harland, R., & Wu, D. K. (1999). Ectopic Noggin blocks sensory and nonsensory organ morphogenesis in the chicken inner ear. *Developmental Biology, 216*, 369–381.

Cotanche, D. A., & Sulik, K. K. (1984). The development of stereociliary bundles in the cochlear duct of the chick embryo. *Developmental Brain Research, 16*, 181–193.

D'Amico-Martel, A., & Noden, D. M. (1983). Contributions of placodal and neural crest cells to avian cranial peripheral ganglia. *American Journal of Anatomy, 166*, 445–468.

Dechesne, C. J., & Pujol, R. (1986). Neuron-specific enolase immunoreactivity in the developing mouse cochlea. *Hearing Research, 21*, 87–90.

Dechesne, C. J., Sans, A., & Keller, A. (1985). Onset and development of neuron-specific enolase immunoreactivity in the peripheral vestibular system of the mouse. *Neuroscience Letters, 61*, 299–304.

Erkman, L., McEvilly, R. J., Luo, L., Ryan, A. K., Hooshmand, F., O'Connell, S. M., Keithley, E. M., Rapaport, D. H., Ryan, A. F., & Rosenfeld, M. G. (1996). Role of transcription factors Brn-3.1 and Brn-3.2 in auditory and visual system development. *Nature, 381*, 603–606.

Fekete, D. M. (1996). Cell fate specification in the inner ear. *Current Opinions in Neurobiology, 6*, 533–541.

Fekete, D. M., Muthukumar, S., & Karagogeos, D. (1998). Hair cells and supporting cells share a common progenitor in the avian inner ear. *Journal of Neuroscience, 18*, 7811–7821.

Frenz, D. A., & Liu, W. (1998). Role of FGF3 in otic capsule chondrogenesis *in vitro*: An antisense oligonucleotide approach. *Growth Factors, 15*, 173–182.

Frenz, D. A., & Van De Water, T. R. (1991). Epithelial control of periotic mesenchyme chondrogenesis. *Developmental Biology, 144*, 38–46.

Frenz, D. A., Galinovic-Schwartz, V., Flanders, K. C., & Van De Water, T. R. (1992). TGF$_1$ is an epithelial-derived signal peptide that influences otic capsule formation. *Developmental Biology, 153*, 324–336.

Frenz, D. A., Liu, W., Williams, J. D., Hatcher, V., Galinovic-Schwartz, V., Flanders, K. C., & Van De Water, T. R. (1994). Induction of chondrogenesis: Requirement for synergistic interaction of basic fibroblast growth factor and transforming growth factor-beta. *Development, 120*, 415–424.

Frenz, D. A., Liu, W., & Capparelli, M. (1996) The role of BMP-2a in otic capsule chondrogenesis. *Annals of the New York Academy of Sciences, 785*, 256–258.

Frenz, D. A., Yoo, H., & Liu, W. (1998). Basilar papilla explants: A model to study hair cell regeneration-repair and protection. *Acta Otolaryngologica, 118*, 651–659.

Gerlach, L. M., Hutso, M. R., Germiller, J. A., Nguyen-Luu, D., Victor, J. C., & Barald, K. F. (2000). Addition of the BMP4 antagonist, noggin, disrupts avian inner ear development. *Development, 127*, 45–54.

Hadrys, T., Braun, T., Rinkwitz-Brandt, S., Arnold, H. H., and Bober, E. (1998). Nkx5-1 controls semicircular canal formation in the mouse inner ear. *Development, 125*, 33–39.

Jahn, A. F. (1988). Bone physiology of the temporal bone, otic capsule, and ossicles. In A. Jahn & J. Santos-Sacchi (Eds.), *Physiology of the ear* (pp. 143–158). New York: Raven Press.

Killackey, H. P., & Belford, G. R. (1979). The formation of afferent patterns in the somatosensory cortex of the neonatal rat. *Journal of Comparative Neurology, 183*, 285–303.

Lanford, P. J., Lan, Y., Jiang, R., Lidsell, C., Weinmaster, G., Gridley, T., & Kelley, M. W. (1999). Notch signaling pathway mediates hair cell development in mammalian cochlea. *Nature Genetics, 21*, 289–292.

Lenoir, M., Puel, J. L., & Pujol, R. (1987). Stereocilia and tectorial membrane development in the rat cochlea: An SEM study. *Anatomy and Embryology (Berl.), 175*, 477–487.

Lewis, E. R., & Li, C .W. (1967). Evidence concerning the morphogenesis of saccular receptors in the bullfrog (*Rana catesbeiana*). *Journal of Morphology, 139*, 351–361.

Li, C. W., Van De Water, T. R., & Ruben, R. J. (1978). The fate mapping of the eleventh and twelfth day mouse ototcyst: An *in vitro* study of the sites of origin of the embryonic inner ear sensory structures. *Journal of Morphology, 157*, 249–268.

Lim, D. J., & Anniko, M. (1985). Developmental morphology of the mouse inner ear: A scanning electron microscopic observation. *Acta Otolaryngologica (Suppl.), 422*, 1–69.

Ma, Q., Sommer, L., Cserjesi, P., & Anderson, D. J. (1997). Mash1 and neurogenin 1 expression patterns define complementary domains of neuroepithelium in the developing CNS and are correlated with regions expressing notch ligands. *Journal of Neuroscience, 17*, 3644–3652.

Ma, Q., Chen, Z., del Barco Barantes, I., de la Pompa, J. L., & Anderson D. J. (1998). Neurogenin-1 is essential for the determination of neuronal precursors for proximal cranial sensory ganglia. *Neuron, 20*, 469–482.

Mansour, S. L., Goddard, J. M., & Capecchi, M. (1993). Mice homozygous for a targeted disruption of the proto-oncogene int-2 have development defects in the tail and inner ear. *Development, 117*, 13–28.

McPhee, J. R., & Van De Water, T. R. (1986). Epithelial–mesenchymal tissue interactions guiding otic capsule formation: The role of the otocyst. *Journal of Embryology and Experimental Morphology, 97*, 1–24.

Morsli, H., Choo, D., Ryan, A. L., Johnson, R., & Wu, D. K. (1998). Development of the mouse inner ear and origin of its sensory organs. *Journal of Neuroscience, 18*, 3327–3335.

Morsli, H., Tuorto, F., Choo, D., Postiglione, M. P., Simeone, A., & Wu, D. K. (1999). Otx1 and Otx2 activities are required for the normal development of the mouse inner ear. *Development, 126*, 2335–2343.

Oh, S. H., Johnson, R., & Wu, D. K. (1996). Differential expression of bone morphogenetic proteins in the developing vestibular and auditory sensory organs. *Journal of Neuroscience, 16*, 6463–6475.

Pedziwiatr, Z. (1971). Morphological data for the theory of temporal bone vibrations. *Polish Medical Journal, 10*, 547–563.

Represa, J., Frenz, D. A., & Van De Water, T. R. (2000). Genetic patterning of embryonic inner ear development. *Acta Otolaryngologica, 120*, 5–10.

Ruben, R. J. (1967). Development of the inner ear of the mouse: A radioautographic study of terminal mitoses. *Acta Otolaryngologica, 220*, 1–44.

Rueda, J., Cantos, R., & Lim, D. J. (1996). Tectorial membrane-organ of Corti relationship during cochlear development. *Anatomy and Embryology, 194*, 501–514.

Rusch, A., Lysakaowski, A., & Eatock, R. A. (1998). Postnatal development of type I and type II hair cells in the mouse utricle: Acquisition of voltage-gated conductances and differentiated morphology. *Journal of Neuroscience, 18,* 7487–7501.

Salminen, M., Meyer, I. B., Bober, E., & Gruss, P. (2000). Netrin 1 is required for semicircular canal formation in the mouse inner ear. *Development, 127,* 13–22.

Tanaka, T., Ozeki, Y., Aoki, T., & Ogura, Y. (1975). Morphological relation of the vestibular sensory hairs to the otolithic membrane and cupula: A scanning electron microscopic study. In M. Marimoto (Ed.), *The Proceedings of the 5th Extraordinary Meeting of the Barany Society* (pp. 403–409). Kyoto: Barany Society.

Torres, M., & Giraldez, F. (1998). The development of the vertebrate inner ear. *Mechanisms of Development, 71,* 5–21.

Torres, M., Gomez-Pardo, E., & Gruss, P. (1996). Pax2 contributes to inner ear patterning and optic nerve trajectory. *Development, 122,* 3381–3391.

Van De Water, T. R. (1986). Determinants of neuron–sensory receptor cell interaction during development of the inner ear. *Hearing Research, 22,* 265–277.

Van De Water, T. R. (1988). Tissue interactions and cell differentiation: Neuron–sensory cell interaction during otic development. *Development, 103,* 185–193.

Van De Water, T. R., & Represa, J. (1991). Tissue interactions and growth factors that control development of the inner ear: Neural tube–otic anlage interaction. In R. J. Ruben, T. R. Van De Water, & K. P. Steel (Eds.), Genetics of hearing impairment, *Annals of the New York Academy of Sciences, 630,* 116–128.

Van De Water, T. R., & Ruben, R. J. (1983). A possible embryonic mechanism for the establishment of innervation of inner ear sensory structures. *Acta Otolaryngologica, 95,* 470–479.

Wang, W., Van De Water, T. R., & Lufkin, T. (1998). Inner ear and maternal reproductive defects in mice lacking the Hmx3 homeobox gene. *Development, 125,* 621–634.

Whitehead, M. C., & Morest, D. K. (1985). The development of innervation patterns in the avian cochlea. *Neuroscience, 14,* 255–276.

Wu, D. K., & Oh, S. H. (1996). Sensory organ generation in the chick inner ear. *Journal of Neuroscience, 16,* 6454–6462.

Xiang, M., Gao, W.-Q., Hasson, T., & Shin, J. J. (1998). Requirement for Brn-3c in maturation and survival, but not in fate determination of inner ear hair cells. *Development, 125,* 3935–3946.

5

GENETIC DEAFNESS

ROBERT J. RUBEN

Departments of Otorhinolaryngology and Pediatrics
Albert Einstein College of Medicine
Yeshiva University
New York, New York

I. INTRODUCTION

The underlying processes that result in hearing loss and deafness are numerous and, in many instances, interact. The most common of these factors is the genetic make-up of the individual. It has been estimated that more than 50% of all hearing losses have a substantial genetic component. This is a low estimate, because for about 25% of those with hearing impairments the etiology is unknown, and many of these will eventually be proven to be genetically derived (see Chapter 1). Additionally, as various acquired causes of hearing loss are prevented, such as congenital rubella and *Haemophilus influenzae* meningitis, the percentage of persons with genetically determined deafness will increase proportionally (Parving & Christensen, 1996). Some of the acquired deafness (e.g., from a standard non-ototoxic dose of aminoglycosides) has now been determined to come about because of genetic predispositions (Fischel-Ghodsian *et al.*, 1993). Another instance of an extrinsic factor that causes a gene to be activated so as to result in hearing loss may be the relationship between otosclerosis and the measles virus (McKenna & Mills, 1989; Niedermeyer & Arnold, 1995). It is anticipated that there will be an increase in the percentage of hearing loss in which a genetic disposition plays a substantial role. Genetic hearing loss is associated with all the different forms of hearing loss whether classified by age, progression, and site of lesion(s) or interactions with extrinsic factors, for example, aminoglycosides (Fischel-Ghodsian *et al.*, 1993).

The information concerning genetics and hearing expands almost daily, and this is expected to continue for the foreseeable future. Much of this new information will have direct utility for the care of patients. These rapid advances are made available in a timely manner through a number of Internet websites. There are two among many (Table 5.1) that both contain substantial information in very usable format and provide links to other pertinent sites.

HISTORY OF THE GENETICS OF HEARING
IMPAIRMENT (Ruben, 1991)

A familial tendency for hearing loss has been recognized at least since the early seventeenth century. Bonet's book (1620), the first printed book concerning the education of the deaf, is based on the education of one child who had numerous hearing-impaired relatives (Plann, 1997). The first work to categorize systematically familial and nonfamilial deafness is Wilde's *Otology* (1853). Wilde's data,

TABLE 5.1   Pertinent Websites for Assessing Current Information Concerning the Genetics of Deafness

HTML	Name	Description
http://www3.ncbi.nlm.nih.gov//	Online Mendelian Inheritance in Man (OMIM)™	Information can be obtained by syndrome, characteristics. Has numerous links to literature. Substantial detail and depth. Excellent search engine.
http://dnalab-www.uia.ac.be/dnalab/hhh	Hereditary Hearing Loss	Gives concise information of the state of the art of the known genes that result in hearing loss

developed before the recognition of Mendel's modes of inheritance, were not widely distributed. Love (1896) and others at the beginning of the twentieth century described and emphasized the role of inheritance as a significant etiology for hearing impairment.

The recognition of familial bases of hearing loss has been used to harm affected individuals through attempts to prevent marriage, sterilize, and exterminate. This tragic aspect of the history of the genetics of hearing impairment begins with A. G. Bell's *On a Deaf Variety of the Human Race* (1880), in which he states that to eliminate deafness the deaf should not marry nor have children. This work, and others of Bell's veiled works (he used sheep breeding as a model for human eugenics) contributed to the early policies of the Nazi regime to sterilize and then exterminate deaf children. These crimes are well documented and published in Biesold's (1988, 1999) *Klagende Hande* (*Crying Hands*).

Although there were some pertinent publications during the first half of the twentieth century, it was not until 1976, with the publication of two books, Fraser's (1976) and the posthumous publication of Konigsmark's work (Konigsmark & Gorlin, 1976), that there was widespread appreciation of the genetics underlying deafness. These works preceded the current enhanced ability to localize genes on chromosomes and to determine the aberrations in the protein sequences. A symposium held in 1990 under the auspices of the New York Academy of Sciences (Ruben *et al.*, 1991) brought together the current information concerning the molecular basis of the genetics of deafness. Since the 1990 meeting, information on the genetics of deafness has vastly increased. During the period 1990 to 2000, the National Library of Medicine (as determined by computer search) has indexed more than 1500 articles that relate to genetics and deafness and/or hearing loss. This growth of information is expected to continue. The present era should be one of defining the molecular abnormalities resulting in deafness and lesser hearing losses, determining how these aberrations affect the hearing mechanisms, and constructing successful interventions to prevent, cure, or ameliorate the effects of the gene action.

II. NOSOLOGY

A. ANATOMICAL

There are numerous ways by which the various genetically based hearing disorders can be classified. The anatomical site(s) of gene action can be used to organize the information in a useful manner. Knowledge of whether the outer ear, external ear canal, middle ear, cochlea, vestibular apparatus, statoacoustic nerve, and/or the central nervous system are affected is useful to the clinician in the care of the specific genetic disorder. One gene may affect a number of sites, and an abnormality at one locus can result in a variety of different anatomical defects.

B. PHENOTYPE

The apparent characteristics of the gene action, the phenotype, are another useful means of classification. There are at least two general phenotypic modes of classification: syndromic and nonsyndromic. The first is defined in terms of whether there are other abnormalities associated with the deafness, such as are found in the various Waardenburg or Usher syndromes. If the deafness is determined to be of genetic etiology and there is no other detectable expression of the gene actions, then these are classified as nonsyndromic.

The second, nonsyndromic phenotypic classification concerns various features of the hearing loss. A time dimension can be applied to classify whether the loss was congenital, early onset, middle life, or presbycusis, thus mapping the presence of progression of the loss. The characteristics of the pure tone audiogram are also used to classify the abnormality. The audiometric profiles can be high tone, low tone, U-shaped audiograms, and others.

C. MODE OF INHERITANCE

The genetically determined hearing losses can be categorized as to whether they are dominant (DFNA#), recessive (DFNB#), X-linked (DFN#), or mitochondrial. (The suffixed numeral refers to the order of identification. Thus, DFNA1 is the first dominant gene to be assigned a locus and DFNB5 is the fifth recessive gene to be.) There are both phenotypic and molecularly defined genetic hearing losses that appear to have more than one mode of inheritance. The difference between a recessive inheritance—carrying two identical abnormal genes or two different abnormal genes (compound heterozygous)—and a dominant mode of inheritance—carrying only one abnormal gene—may appear as a difference in the amount of the hearing impairment (Zlotogora, 1997).

D. MOLECULAR ABERRATIONS: CHANGES IN NUCLEAR DNA AND MITOCHONDRIAL DNA (mtDNA)

There are several types of abnormalities in the structure of an individual's DNA that result in a symptomatic form of hearing impairment. These consist of deletions or insertions of a portion of the DNA; substitution of one or more nucleic acids in a segment of DNA; a translocation, in which a piece of the DNA is exchanged for another piece of the DNA; and inversions, in which the orientation of a segment of DNA is flipped; or duplication of a stretch of DNA (see Gerber, 1998). Additionally, there may abnormalities in chromosome number.

Mitochondria, the energy-producing organelles, contain their own genetic material. Changes in mtDNA occur in a number of syndromic and nonsyndromic hearing impairments. The mitochondrial disorders are transmitted from the mother to the child.

III. SYNDROMIC HEARING IMPAIRMENT

There are numerous forms of syndromic deafness and hearing impairments. The 10 for which the gene is known are listed in Table 5.2. There are many other forms of syndromic hearing impairment that have substantial impact on the individual, and the number of individuals whom they affect, that have not been localized on a chromosome. A list of these with descriptions is obtained from the URLs listed in Table 5.1. The nomenclature for Online Mendelian Inheritance in Man (OMIM) is given in Table 5.3. A search of OMIM using the word *hearing* produced 457 entries. Supplemental to the ones discussed below are three others that, because of their ubiquity and/or morbidity, need to be noted.

The first of these is one of the most common of hearing impairments in the young, that caused by otitis media. The data of Casselbrant *et al.* (2000), based on a large twin study, indicate that there is a strong genetic component to the amount of time with middle ear effusion and episodes of middle ear effusion and acute otitis media in children.

TABLE 5.2   Ten Syndromic Forms of Hearing Impairment (Van Camp & Smith, 2000)

Alport syndrome
Branchio-oto-renal syndrome
Jervell and Lange–Nielsen syndrome
Mitochondrial syndromes
Norrie disease
Pendred syndrome
Stickler syndrome
Treacher Collins syndrome
Usher syndrome
Waardenburg syndrome

TABLE 5.3   Numbering and Symbols (McKusick, 2000)

Each entry is given a unique six-digit number whose first digit indicates the mode of inheritance of the gene involved:

1——	(100000–)	Autosomal dominate (entries created before 15 May 1994)
2——	(200000–)	Autosomal recessive (entries created before 15 May 1994)
3——	(300000–)	X-linked loci or phenotypes
4——	(400000–)	Y-linked loci or phenotypes
5——	(500000–)	Mitochondrial loci or phenotypes
6——	(600000–)	Autosomal loci or phenotypes (entries created after 15 May 1994)

The second is Shprintzen (velocardiofacial) syndrome (Shprintzen *et al.*, 1981) (OMIM Link 192430; this link is the reference code from Online Mendelian Inheritance in Man). The locus for this syndrome is at 22q11 and is similar to the DiGeorge syndrome. Shprintzen syndrome consists of cleft palate, pharyngeal hypotonia, medial displacement of the internal carotid arteries, cardiac anomalies, typical facies, learning disorders, slender hands and digits, umbilical hernia, hypospadias, and, in adolescents and adults, psychotic illness. Conductive hearing loss is found in 47% and a sensory–neural loss in 17% of patients with Shprintzen syndrome (Reyes *et al.*, 1999; Shprintzen *et al.*, 1981; ID:14). These patients need to be identified so as to avoid inappropriate adenoidectomy (and the possibility of damage to the internal carotid artery) and the exacerbation of their velo-pharyngeal insufficiency. Their hearing impairments need to be recognized and cared for.

The third is neurofibromatosis, type II (NFII) (OMIM Link 101000) whose locus is at 22q12.2. These patients have the central form of neurofibromatosis, which is characterized by tumors of both statoacoustic nerves, and meningiomas and schwannomas of the dorsal roots of the spiral ganglia. There is often associated posterior capsular lens opacity. Almost half of these individuals will present with unilateral or bilateral hearing loss in the first two decades of life. Individuals will present in the first decade with severe morbidity due to the intracranial tumors and the subsequent loss of hearing, vestibular response, and, in some cases, blindness. Many of these patients' morbidities are the probable result of spontaneous mutation. The diagnosis of NFII should be considered in cases of asymmetrical hearing loss or those with poor discrimination. MRI is for diagnosis, and reveals small asymptomatic tumors in the statoacoustic nerve.

A. ALPORT SYNDROME (OMIM Link 104200)

This syndrome consists of nephritis, which can progress to renal failure. The hearing loss is sensory–neural, varying from modest to severe, and is usually progressive. Males are more severely affected than females (Admiraal, 1970; Turner, 1970). There are three forms of genetic inheritance: autosomal dominant, recessive at 2q36–37, and sex-linked at Xq22. All forms have variable penetrance.

B. BRANCHIO-OTO-RENAL (BOR) SYNDROME (OMIM Link 113560)

BOR consists of a number of variable anomalies of the face and neck, which may include abnormalities of cup-shaped and/or anteverted pinnae; bilateral pre-helical pits; bilateral bronchial fistulae; and bilateral renal dysplasia with anomalies of the collecting system. Additionally, there have been reported polycystic kidneys and abnormalities of the lachrymal ducts including stenosis and/or aplasia. The hearing loss may be conductive, mixed, or sensory neural (Cremers & Fikkers-van Noord, 1980). Many, if not most, of these patients have a spectrum of abnormalities of the bony labyrinth ranging from aplasia to deficient coils of the cochlea. The genetic transmission is dominant, and the gene has been located on 8q13.3.

C. JERVELL AND LANGE–NIELSEN SYNDROME (OMIM Link 220400)

The Jervell and Lange–Nielsen syndrome consists of a cardiac conduction abnormality characterized by a prolonged QT interval. This is associated with syncopal attacks in the affected individual. The cardiac symptoms appear during the first 2 to 3 years of life and, if uncared for, can result in death (Cusimano *et al.*, 1991). The hearing loss is typically a congenital severe to profound sensory–neural deafness. The mode of inheritance is recessive and there are two different gene locations: 11p15.5 and 21q22.1–22.2.

D. MITOCHONDRIAL SYNDROMES

Several forms of mitochondrial hearing loss with other associated defects have been reported. These are myoclonic epilepsy and ragged red fibers (MERRF) on tRNAlys at 8344>G. These patients have severe neurological symptoms including blindness and a variable amount of hearing loss. There is a variant of MERRF that occurs on tRNAlys but at 8356T>C that has an associated postlingual progressive deafness. Another is mitochondrial encephalopathy, lactic acidosis, and stroke-like episodes (MELAS). The locus is on tRNAleu (UUR) at 3243A>G. About 30% of these patients will have an associated hearing loss. Kearns–Sayre syndrome (KSS) consists of external ophthalmoplegia and retinopathy that begin by age 20. Additionally, there is an associated ataxia, heart block, and hearing loss. This hearing loss is thought to be central, based on auditory evoked potential data (Korres *et al.*, 1999). The defects on the mitochondria are large and are found on several genes.

E. NORRIE DISEASE (OMIM Link 310600)

This is an X-linked disorder that has congenital ocular symptoms, including retinal pseudotumor and necrosis of the inner layer of the retina, cataracts, and blindness (Black & Redmond, 1994). There is a progressive sensory–neural hearing loss and mental retardation in half of the patients. This disease begins with blindness, and the hearing loss comes on later in life. This is the reverse of most of the Usher disease variants. The gene is located at Xp11.3 (Berger *et al.*, 1992).

F. PENDRED SYNDROME (OMIM Link 274600)

Pendred syndrome is a recessive disorder associated with a mild form of thyroid disease in that there can be a clinical goiter; it was first described by Vaughn Pendred in 1896, and a century later the gene was mapped to chromosome 7 (Coyle *et al.*, 1996). There is a reasonably specific test for this condition in that an affected patient will show only a partial discharge of iodine when thiocyanate or perchlorate is given. The histology of the affected thyroid gland is unusual and can be mistaken for cancer; cancers have been reported, however, in these patients.

The hearing loss may be either a congenital or progressive sensory–neural loss and may be associated with defective vestibular function. The bony labyrinth of these patients may be abnormal, as has been seen in temporal bone histology and imaging. Many of these patients have an enlarged vestibular aqueduct (Cremers *et al.*, 1998). The gene is located at 7q21–34, and there is a number of allelic variants.

G. STICKLER SYNDROME (OMIM Links 108300, 184840, and 121028)

There are three forms of this dominant syndrome reported (Table 5.4); the most common is STL1 located at 12q13.11–q13.2. The classic syndrome consists of progressive myopia, vitreoretinal degeneration, premature joint degeneration with abnormal epiphyseal development, midfacial hypoplasia, irregularities of the vertebral bodies, and cleft palate, and many will have a sensory–neural hearing loss that can be exacerbated by the concomitant chronic or intermittent otitis media with effusion (Ruben & Math, 1978). Stickler syndrome affects vision and hearing, and these are less-than-total losses of either sensory modality. Additionally, it affects the expressive aspect of spoken language because of the cleft palate. Some of these children will have a tracheal or laryngeal stenosis, which further decreases the expressive faculties as they may have a tracheotomy in place for some time during their language formative years (Nowak, 1998).

TABLE 5.4   Three Forms of Stickler Syndrome (Van Camp & Smith, 2000)

Locus name	Location	Gene	Entry
STL1	12q13.11–q13.2	COL2A1	108300
STL2	6p21.3	COL11A2	184840
STL3	1p21	COL11A1	121028

H. TREACHER COLLINS–FRANCESCHETTI SYNDROME
(OMIM Link 154500)

The features of this autosomal-dominant syndrome are an antimongoloid slant of the eyes, coloboma (fissure) of the lower eyelid, micrognathia, hypoplastic zygomatic arches, macrostomia, and microtia. Most of these patients have an asymmetric hearing loss worse than moderate. All those with hearing loss have a conductive component, and about 10 to 20% have a mixed loss (Pron *et al.*, 1993; Jahrsdoerfer & Jacobson, 1995). The conductive loss is due to malformation of one or more of the ossicles. There are more than 35 different mutations at the locus 5q32–q33.1.

I. USHER SYNDROME (OMIM Links 276900, 276903, 276904, 601067, 602097, 602083, 2376901, 276905, 276902; Table 5.5)

Usher syndrome affects vision and hearing. There are three clinical types (Table 5.5) (Wagenaar, 2000). It is marked by a retinitis pigmentosa with a progressive loss of vision during the first decades of life and with either a congenital or progressive hearing loss of variable degree. Additionally, many of these patients will have a loss of vestibular function. The most common variety is Type I. These

TABLE 5.5   Usher Syndrome: Clinical Classification (Wagenaar, 2000)

	Hearing impairment	Visual impairment	Vestibular function
Usher Type I	Congenital, Severe to profound	RP starts before puberty	Areflexia, Variable
Usher Type II Normal	Congenital, mild to moderate; can be progressive	RP starts before or after puberty	
Usher Type III	Congenital, Progressive	RP starts before or after puberty	Variable

patients should be identified as early as possible, for their disease affects three sensory systems: hearing, balance, and vision. Usher syndrome is one of the main reasons for ophthalmological screening of all hearing-impaired infants and children (see section III.L.7). The vestibular impairment will manifest itself as late walking that can be mistakenly interpreted as developmental delay, especially in a hearing- and visually impaired child. Understanding of the molecular bases of Usher syndrome is still evolving. There are at least ten different variations on six different chromosomes (Table 5.6) that are phenotypically classified as Usher syndrome. As with many forms of inherited deafness, there is a mouse model that is being used to further understand the molecular pathology (Saw et al., 1997; ID:6). The ten forms are all recessive, and are located at 1q41, 3p23–24.2, 3q21–q25, 5q14.3–q21–23, 10, 10q, 11p15.1, 11q13.5, 14q32, and 21q.

J. WAARDENBURG SYNDROME (OMIM Links 193500, 193510, 148820, 277850)

Waardenburg syndrome is presently classified into four types (Table 5.7), all with considerable variability of pigmentary and hearing abnormalities. Their pigmentary and facial features phenotypically and clinically identify these pa-

TABLE 5.6   Usher Syndrome: Molecular Classification (Van Camp & Smith, 2000)

Locus name	Location	Gene	Screening markers	Entry
USH1A	14q32	Unknown	D14S250, D14S260, D14S292, D14S78	276900
USH1B	11q13.5	MYO7A	D11S906, D11S911, D11S52, OMP-CA	276903
USH1C	11p15.1	Unknown	D11S902, D11S921, D11S899, D11S861	276904
USH1D	10q	Unknown	D10S529, D10S202, D10S573	601067
USH1E	21q	Unknown	D21S1884, D21S1257, D212S265, D21S1258	602097
USH1F	10	Unknown	D10S199, D10S578, D10S596	602083
USH2A	1q41	USH2A	D1S229, D1S490, D1S237, D1S474	276901
USH2B	3p23–24.2.	Unknown	D3S1578, D3S3647, D3S3658	276905
0USH2C	5q14.3–q21.3	Unknown	D5S428, D5S421	
USH3	3q21–q25	Unknown	D3S1299, D3S1555, D3S1280, D3S1279	276902

TABLE 5.7   Waardenburg Syndrome: Clinical Classification (Van Camp & Smith, 2000)

Type I	Dystopia canthorum
Type II	No dystopia canthorum
Klein–Waardenburg syndrome (type III)	Type I and upper limb abnormalities
Waardenburg–Shah syndrome (type IV)	Type II and Hirschsprung disease (autosomal recessive inheritance)

tients. Many will have some combination of dystrophia canthorum (lateral displacement of the inner canthus of each eye), a white forelock, and heterochromia of the iris (Read & Newton, 1997; ID:12). Additionally, they may have cleft palate or a submucosal cleft of the palate, and there is an association with Hirschsprung disease and upper limb abnormalities. The range of hearing will be from bilateral congenital profound loss to normal, with other varieties of sensory–neural losses including unilateral losses (DeStefano *et al.*, 1998; Lalwani *et al.*, 1996; Liu *et al.*, 1995; Morell *et al.*, 1997). There are six different molecular types (Table 5.8).

TABLE 5.8   Waardenburg Syndrome: Molecular Classification (Van Camp & Smith, 2000)

Type	Location	Gene	Entry
WS type I (WS1)	2q35	PAX3	*193500*
WS type II (WS2)	3p14.1–p12.3	MITF (: *156845*)	*193510*
WS type III	2q35	PAX3	*148820*
WS type IV	13q22	EDNRB (: *131244*)	*277850*
WS type IV	20q13.2–q13.3	EDN3 (: *131242*)	*277580*
WS type IV	22q13	SOX10 (: *602229*)	*277580*

The mode of inheritance is dominant, three of the types with gene loci at 2q35 and 3p14.1–p12.3, and three types that are recessive with loci at 13q22, 20q13.2–q13.2, and 22q13.

K. NONSYNDROMIC HEARING IMPAIRMENT

There is dominant, recessive, sex-linked, and mitochondrial transmission of nonsyndromic hearing impairments.

1. Dominant

The loci for the 31 DFNA hearing impairments are listed in Table 5.9. Each of these syndromes represents either one or just a few kindred. The forms of DFNA vary between and within each of the separate entities. There can be early-onset impairment (Kunst *et al.*, 1999) or impairments later in life with progression (Van Camp *et al.*, 1999), with many other variations. It is critical to make a genetic diagnosis, because at least one of these DFNA syndromes may be treatable with medication (Fukushima *et al.*, 1999). It is expected that there will be many specific and generic effective interventions for the various forms of genetic hearing impairments as understanding of the molecular abnormalities increases.

2. Recessive

The loci for the 28 DFNB are listed in Table 5.10. The DFNBs manifest themselves similarly to the DFNAs in that there is heterogeneity of phenotype as to time of onset, progression, and severity. DFNB1—Connexin 26 (URL http://www.iro.es/cx26deaf.html)—is the most prevalent cause of all genetic hearing impairments. The abnormal gene is found in 3.01%, with a probable range of

TABLE 5.9   Nonsyndromic Hearing Impairment, Autosomal Dominant Loci (DFNA) (Van Camp & Smith, 2000)

Locus name	Location	Gene	OMIM entry
DFNA1	5q31	*HDIA1*	*124900*
DFNA2	1p34	*GJB3*	600101
		KCNQ4	
DFNA3	13q12	*GJB2*	*601544*
		GJB6	
DFNA4	19q13	Unknown	*600652*
DFNA5	7p15	*DFNA5*	*600994*
DFNA6	4p16.3	Unknown	*600965*
DFNA7	1q21–q23	Unknown	*601412*
DFNA8	11q22–24	*TECTA*	*601543*
DFNA9	14q12–q13	*COCH*	*601369*
DFNA10	6q22–q23	Unknown	*601316*
DFNA11	11q12.3–q21	*MYO7A*	*601317*
DFNA12	11q22–q24	*TECTA*	*601842*
DFNA13	6p21	Unknown	*601868*
DFNA14	4p16	Unknown	Unknown
			602459
DFNA15	5q31	*POU4F3*	
			602460
DFNA16	2q24	Unknown	Unknown
DFNA17	22q	Unknown	Unknown
DFNA18	3q22	Unknown	Unknown
DFNA19	10 (pericentr.)	Unknown	Unknown
DFNA20	17q25	Unknown	Unknown
DFNA21			
DFNA22			
DFNA23	14q	Unknown	Unknown
DFNA24	4q	Unknown	Unknown
DFNA25	12q21–24	Unknown	Unknown
DFNA26	17q25	Unknown	Unknown
DFNA27	4q12	Unknown	Unknown
DFNA28	8q22	Unknown	Unknown
DFNA29			
DFNA30	15q26	Unknown	
DFNA31			

TABLE 5.10   Nonsyndromic Hearing Impairment, Autosomal-Recessive Loci (Van Camp & Smith, 2000)

Locus name	Location	Gene	OMIM entry
DFNB1	13q12	GJB2	220290
DFNB2	11q13.5	MYO7A	600060
DFNB3	17p11.2	MYO15	600316
DFNB4	7q31	PDS (see note 2)	600791
DFNB5	14q12	Unknown	600792
DFNB6	3p14–p21	Unknown	600971
DFNB7	9q13–q21	Unknown	600974
DFNB8	21q22	Unknown	601072
DFNB9	2p22–p23	OTOF	601071
DFNB10	21q22.3	Unknown	see DFNB8
DFNB11	9q13–q21	Unknown	see DFNB7
DFNB12	10q21–q22	Unknown	601386
DFNB13	7q34–36	Unknown	603098
DFNB14	7q31	Unknown	603678
DFNB15	3q21–q25 19p13	Unknown	601869
DFNB16	15q21–q22	Unknown	603720
DFNB17	7q31	Unknown	603010
DFNB18	11p14–15.1	Unknown	602092
DFNB19	18p11	Unknown	Unknown
DFNB20	11q25–qter	Unknown	604060
DFNB21	11q	TECTA	603629
DFNB22			
DFNB23	10p11.2–q21	Unknown	Unknown
DFNB24	11q23	Unknown	Unknown
DFNB25	4p15.3–q12	Unknown	Unknown
DFNB26	4q2 modif. 1q22–23	Unknown	Unknown
DFNB27			
DFNB28	22q13	Unknown	Unknown

2.5 to 3.5% of the population in the Midwestern United States (Green *et al.*, 1999). It is found more frequently in populations whose origins are from the Mediterranean, and especially in Jewish populations of Ashkenazi origin (Morell *et al.*, 1998), who have been found to have a tendency for a rare mutation of the gene 167delT, and an observed carrier rate of 4.03% (95% confidence interval of 2.5 to 6.0%). Connexin 26 appears to be associated with at least 50% of all nonsyndromal deafness (Murgia *et al.*, 1999). The hearing loss, sensory–neural, is characterized by being either congenital or early onset; it can be progressive, asymmetrical, and of varying degree (Cohn *et al.*, 1999). This common, severe genetic disorder should be screened for as a part of a newborn hearing-screening program, because it is probable that neonates with Connexin 26 mutation who display early progressive loss would not be identified by the physiological techniques presently in use.

3. X-Linked

The loci for the five DFNs are listed in Table 5.11. These syndromes are similar to the other nonsyndromic hearing disorders in that they present with a myriad of phenotypes, most often but not exclusively in the male (Cremers & Huygen, 1983; Papadaki *et al.*, 1998). The most common of these is DFN3: deafness mixed with perilymphatic gusher or Nance syndrome (Nance *et al.*, 1970). These patients, primarily males, may have a progressive mixed hearing loss and a characteristic dilatation of the internal auditory meatus (Cremers *et al.*, 1985). Attempts to repair the conductive loss with manipulation of the footplate of the stapes has resulted in a pouring out of perilymph—a gusher—and a resultant loss of hearing in the

TABLE 5.11   Nonsyndromic Hearing Impairment, X-Linked Recessive Loci (Van Camp & Smith, 2000)

Locus name	Location	Gene	Screening markers	OMIM entry
DFN1	Xq22	DDP	*DXS101*	*304700*
DFN2	Xq22	Unknown	*COL4A5*	*304500*
DFN3	Xq21.1	*POU3F4*	*DXS26* *DXS995* *DXS232*	*304400*
DFN4	Xp21.2	Unknown	*DXS997* DXS992	*300030*
DFN5	Xp22	Unknown	*DXS8036* *DXS8022* DXS8019	*300066*

operated ear. The presence of a progressive conductive or mixed hearing loss can be associated with a stapedial reflex in these patients (Snik *et al.*, 1995), and this observation may be used so that interventions other than surgery are utilized for the restoration of hearing.

4. Mitochondrial

The loci for the two nonsyndromic mitochondrial based hearing impairments are listed in Table 5.12. One of these, 12S rRNA, which results in an increased susceptibility to aminoglycosides (entry nos. 580000 and 561000), is caused by a mitochondrial mutation in gene 12S rRNA, and the mutation is 1555A>G (Fischel-Ghodsian *et al.*, 1993). Individuals carrying this mutation will experience ototoxicity at dosage levels that will not cause a hearing loss in a normal individual. As there is now no screen for these mutations, a history should be obtained as to whether there has been hearing loss in the family following aminoglycoside therapy. In many instances, however, there has been no familial exposure to an aminoglycoside and the patient may be the first affected of that family. The rarity of this condition should be considered in torts in which hearing impairment has seemingly resulted, usually but not exclusively in newborns, when the patient received a standard dosage of the aminoglycoside.

TABLE 5.12   Nonsyndromic Hearing Impairment, Mitochondrial Genes Loci (Van Camp & Smith, 2000)

Gene	Mutation	OMIM entry
12S rRNA	1555A>G	*580000* *561000*
tRNA–Ser(UCN)	7445A>G	*590080*

L. CLINICAL APPLICATION

The advances in genetics now enable the clinician to care for the hearing impaired with increased effectiveness. The new information mandates a high level of accuracy and continuous attention to ethical tenets.

1. Diagnosing

The process of establishing a diagnosis entails an evaluation of the patient and often of a number of the first- and second-degree relatives.

2. History

Information should be acquired concerning the time of onset of the hearing loss, specific information about potential acquired causes such as ototoxic medications, especially salicylates, and sound trauma. A detailed family–genetic history is obtained for all hearing loss that is not obviously acquired. The genetic history should include siblings, children, and as many relatives as possible for two previous generations. Specific data are obtained about these relatives, not only concerning the hearing and whether there are any apparent physical signs— for example, different colored eyes as found in the Waardenburg syndrome—but also what their last names may have been in the past and from which cities or region they and their progenitors came from. The ascertainment of last name and region of origin many times will indicate a possible relatedness of the parent of the affected individual. Health care providers working for patients who are members of circumscribed communities need to have knowledge of families that carry various genes for hearing impairment. The genetic history is obtained in the course of several visits. On the first visit, an outline is made and the person responsible for the patient—either the patient or a caregiver—is given the task of inquiring in detail about other members of the family. At a second visit, it is usually helpful, if possible, to have a member of the family from an older generation aid in the process of providing the pertinent history.

3. Functional Testing

Each patient requires a complete assessment of the auditory–vestibular system to include middle ear, inner ear, and the statoacoustic nerve. The techniques used depend on the age of the patient. Infants less than 6 months of age will be assessed with physiological measures that include middle ear impedance, cochlear emissions, and frequency-specific air and bone conduction auditory evoked potentials (Stapells & Ruben, 1989). Many infants and toddlers older than 6 months can be assessed with behavioral audiograms (Gravel & Traquina, 1992), in addition to the cochlear emissions and impedance measures. The initial hearing assessment must be accurate at all frequencies and, where appropriate, in discriminatory ability, as this evaluation serves to establish the extent of the loss and is the standard by which the patient is monitored for progression of the hearing impairment.

Audiometric testing of relatives, especially younger siblings, is carried out, as this will reveal other affected members. Many cases of hearing impairment will be nonsyndromal and have no obvious family history to indicate that the cause is genetic. Hearing evaluations of parents, siblings, or children may suggest a probable genetic origin, in that there can be frequency-specific notches in the transient evoked cochlear emission and/or the audiogram. This assessment appears to be more accurate in people carrying an autosomal dominant in which there is low penetrance, for example, Waardenburg syndrome (Liu et al., 1995), than in obligate carriers of recessive genes (Lina-Granade et al., 1998). Although there is less accuracy in the recessive carriers, the finding in a parent, sibling, or child of a propositus of a hearing loss that is not predicted based on the individual's age or hearing history is useful. It will indicate other possible investigations, and will benefit the presumably affected person who should be audiometrically monitored.

4. Serology

Viral and serological studies can be done for congenital infection. The incidence of congenital rubella and syphilis appears to be relatively rare. These studies should be obtained when the history and/or the physical examination indicate that such infection may be a possibility. Two hallmarks of congenital rubella are abnormalities of the retina and/or small infant size. Currently, the most common form of congenital infection is from cytomegalovirus (CMV), which, in some cases, can result in a progressive early-onset hearing loss (Ahlfors, Ivarsson, & Harris, 1999; Fowler et al., 1999).

5. Imaging

The CT will yield information on the bony structure of the ear. This is especially important in the diagnosis of labyrinthine malformations; such findings are used both to substantiate a diagnosis—for example, BOR, Pendred, Treacher Collins, DFN3 gusher—and to direct care with regard to the possibility of a perilymphatic fistula. MRI is used to evaluate patients with progressive unilateral or asymmetric losses, especially those with decreased speech discrimination.

6. Dysmorphology

Evaluation of the patient's facial features, pigmentation, and overall physical structure will add to the information necessary for diagnosis. Included in the routine assessment should be the intercanthal distance, the status of the palate, limb and digital morphology, and other facial features.

7. System Evaluation

The visual system needs to be evaluated to ensure that the patient has optimal visual acuity and/or to make a specific diagnosis (e.g., Usher disease) and/or to provide for a care plan that would include a static or progressive visual impairment. Early diagnosis of Usher disease is critical and is facilitated by the use of the electroretinogram. This may not be accurate in a young child and is most sensitive at age 3–4 years. It has been found to be positive in a child of 18 months (Smith et al., 1998). The ophthalmologic evaluation can give information concerning congenital infections, such as rubella, toxoplasmosis, and so on. An important consideration is the greater adverse effect that a visual impairment will have on a person burdened with an auditory deficiency. The hearing-impaired individual is even more dependent on vision than others and needs vision to function optimally. The early diagnosis of myopia, astigmatism, or strabismus will be of considerable advantage to the hearing impaired, especially the young child. Ophthalmologic examination is required, for this author, in every case of static or progressive childhood hearing impairment.

The genital–urinary system is evaluated for anatomic malformation, with the use of ultrasound, in all patients with external and/or middle ear malformation, because of the high incidence of renal abnormalities found in these patients.

Renal function is assessed through the measure of creatinine and blood urea nitrogen in patients suspected of having Alport syndrome. Evaluation of thyroid function with the use of the perchlorate test is indicated if there is an indication of Pendred disease. The recording of an electrocardiogram is carried out for those who are suspected of having Jervell and Lange–Nielson disease. Most often there will be no indication that an individual will have any of the three above-mentioned disorders. It is suggested that these evaluations be carried out not as a screen but when there is information to suggest autosomal recessive inheritance, or when the patient and/or family show some finding that would indicate that there is a possibility of the disorder. The electrocardiogram and the renal function studies are the least invasive, whereas the thyroid studies are more invasive.

Vestibular studies are useful in establishing a diagnosis of Usher disease. They also contribute to the management of an infant in that they aid in better understanding of why motor development may be delayed. Patients who have no vestibular function and their caregivers need to be cautioned concerning swimming, as they have a decreased ability to orient in water. There have been drownings, which are thought to be attributable to the lack of vestibular function.

Patients with hearing impairment with onset during the period of language development should undergo a complete evaluation of expressive and receptive language functions and of their speech abilities. These data will provide a baseline for evaluations of therapy and are also useful in directing habilitation. There is also the possibility that the patient may have a specific language disorder (see Chapter 6), which will be exacerbated by the hearing impairment. Those who appear to be cognitively delayed, with or without other neurological signs, require an appropriate neurological evaluation.

8. Molecular DNA and RNA Testing

Genetic disorders can be accurately and precisely diagnosed by molecular evaluation; presently, however, there is only limited availability for this testing. Each medical center has a number of genes that it may test. Many professionals will cooperate with one another to test samples. It is expected that, with the development of gene chip technology, there will be genetic tests widely available for many of the known genetic disorders of hearing impairment. These evaluations will be used to determine, in regard to a given patient, who in the family is affected or are carriers, and may be used to screen initially for abnormal genes.

M. MANAGEMENT

There are several special areas of patient management that are obligated when a diagnosis of a genetic basis for a hearing impairment is established.

1. Follow-Up

Many genetic disorders are characterized by a progression of the hearing impairment and/or another clinical deficit. These patients require periodic evaluations so that appropriate care can be provided. The periodicity—duty cycle—of follow-up in some instances will be determined by previous reported experience with a particular genetic syndrome. If this information is not available, then periodicity of follow-up is determined by population studies (Ruben & Fishman, 1980). The rapid advances in medical genetics in the areas of diagnosis and, now, intervention, must be applied to patients who have been diagnosed. The new information is used as part of the continual care of the patient. Each patient should be aware of his or her diagnosis and be enabled to access the new developments, for example, through the use of the Internet.

2. Counseling

The action of the gene over time is an important dimension in the care of genetic disorders. There are two different aspects. The first is the way in which the gene will affect the individual. These issues are attended to both in the informing interview and at the periodic follow-up visits. The second concerns potential transmission of the gene to the patient's children, and how this may affect the progeny. Once the mode of inheritance is established, and the degree of penetrance is known, then a reasonable estimate of transmission can be communicated to the patient or the parents. Dominant genes will affect half of the progeny with usually variable penetrance. The recessive genes differ. If another child from the same couple is affected, then, in the main, 25% of the progeny will be homozygous. The offspring of a known recessive homozygote may or may not have a significantly increased probability of being affected, depending on the gene causing the impairment. The children of a homozygote or a compound heterozygote for Connexin 26 would be at a higher risk for hearing impairment because of the ubiquity of the abnormal Connexin gene. A child of a homozygote recessive, a rare recessive, would be at somewhat greater risk for impairment than the normal population if there were no assorted matings. Similarly, a hearing impairment with unknown etiology cannot be designated as not genetic; furthermore, children of this patient will be at a greater risk. The probability of having an affected child is greater than for the previous population based risk of 10% (Fraser, 1976), but less than the 25% of a known recessive.

3. Screening

Techniques are currently available to screen for a number of the genetic hearing impairments. These screening techniques have the potential to affect several purposes. One would be to screen all newborns for the disorders that are the most common and/or those with high morbidity, in the way the various hormonal screens are carried out, such as those for PKU and hypothyroidism. Such information would be beneficial for instituting prompt and effective care and effective preventive interventions. Other uses of a screen may or may not affect the conduct of a person's life, and thus bring ethical issues strongly into play. The screen could be used, for example, to determine who in a family carried a recessive gene, or whether a potential mate carried a gene synergetic for hearing impairment. There is also the potential use of a screen to determine the genetic makeup of a fetus.

4. Ethics

There is a population of people whose language is visual, because they have little or no access to auditory communication. Many of these individuals whose language is based on vision do not consider their lack of use of sound as an abnormality nor as a disease. From the end of the nineteenth century to the middle of the twentieth, there had been a number of programs directed not only at extinguishing their language, and in some cases their subculture, but also with the thrust of euthanizing, sterilizing, or prohibiting marriage so that those genetically so affected would cease to exist (Bell, 1883; Biesold, 1999; Ruben, 1991). This history underscores the importance of a critical tenet of self-determination, autonomy, in the ethics of genetic medicine. Individuals have the right to determine whether they will utilize any given intervention. The governing bodies can provide information, as from a screening program, but they cannot mandate a particular course of a biological therapy. In the case of hearing impairment and deafness, options exist that are sufficient to enable a person to achieve a normal life in the culture at large, and in a longstanding and recognized subculture of visually based language. Fetal testing for hearing-impairment genes raises an ethical issue. In assessing these, it must be kept in mind that the advent of gene therapies or other specific therapies directed at preventing or reversing deleterious gene action, should become a means to cure and to prevent, and not to destroy (see Chapter 11). The power that a deepening understanding of genetics provides cannot be used to eliminate any human group. Although such a statement may seem gratuitous, it is sobering to consider that past and recent history indicate the need for maintaining that idea in the forefront of awareness.

REFERENCES

Admiraal, R. J. (1970). Hereditary hearing loss with nephropathy (Alport's syndrome). *Acta Otolaryngologica, Suppl., 271*, 7–26.

Ahlfors, K., Ivarsson, S. A., & Harris, S. (1999). Report on a long-term study of maternal and congenital cytomegalovirus infection in Sweden: Review of prospective studies available in the literature. *Scandinavian Journal of Infectious Diseases, 31*, 443–457.

Bell, A. G. (1880). *On a deaf variety of the human race.* Washington, DC: National Academy of Sciences.

Bell, A. G. (1883). Memoir upon the formation of a deaf variety of the human race. *Proceedings of the National Academy of Sciences*, pp. 1–86.

Berger, W., Meindl, A., van de Pol, T. J., Cremers, F. P., Ropers, H. H., Doerner, C., Monaco, A., Bergen, A. A., Lebo, R., & Warburg, M. (1992). Isolation of a candidate gene for Norrie disease by positional cloning. *Nature Genetics, 1*, 199–203. [Published erratum appears in *Nature Genetics*, 1992, 2, 84.]

Biesold, H. (1988). *Klagende hande.* Germany: Solms.

Biesold, H. (1999). *Crying hands: Eugenics and deaf people in Nazi Germany.* Washington, DC: Gallaudet University Press.

Black, G., & Redmond, R. M. (1994). The molecular biology of Norrie's disease. *Eye, 8*(Pt. 5), 491–496.

Bonet, J. P. (1620). *Reduction de las letras y arte para enseñar a abler las mudos.* Madrid: Francisco Abarca de Angulo.

Casselbrant, M. L., Mandel, E. M., Fall, P. A., Rockette, H. E., Kurslasky, M., Bluestone, C. D., & Ferrell, R. E. (2000). The heritability of otitis media: A twin and triplet study. *Journal of the American Medical Association, 282*, 2125–2130.

Cohn, E. S., Kelley, P. M., Fowler, T. W., Gorga, M. P., Lefkowitz, D. M., Kuehn, H. J., Schaefer, G. B., Gobar, L. S., Hahn, F. J., Harris, D. J., & Kimberling, W. J. (1999). Clinical studies of families with hearing loss attributable to mutations in the connexin 26 gene (GJB2/DFNB1). *Pediatrics, 103*, 546–550.

Coyle, B., Coffey, R., Armour, J. A., Gausden, E., Hochberg, Z., Grossman, A., Britton, K., Pembrey, M., Reardon, W., & Trembath, R. (1996). Pendred syndrome (goiter and sensorineural hearing loss) maps to chromosome 7 in the region containing the nonsyndromic deafness gene DFNB4. *Nature Genetics, 12*, 421–423.

Cremers, C. W., & Fikkers-Van Noord, N. M. (1980). The earpits-deafness syndrome. Clinical and genetic aspects. *International Journal of Pediatric Otorhinolaryngology, 2*, 309–322.

Cremers, C. W., & Huygen, P. L. (1983). Clinical features of female heterozygotes in the X-linked mixed deafness syndrome (with perilymphatic gusher during stapes surgery). *International Journal of Pediatric Otorhinolaryngology, 6*, 179–185.

Cremers, C. W., Hombergen, G. C., Scaf, J. J., Huygen, P. L., Volkers, W. S., & Pinckers, A. J. (1985). X-linked progressive mixed deafness with perilymphatic gusher during stapes surgery. *Archives of Otolaryngology, 111*, 249–254.

Cremers, C. W., Marres, H. A., & van Rijn, P. M. (1991). Nonsyndromal profound genetic deafness in childhood. In R. J. Ruben, T. R. Van De Watter, & K. P. Steel (Eds.), Genetics of hearing impairment. *Annals of the New York Academy of Sciences, 630*, 191–196.

Cremers, C. W., Bolder, C., Admiraal, R. J., Everett, L. A., Joosten, F. B., VanHauwe, P., Green, E. D., & Otten, B. J. (1998). Progressive sensorineural hearing loss and a widened vestibular aqueduct in Pendred syndrome. *Archives of Otolaryngology—Head & Neck Surgery, 124*, 501–505.

Cusimano, F., Martines, E., & Rizzo, C. (1991). The Jervell and Lange–Nielsen syndrome. *International Journal of Pediatric Otorhinolaryngology, 22*, 49–58.

DeStefano, A. L., Cupples, L. A., Arnos, K. S., Asher, J. H. J., Baldwin, C. T., Blanton, S., Carey, M. L., da Silva, E. O., Friedman, T. B., Greenberg, J., Lalwani, A. K., Milunsky, A., Nance, W. E., Pandya, A., Ramesar, R. S., Read, A. P., Tassabejhi, M., Wilcox, E. R., & Farrer, L. A. (1998). Correlation between Waardenburg syndrome phenotype and genotype in a population of individuals with identified PAX3 mutations. *Human Genetics, 102*, 499–506.

Fischel-Ghodsian, N., Prezant, T. R., Bu, X., & Oztas, S. (1993). Mitochondrial ribosomal RNA gene mutation in a patient with sporadic aminoglycoside ototoxicity. *American Journal of Otolaryngology, 14*, 399–403.

Fowler, K. B., Dahle, A. J., Boppana, S. B., & Pass, R. F. (1999). Newborn hearing screening: Will children with hearing loss caused by congenital cytomegalovirus infection be missed? *Journal of Pediatrics, 135*, 60–64.

Fraser, G. F. (1976). *The causes of profound deafness in childhood.* Baltimore: The Johns Hopkins University Press.

Fukushima, K., Kasai, N., Ueki, Y., Nishizaki, K., Sugata, K., Hirakawa, S., Masuda, A., Gunduz, M., Ninomiya, Y., Masuda, Y., Sato, M., McGuirt, W. T., Coucke, P., VanCamp, G., & Smith, R. J. (1999). A gene for fluctuating, progressive autosomal dominant nonsyndromic hearing loss, DFNA16, maps to chromosome 2q23–24.3. *American Journal of Human Genetics, 65*, 141–150.

Gerber, S. E. (1998). *Etiology and prevention of communicative disorders.* San Diego: Singular.

Gravel, J. S., & Traquina, D. N. (1992). Experience with audiologic assessment of infants and toddlers. *International Journal of Pediatric Otolaryngology, 23*, 59–71.

Green, G. E., Scott, D. A., McDonald, J. M., Woodworth, G. G., Sheffield, V. C., & Smith, R. J. (1999). Carrier rates in the midwestern United States for *GJB2* mutations causing inherited deafness. *Journal of the American Medical Association, 281*, 2211–2216.

Jahrsdoerfer, R. A., & Jacobson, J. T. (1995). Treacher Collins syndrome: Otologic and auditory management. *Journal of the American Academy of Audiology, 6*, 93–102.

Konigsmark, B. W., & Gorlin, R. J. (1976). *Genetic and metabolic deafness.* Philadelphia: Saunders.

Korres, S. G., Manta, P. B., Balatsouras, D. G., & Papageorgiou, C. T. (1999). Audiological assessment in patients with mitochondrial myopathy. *Scandinavian Audiology, 28*, 231–240.

Kunst, H., Marres, H., Huygen, P., Ensink, R., VanCamp, G., VanHauwe, P., Coucke, P., Willems, P., & Cremers, C. (1998). Nonsyndromic autosomal dominant progressive sensorineural hearing loss: Audiologic analysis of a pedigree linked to DFNA2. *Laryngoscope, 108*, 74–80.

Lalwani, A. K., Mhatre, A. N., San Agustin, T. B., & Wilcox, E. R. (1996). Genotype-phenotype correlations in type 1 Waardenburg syndrome. *Laryngoscope, 106*, 895–902.

Lina-Granade, G., Kreiss, M., Gelas, T., Collet, L., & Morgan, A. (1998). Cochlear irregularities in obligate carriers of recessive genetic hearing impairment and in control subjects. In D. Stephens, A. Read, & A. Martini (Eds.), *Developments in genetic hearing impairment* (pp. 68–76). London: Whurr.

Liu, X. Z., Newton, V. E., & Read, A. P. (1995). Waardenburg syndrome type, II: Phenotypic findings and diagnostic criteria. *American Journal of Medical Genetics, 55*, 95–100.

Love, J. K. (1896). *Deaf mutism: A clinical and pathological study.* Glasgow: James MacLehose and Sons.

McKenna, M. J., & Mills, B. G. (1989). Immunohistochemical evidence of measles virus antigens in active otosclerosis. *Otolaryngology–Head and Neck Surgery, 101*, 415–421.

McKusick, V. A. (2000). *Mendelian inheritance in man* [online]. 4-29-2000. Internet Communication.

Morell, R., Friedman, T. B., Asher, J. H. J., & Robbins, L. G. (1997). The incidence of deafness is nonrandomly distributed among families segregating for Waardenburg syndrome type 1 (WS1). *Journal of Medical Genetics, 34*, 447–452.

Morell, R. J., Kim, H. J., Hood, L. J., Goforth, L., Friderici, K., Fisher, R., VanCamp, G., Berlin, C. I., Oddoux, C., Ostrer, H., Keats, B., & Friedman, T. B. (1998). Mutations in the connexin 26 gene (GJB2) among Ashkenazi Jews with nonsyndromic recessive deafness. *New England Journal of Medicine, 339*, 1500–1505.

Murgia, A., Orzan, E., Polli, R., Martella, M., Vinanzi, C., Leonardi, E., Arslan, E., & Zacchello, F. (1999). Cx26 deafness: Mutation analysis and clinical variability. *Journal of Medical Genetics, 36*, 829–832.

Nance, W. E., Sweeney, A., McLeod, A. C., & Cooper, M. C. (1970). Hereditary deafness: A presentation of some recognized types, modes of inheritance, and aids in counseling. *Southern Medical Bulletin, 58*, 41–57.

Niedermeyer, H. P., & Arnold W. (1995). Otosclerosis: A measles virus associated inflammatory disease. *Acta Otolaryngologica, 115*, 300–303.

Nowak, C. B. (1998). Genetics and hearing loss: A review of Stickler syndrome. *Journal of Communication Disorders, 31*, 437–453.

Papadaki, E., Prassopoulos, P., Bizakis, J., Karampekios, S., Papadakis, H., & Gourtsoyiannis, N. (1998). X-linked deafness with stapes gusher in females. *European Journal of Radiology, 29*, 71–75.

Parving, A., & Christensen, B. (1996). Epidemiology of permanent hearing impairment in children in relation to costs of a hearing health surveillance program. *International Journal of Pediatric Otorhinolaryngology, 34*, 9–23.

Phelps, P. D., Coffey, R. A., Trembath, R. C., Luxon, L. M., Grossman, A. B., Britton, K. E., Kendall-Taylor, P., Graham, J. M., Cadge, B. C., Stephens, S. G., Pembrey, M. E., & Reardon, W. (1998). Radiological malformations of the ear in Pendred syndrome. *Clinical Radiology, 53*, 268–273.

Plann, S. (1997). *Silent minority: Deaf education in Spain, 1550–1835.* Berkeley: University of California Press.

Pron, G., Galloway, C., Armstrong, D., & Posnick, J. (1993). Ear malformation and hearing loss in patients with Treacher Collins syndrome. *Cleft Palate and Craniofacial Journal, 30*, 97–103.

Read, A. P., & Newton, V. E. (1997). Waardenburg syndrome. *Journal of Medical Genetics, 34*, 656–665.

Reyes, M. R., LeBlanc, E. M., & Bassila, M. K. (1999). Hearing loss and otitis media in velo-cardio-facial syndrome. *International Journal of Pediatric Otorhinolaryngology, 47*, 227–233.

Ruben, R. J. (1991). The history of the genetics of hearing impairment. *Annals of the New York Academy of Sciences, 630*, 6–15.

Ruben, R. J., & Fishman, G. (1980). Otological care of the hearing impaired child. In G. T. Mencher & S. E. Gerber (Eds.), *Early management of hearing loss* (pp. 105–120). New York: Grune & Stratton.

Ruben, R. J., & Math, R. (1978). Serous otitis media associated with sensorineural hearing loss in children. *Laryngoscope, 88*, 1139–1154.

Ruben, R. J., Van De Water, T. R., & Steel, K. P. (Eds.) (1991). *Genetics of hearing impairment.* New York: New York Academy of Sciences.

Saw, D. J., Steel, K. P., & Brown, S. D. (1997). Shaker mice and a peek into the House of Usher. *Experiments in Animals, 46*, 1–9.

Sheffield, V. C., Kraiem, Z., Beck, J. C., Nishimura, D., Stone, E. M., Salameh, M., Sadeh, O., & Glaser, M. (1996). Pendred syndrome maps to chromosome 7q21–34 and is caused by an intrinsic defect in thyroid iodine organification. *Nature Genetics, 12*, 424–426.

Shprintzen, R. J., Goldberg, R. B., Young, D., & Wolford, L. (1981). The velo-cardio-facial syndrome: A clinical and genetic analysis. *Pediatrics, 67*, 167–172.

Smith, S. D., Kimberling, W. J., Schaefer, G. B., Horton, M. B., & Tinley, S. (1998). Medical genetic evaluation for the etiology of hearing loss in children. *Journal of Communication Disorders, 31*, 371–389.

Snik, A. F., Hombergen, G. C., Mylanus, E. A., & Cremers, C. W. (1995). Air-bone gap in patients with X-linked stapes gusher syndrome. *American Journal of Otology, 16*, 241–246.

Stapells, D. R., & Ruben, R. J. (1989). Auditory brain stem responses to bone-conducted tones in infants. *Annals of Otology, Rhinology and Laryngology, 98*, 941–949.

Turner, J. S. (1970). Hereditary hearing loss with nephropathy (Alport's syndrome). *Acta Otolaryngologica, Suppl., 271*, 7–26.

Van Camp, G., & Smith, R. J. H. (2000). Hereditary hearing loss homepage [online]. Internet Communication.

Van Camp, G., Kunst, H., Flothmann, K., McGuirt, W., Wauters, J., Marres, H., Verstreken, M., Bespalova, I. N., Burmeister, M., VandeHeyning, P. H., Smith, R. J., Willems, P. J., Cremers, C. W., & Lesperance, M. M. (1999). A gene for autosomal dominant hearing impairment (DFNA14) maps to a region on chromosome 4p16.3 that does not overlap the DFNA6 locus. *Journal of Medical Genetics, 36,* 532–536.

Wagenaar, M. (2000). *The Usher syndrome: A clinical and genetic correlation.* Den Haag: CIP—gegevens koninklijke bibliotheek.

Wilde, S. W. R. W. (1853). *Particle observations on aural surgery and the nature and treatment of diseases of the ear with illustrations.* Philadelphia: Blanchard & Lea.

Zlotogora, J. (1997). Dominance and homozygosity. *American Journal of Medical Genetics, 68,* 412–416.

6

GENETIC LANGUAGE DISORDERS

JULIE WILLIAMS

Department of Psychological Medicine
University of Wales College of Medicine
Cardiff, United Kingdom

JIM STEVENSON

Department of Psychology
University of Southampton
Southampton, United Kingdom

A variety of disorders reflects abnormalities in the processing of language. Genetic research has concentrated on two of the main categories of language impairment disorders, focusing on specific language impairment (SLI) and specific reading disability (SRD). Current quantitative and molecular research in this area is

The Handbook of Genetic Communicative
Disorders

producing many interesting findings that show strong evidence of the presence of a number of genes contributing to these disorders. This chapter reviews these areas of research and provides a perspective on the recent advances in our knowledge of the genetic components of language disorders.

I. SPECIFIC LANGUAGE IMPAIRMENT (SLI)

Specific language impairment can be defined broadly as a significant difficulty in the acquisition of spoken language that occurs in the context of normal hearing and nonverbal intelligence and not associated with other developmental disorders. It needs to be distinguished from acquired language impairments that arise after normal language ability has been acquired and that are a consequence of neurological damage or deterioration. The latter are more often seen in adults. The definition also differentiates SLI from language delay or disability that is part of a global deficit in cognitive ability, such as Down syndrome, and from developmental disorders such as autism, where language impairment is part of the pattern of symptoms defining the condition.

This definition is based on relative underachievement of language skills compared to that expected from general ability measures. The operationalization of this definition can either be the use of a regression procedure whereby a language measure is regressed onto nonverbal intelligence and the residual obtained for each child, that is, the difference between observed and expected language scores. This more rigorous approach to the identification of SLI requires that the regression relationship be known for the general population. This knowledge may not be available, and an alternative is to identify SLI as a language age that is below chronological age but where the child has a nonverbal IQ above 85. In either approach to identifying SLI, there is an issue of how to specify the required degree of impairment. In practice, most measures of spoken language that are between one and two standard deviations below age expectations are used to define SLI (Tomblin *et al.*, 1992).

A. EPIDEMIOLOGY

Epidemiological studies of SLI have produced a variety of prevalence estimates ranging from 0.57 to 7.4% (Dale *et al.*, 1998; Fundudis *et al.*, 1997; Randall *et al.*, 1974; Stevenson & Richman, 1996; Tomblin, 1996). The lower estimates of prevalence relate to studies with either more stringent definitions of SLI—such as language skills at least two standard deviations below those predicted (Randall *et al.*, 1974)—or where the definition was limited to specific forms of language impairment, for example, severe specific expressive language impairment (which was found in 0.57% of a sample of 705 children studied by Stevenson and Richman, 1976). On the other hand, Tomblin (1996) and Rice (1997) reported a prevalence rate of 7.4% overall in boys and 6% in girls. Their sample of 849 kindergarten children was screened for a broad range of language skills, including vocabulary, grammar, narrative, receptive, and expressive language, which were used to produce a criterion for SLI that aimed to reflect clinical diagnosis. Tomblin also observed that 80% of the children with deficits displayed both expressive and receptive language problems, and the majority showed evidence of selective deficit in grammar development, but few showed deficits in speech impairment.

B. FAMILY STUDIES

Most studies of familiality have focused on single families with multiple cases of language impairment (Arnold, 1961; Borges-Osorio & Salzano, 1985; Hurst *et al.*, 1990; McReady, 1926; Samples & Lane, 1985). However, it is likely that these studies may have limited generalizability, because many cases of SLI do not show such strong within-family transmission. Another strategy has been to estimate the frequency of language impairment among the relatives of language-impaired probands (Bishop & Edmundson, 1986; Byrne *et al.*, 1974; Hier & Rosenberger, 1980; Ingram, 1959; Luchsinger, 1970). These studies generated estimates of language impairment rates in relatives ranging from 24 to 63% when probands had a positive family history for SLI. However, these studies were performed without matched control families unaffected by SLI. More recently, family studies have included matched control families in their designs. They have also reported high rates of language impairment in first degree relatives (2- to 7-fold increase) that ranged between 17 and 43% (Lewis, 1992; Neils & Aram, 1986; Rice, 1997; Spitz *et al.*, 1997; Tallal *et al.*, 1989; Tomblin, 1989, 1996; Van der Lely & Stollwerck, 1996).

Van der Lely and Stollwerck studied the familiality of SLI characterized by persistent and disproportionate impairment of grammatical comprehension and expressive language. They observed that 77.8% of children with SLI had a positive family history of language impairment compared with 28.5% of control children. Lewis (1992), in contrast, studied the first-degree relatives of probands with phonological disorders and found rates of language and/or speech disorders ranging between 12 and 31%. In a prospective study of language development (16–26 months), Spitz and colleagues (1997) found 50% of children with a positive family history demonstrated language delay, whereas none of the children with a negative family history experienced delay. In 1996, Tomblin estimated the risk of SLI in first-degree relatives to be 21%, and in same-sex family members to be 28%, which rose to 33% in same-sex dizygotic twins, and finally to 71% in monozygotic twins. More recently, Rice (1997) studied the affectedness rates of a wide range of relatives of SLI probands. She observed that the percentage of affectedness in relatives of probands was 26% in brothers and 29% in sisters, in contrast to controls, who displayed rates of 3 and 4%, respectively. Fathers showed affectedness rates of 29%, mothers 7%, paternal aunts 21%, paternal uncles 27%, paternal grandparents 10%, maternal aunts 22%, maternal uncles 15%, and maternal grandparents between 0 and 7%.

In summary, SLI appears to be highly familial, although the rates appear to change with the definition of SLI used. Although familiality suggests a genetic contribution to SLI, it cannot be taken as definitive proof, as family similarities can stem from common environmental influences. Clearer evidence can come only from other studies that attempt to dissect the general influences of genetic and environmental factors. Twin studies are the main example of this type of approach.

C. TWIN STUDIES

There are few large twin studies of SLI, although twin studies of global language impairments have shown good evidence of moderate heritability (Aoki & Asaka, 1993; DeFries & Plomin, 1983; Hardy-Brown, 1983; Hardy-Brown & Plomin, 1985; Hardy-Brown et al., 1981; Hay et al., 1987; Locke & Mather, 1989; Matheny & Bruggemann, 1973; Mather & Black, 1984; Munsinger & Douglass, 1976; Osborne et al., 1968; Plomin, 1986; Plomin et al., 1988; Scarr & Carter-Saltzman, 1983). Tomblin (1996), Tomblin and Buckwalter (1998), and Lewis and Thompson (1992) studied 43 twin pairs in which at least one twin had SLI. They found a proband concordance rate for history of speech and/or language therapy of 0.86 in monozygotic (MZ) twins and 0.48 in dizygotic (DZ) twins. Recognizing the need for more powerful twin studies, Bishop and colleagues (1995) studied 90 twin pairs where at least one twin met strict criteria for the development of speech and language disorder. Using DSM-IIIR criteria and operational definitions, they found that only 8 (ca. 30%) of the 27 DZ pairs were concordant for developmental articulation disorder, whereas 34 (ca. 54%) of the 63 MZ twins were concordant. They reported a proband-wide concordance rate of 46% for DZ twins and 70% for MZ twins for male twin pairs. However, they observed little difference between the small groups of female twins (MZ = 43%, DZ = 44%). In 1994, Stromswold performed a meta-analysis of 188 MZ twin pairs and 94 DZ pairs and found a pairwise concordance rate of 72.9% for MZ and 35.1% for DZ twins. From these data, he calculated a heritability estimate of 0.76 and a phenotype penetrance of 0.8.

More recently, Dale and colleagues (1998) performed a twin study on the first signs of language problems in children aged 2 years. They performed an extremes analysis (lowest 5%) of a sample of 6,862 2-year-old twins from a potential sample of 15,512 assessed for productive vocabulary (measured by the MacArthur Communicative Development Inventory; Fenson et al., 1994). From a final sample of 3,000 twins, they found a group difference heritability (lowest 5%) of 73% for productive vocabulary scores, with a shared environment accounting for 18% of the variance. However, almost the opposite pattern was observed for productive vocabulary in the whole sample, with heritability estimates in the region of 25% and shared environment accounting for the majority of the variance (69%). This is an extremely interesting result, because it strongly suggests that the genetic etiology of productive vocabulary performance is different at the extreme low end of the dimension. It thus appears that genes play a significant role in the development of severe productive vocabulary impairment but play little role in the normal variation of this trait. This argues against a continuum in the phenotypic–genotypic relationship and supports a more categorical perspective.

D. MODE OF TRANSMISSION

A number of studies has attempted to calculate how genes are transmitted through pedigrees. However, with a variety of different definitions of SLI and the different types of samples collected, it is difficult to get a clear picture of the mode of inheritance. In addition, in common disorders such as SLI, it is likely that a number of genes play a role, which makes estimating the specific modes of inheritance of each gene extremely difficult. In a segregation analysis of speech and language disorders, Lewis et al., (1993) were unable to distinguish between a major gene model and a multifactorial transmission model for SLI. However, Van der Lely and Stollwerck (1996) supported an autosomal-dominant mode of inheritance. The high rates of affection in first-degree relatives of probands with SLI have also been considered to be consistent with a common autosomal recessive allele.

E. MOLECULAR GENETIC STUDIES

Molecular genetic research of SLI is still in its early stages, but has already produced significant evidence of linkage. Fisher and colleagues (1998) identified a region on chromosome 7 that co-segregated with speech and language disorder in a large three-generation family, where half the members were affected (i.e., 15 of the 30 relatives). Their findings resulted from a full genome scan, which initially identified a 27.4-cM region of linkage on chromosome 7 between genetic markers D7S527 and D7S530. Fine mapping of this region using additional markers showed a peak multipoint LOD score (see Chapter 3) of 6.62 in a 3.8-cM interval between D7S2425 and CFTR (the gene coding for cystic fibrosis). An LOD score of >3.3 indicates significant linkage in complex disorders (Terwilleger & Ott, 1994). We estimate that this region is likely to contain at least 100 genes based on current estimates (Dunham et al., 1999). Fisher and colleagues (1998) have also suggested several possible candidate genes within this region of linkage, including a gene-protein-activated phosphoinositide-3 kinase, the interferon-related protein PC4 (which may be significant in neurodevelopment), Bravo/Nr-CAM (a neuronal cell adhesion molecule), and WNT-2 (a putative signalling molecule involved in development). It is also noteworthy that this region of linkage lies within a larger region of linkage to autism, which has a high prevalence of language delay (Bailey, 1998).

However, it should be noted that the language disorder segregating in the family mentioned above is not typical of SLI and is characterized by deficient grammatical ability and expressive language, and grossly defective articulation manifest as a severe speech dyspraxia (Vargha-Khadem & Passingham, 1990) and orofacial dyspraxia (Vargha-Khadem *et al.*, 1995) in addition to language delay. Gopnik (1990) and Gopnik and Crago (1991) have suggested that the disorder is an impairment of word generation specifically of word endings in accordance with grammatical rules and have cited the linkage as evidence supporting genes related to specific aspects of grammar processing (Maynard-Smith & Szathmary, 1995). However, there is also evidence of extensive cognitive impairment in affected family members with nine individuals having IQs below 82 (Watkins *et al.*, 1999). In addition, brain imaging studies of this family (Fisher *et al.*, 1998) suggest functional abnormalities in areas of the frontal lobe related to motor activity and also observe anatomical abnormalities in several brain regions including the neostriatum. It is significant to note that phenotypic–genotypic relationships that tie brain areas and specific cognitive functions to gene products may improve our understanding of language processing and brain development and form an exciting new prospect for future neuroscience research.

II. THE GENETICS OF SPECIFIC READING DISABILITY (SRD)

Understanding how language is processed in the brain is one of the major challenges for neuroscience research today. Identifying genes that contribute to the processes underlying the way written language is manipulated cognitively may provide important insights into how language is processed in general. Reading is a complex task that aims to extract meaning from the written word. Specific reading disability, or developmental dyslexia, is characterized as a gross difficulty in reading and writing that is not attributable to a general intellectual impairment or to a lack of exposure to an appropriate educational environment. Specific reading disability (SRD) is usually characterized as a deficit of at least 2 years in reading age compared to that predicted from chronological age. However, as with SLI, measures of reading ability differ considerably among studies, and, as yet, there are no universal operational definitions of reading disability to allow proper generalizability across studies.

A variety of cognitive components have been implicated in the development of SRD. These include deficits of visual processing (Stein, 1993), deficits in the language processing system (Shankweiler *et al.*, 1979), and deficits in temporal processing (Stein & Walsh, 1997). However, most evidence suggests that deficits in phonological processing are central to the development of SRD. The functional unit of phonological processing is the phoneme, the smallest discernible segment of speech. Phonological processing includes phoneme awareness, decoding, storage, and retrieval. Another component of the reading process is the visual appearance or shape (orthographic information) of a written word (Olson *et al.*, 1994). In addition, the speed at which language-based information is processed may also be of importance (Wolf & Bowers, 1999). Indeed, our own work (Robinson *et al.*, 2000) has identified three factors that describe severe SRD (children with at least 2½ years deficit in reading age compared to chronological age; $N = 250$) as comprising phonologic, orthographic, and rapid-naming dimensions. Within this population, each factor accounts for a maximum of 18% of the variance.

A. FAMILY STUDIES

In an early family study of SRD, Rutter, Tizard, and Whitmore (1970) observed that 34% of children with specific reading retardation had a parent or sibling with a reading problem compared to 9% of control children. Other early studies also supported the familiality of SRD (Hallgren, 1950; Owen *et al.*, 1971; Walker & Cole, 1965; Yule & Rutter, 1975). Indeed, four of the major family studies undertaken have reported consistently high sibling recurrence risks of 40.8% ($N = 174$, Hallgren, 1950), 42.5% ($N = 40$, Finucci *et al.*, 1976), 43% ($N = 168$, Vogler *et al.*, 1985), and 38.5% ($N = 52$, Gilger *et al.*, 1991). Gilger and colleagues studied the probability of a mother or father being affected, given an affected or control male or female offspring, in three separate population samples. The Iowa and Colorado population samples probably provide the best estimates for the normal population. Gilger *et al.* (1991) found that these showed that, for male probands, the risk in fathers ranged between 30 and 35% and between 12 and 15% for mothers, whereas the risk for female probands to fathers ranged from 17 to 41% and from 30 to 42% for mothers. The risk of SRD in fathers or mothers of a normal control proband was 4 and 3%, respectively. Although there is variation in estimates of population frequency of SRD, reasonable estimates range between 5 and 10% (Pennington, 1990).

B. TWIN STUDIES

Early twin studies of SRD that showed significantly greater MZ than DZ concordance for specific reading disability suffered method problems, especially ascertainment bias and the inconsistent use of operational definitions of SRD (Bakwin, 1973; Zerbin-Rudin, 1967). The first systematic evidence that the high familiality of SRD was due to genetic, rather than social, factors came in the 1980s. During this time, two important twin studies were published: The Colorado Twin Reading Study (DeFries & Fulker, 1987; DeFries *et al.*, 1987) and the London Twin Study (Stevenson *et al.*, 1987). Both provided strong evidence for the role of genes in SRD.

These studies differed in some aspects of method. The Colorado study used twins where one member of each twin pair was reading disabled, whereas the

London study selected twins from the normal population who represented the full range of reading ability. Nevertheless, there was convergent evidence from the two studies about the heritability of reading and spelling. The twins for the Colorado study were obtained from schools where at least one member of the twin pair was suspected by the teachers as having a reading disability. The reading ability of both twins was then assessed by a standard battery of tests that had been shown previously to discriminate between reading-disabled and normal readers. The study is ongoing, and the number of twin pairs recruited was 382 MZ and 262 DZ pairs (in 1996), of whom half were control pairs and half had at least one twin with SRD. The London study was of 285 twin pairs identified from the general population on the basis of birth records and from the registers of schools in the London area. Although the number of reading-disabled twins was far fewer than was available in the Colorado study, the London study was able to investigate genetic and environmental influences on the full range of reading and spelling ability.

The Colorado study found substantial heritable components to reading (44%) and spelling (62%). They also observed highly heritable deficits in phonological processing as indicated by nonword reading (75%), but did not detect a significant heritable component for orthographic processing (31%). Common family environment was also shown to have a significant influence (48%). The London Twin Study, in contrast, found no evidence supporting heritability of reading per se. However, it produced strong evidence for some aspects of reading disability. Phonological coding (nonword reading) showed heritability of 82% where probands had evidence of specific reading disability, and homophone recognition showed heritability of 67% in the normal range, which was not significant when probands showed evidence of SRD. Stevenson (1991) also observed significant heritability for impaired spelling (62%) and a greater pattern of heritability for deficits in phonological processing than for deficits in orthographic coding.

Olson and colleagues have extended their analysis of phonological and orthographic dimensions within the Colorado Twin Study (Gayan et al., 1994, 1997; Olson et al., 1994). They observed significant heritability for orthographic coding (56%), which was approximately the same as that observed for phonological coding (59%). Similarly, Castles and colleagues (1999) studied orthographic and phonological subgroups that were adjusted to be independent of overall reading ability to provide a clearer measure of associated skills. Their study involved 592 pairs of twins—272 MZ and 320 DZ—in which at least one twin fell within the SRD category. Children whose subtype scores fell in the top third of the distribution (i.e., their standardized scores on the phonological processing measure were higher than their scores on the orthographic processing measure) were allocated to the orthographic group. Children whose subtype scores fell in the bottom third of the distribution were allocated to the phonological dyslexia group. They observed a highly significant heritable component for word recognition (67%) for the phonological subgroup that became more significant for the extreme form of the subtype (lower fifth of the distribution, heritability = 78%). They also found a significant heritable component for word recognition deficit in the orthographic group (heritability of 31%), although, interestingly, a greater environmental component to word recognition deficit was observed in the orthographic group.

C. MODE OF TRANSMISSION

Pennington and colleagues (1991) have performed the most extensive complex segregation analysis of SRD. They examined the relatives of SRD probands in four independent samples from the states of Colorado (rural and urban), Washington, and Iowa, producing a sample of 204 families and 1,698 individuals. Their results supported a major locus transmission in three of the four samples and a polygenic transmission in the fourth. There was also evidence of sex differences in penetrance rates, with females showing lower estimates of penetrance in the autosomal-dominant family. It is possible that this might go some way to explain the slight excess of males observed in SRD (i.e., sex ratio of 1.5 to 1 male:female) (Shaywitz et al., 1990; Wadsworth et al., 1992), although the higher ratio of males to females could also be attributed to an artefact of clinical ascertainment (Shaywitz et al., 1990). Pennington and colleagues (1991) have also shown that the slight excess of males is unlikely to be due to classic X-linked transmission. There was no robust evidence of transmission from fathers to sons or for mitochondrial transmission, as transmission rates from each parental sex were essentially equal (0.34 for fathers and mothers, Colorado sample), or for imprinting, for the above reasons and also that there was no observed effect of parental sex on the severity of SRD in the offspring.

D. MOLECULAR GENETICS

Molecular genetic research of SRD has already produced strong evidence of linkage to chromosome 6p (Cardon et al., 1994, 1995; Fisher et al., 1999; Gayan et al., 1999; Grigorenko et al., 1997, 2000), significant evidence of linkage to chromosome 15 (Grigorenko et al., 1997; Schulte-Korne et al., 1998; Smith et al., 1983), significant linkage to chromosome 2 (Fagerheim et al., 1999; Petryshen et al., 2000b), and suggestive evidence of linkage to chromosome 1 (Rabin et al., 1993). In addition, studies using linkage disequilibrium mapping have fine mapped the region on chromosomes 6 and 15 to areas of approximately 1–6 cM, which show good evidence to contain the putative genes (Morris et al., 2000; Turic et al., 2000).

The observation of elevated risk for autoimmune disease in relatives of SRD probands focused molecular genetic research on the human leukocyte antigen (HLA) region of chromosome 6p (Hugdahl et al., 1990; Pennington et al., 1987). Cardon and colleagues (1994) were the first to report linkage between SRD and chromosome 6. They detected significant linkage ($p = 0.0002$) implicating a region at 6p21.3 in a sample of 114 sibling pairs from 19 families and a sample of DZ twins taken from the Colorado Twin Register (50 pairs). Their measure of SRD was based on a composite score of reading ability, which they treated as a quantitative variable to test for linkage. Although the results of the original study were later amended to take account of MZ twins included by mistake, the linkage remained significant (twins $p = 0.009$; siblings $p = 0.0003$: Cardon et al., 1995).

Grigorenko and colleagues (1997, 2000) used samples of large multiplex families (six, later expanded to eight) and found significant evidence of linkage to 6p21.3 in a region spanned by markers D6S464 and D6S273. In the 1997 study, they appeared to show strongest evidence of linkage to a phenotype characterized as phonemic awareness, although significant linkage was also observed with phonological decoding and single-word reading. However, their extended study (2000) produced a less clear relationship showing linkage to single-word reading, vocabulary, and spelling with phonemic awareness and phonological decoding showing little evidence of a relationship. However, it must be noted that the evidence for relationships with specific RD phenotypes or dimensions may be influenced by the methods of ascertainment, phenotypic definition, and the frequency of the phenotypes in the sample studied. For example, in one Grigorenko study, 38% of individuals were categorized as having a phonemic-awareness deficiency while only 18% had a vocabulary deficit. Furthermore, as most of these phenotypes show significant correlation with each other—which results in many individuals having numerous phenotypes—clear relationships, if they exist, may be difficult to establish. In addition, studies that have attempted to explore relationships with subphenotypes or phenotypic dimensions have varied in their approaches both to the phenotypic definitions and in the assumptions underlying analysis—namely, whether the phenotype is viewed as a categorical variable (as is the case in the Grigorenko studies) or whether the phenotype is viewed as a continuous dimension (e.g., by Cardon et al., 1994).

Fisher and colleagues (1999) studied a sample of 181 sibling pairs in which one member of each pair was selected for SRD. They observed evidence of linkage with phonological (nonword reading, $p = 0.0035$) and orthographic processing (irregular-word reading, $p = 0.0035$), with a peak around markers D6S276 and D6S105. Similarly, Gayan and colleagues (1999) tested 79 sibships including 180 individuals not included in previous studies in which at least one sibling had evidence of SRD. They observed evidence for linkage to orthographic (LOD = 3.1) and phonologic (LOD = 2.42) deficits that peaked at marker D6S461 for the former and 2–3 cM proximal to this for the latter. However, Field and Kaplan (1998) and Petryshen et al. (2000b) found no evidence of linkage with SRD with markers in the region 6p23–6p21.3 using either qualitative or quantitative measures of the SRD phenotype. The design of their study differed from previous approaches. They used families who contained at least two individuals with severe phonological reading deficits, and they have speculated that their families may have a different balance of SRD subtypes within them that may not be strongly linked to the region studied. We mapped the region of putative linkage (D6S109–D6S1538) for linkage disequilibrium. We identified a region between D6S109 and D6S1260 that showed significant evidence of haplotype association with SRD in two independent samples of parent-proband trios (Turic et al., 2000).

Smith *et al.* (1983) were the first to report some evidence of linkage between SRD and chromosome 15. Their study used a limited number of chromosomal heteromorphisms and produced an LOD score of 3.2. Subsequently, Smith and colleagues (1986, 1990) showed that the positive linkage result was due to 20% of the families studied. However, Bisgaard and colleagues (1987) failed to show linkage between SRD and chromosome 15 heteromorphisms. However, the assessment method for SRD was far less rigorous and involved no direct testing, only questionnaires and interviews. In 1997, Grigorenko and colleagues reported significant evidence of linkage (LOD score = 3.15) with marker D1S143 and single-word reading in six extended families, each of which contained four individuals with significant reading disability. No significant linkage was observed with phonological phenotypes, although phonological awareness was found to be linked to chromosome 6 in the same families. Schulte-Korne *et al.* (1998) also reported suggestive evidence of linkage (maximum LOD score = 1.78: D15S132–D1S143) to chromosome 15 for spelling disability in seven multiplex families. More recently, we observed an association with SRD and haplotypes resulting from the combination of microsatellite markers D15S146/D15S214/D15S994 using a two-stage, family-based, linkage disequilibrium mapping design (Morris *et al.*, 2000). We observed a significant haplotypic association ($p < 0.001$) in both stage 1 (101 parent-RD proband trios) and stage 2 samples (77 trios). Twenty genes have been identified within this region of association, of which three are involved in regulating neurotransmission and one is a member of a gene family with another family member mapping to our candidate region for SRD on chromosome 6.

Other chromosomal regions have been identified as possibly containing genes contributing to SRD. In 1993, Rabin and his colleagues reported suggestive evidence of linkage ($Z_{max} = 21.95$, 1p34–p36) in a series of families, a proportion of whom had been linked previously to chromosome 15 (Smith *et al.*, 1983). Coincidentally, Froster *et al.* (1993) identified a family in whom SRD appeared to co-segregate with a balanced translocation [t(1;2)(p22:q31)], suggesting linkage to a gene on the distal region of 1p or 2q. It is interesting, therefore, that Fagerheim *et al.* (1999) reported linkage in a large Norwegian family to a region with maximum LOD scores of 3.54, 2.92, and 4.32 for three diagnostic models. These findings were the result of a genome-wide search for linkage using a 20-cM marker map in 36 members of a family of more than 80 identified members and implicated a region on chromosome 2p15–16 that appears to show evidence of replication in an independent sample (Petryshen *et al.*, 2000a). However, this region is different from that implicated by Froster and colleagues.

III. CONCLUSIONS

Genes play a significant role in the development of language disorders as demonstrated by specific language impairment and specific reading disability.

Indeed, advances have identified chromosomal regions that show good evidence of containing susceptibility genes. As the pace of this research increases, there is great optimism that genes will soon be found and our understanding of the origins of these disorders will truly begin.

REFERENCES

Aoki, S., & Asaka, A. (1993). *Genetic analysis of motor development, language development and some behavior characteristics in infancy.* Paper presented at the annual meeting of the Behavior Genetics Association.

Arnold, G. E. (1961). The genetic background of developmental language disorders. *Folia Phoniatrica, 13,* 246–254.

Bailey, A. (1998). A full genome screen for autism with evidence for linkage to a region of chromosome 7q [on behalf of the International Molecular Genetic Study of Autism Consortium]. *Human Molecular Genetics, 7,* 571–578.

Bakwin, H. (1973). Reading disability in twins. *Developmental Medicine and Child Neurology, 15,* 184–187.

Bisgaard, M. L., Eiberg, H., Moller, N., Niebuhr, E., & Mohr, J. (1987). Dyslexia and chromosome 15 heteromorphism: Negative LOD in a Danish material. *Clinical Genetics, 32,* 118–119.

Bishop, D. V. M., & Edmundson, A. (1986). Is otitis media a major cause of specific developmental language disorders? *British Journal of Disorders of Communication, 21,* 321–338.

Bishop, D. V. M., *et al.* (1995). Genetic basis of specific language impairment: Evidence from a twin study. *Developmental Medicine and Child Neurology, 37,* 56–71.

Borges-Osorio, M. R., & Salzano, F. M. (1985). Language disabilities in 3 twin pairs and their relatives. *Acta Geneticae Medicae et Gemellologiae, 34,* 95–100.

Byrne, B., Willerman, L., & Ashmore, L. (1974). Severe and moderate language impairment: Evidence for distinctive etiologies. *Behavioral Genetics, 4,* 331–345.

Cardon, L. R., Smith, S. D., Fulker, D. W., Kimberling, B. F., & DeFries, J. C. (1994). Quantitative trait locus for reading disability on chromosome 6. *Science, 266,* 276–279.

Cardon, L. R., Smith, S. D., Fulker, D. W., Kimberling, B. F., Pennington, B. F., & DeFries, J. C. (1995). Quantitative trait locus for reading disability. *Science, 268,* 1553.

Castles, A., Datta, H., Gayan, J., & Olson, R. K. (1999). Varieties of developmental reading disorder: Genetic and environmental influences. *Journal of Experimental Child Psychology, 72,* 73–94.

Dale, P. S., Simonoff, E., Bishop, D. V. M., Eley, T. C., Oliver, B., Price, T. S., Purcell, S., Stevenson, J., & Plomin, R. (1998). Genetic influence on language delay in two-year-old children. *Nature Neuroscience, 1,* 324–328.

DeFries, J. C., & Plomin, R. (1983). Adoption designs for the study of complex behavioral characteristics. In C. L. Ludlow & J. A. Cooper (Eds.), *Genetic aspects of speech and language disorders* (pp. 131–138). New York: Academic Press.

DeFries, J. C., Fulker, D. W., & LaBuda, M. C. (1987). Evidence for a genetic aetiology in reading disability of twins. *Nature, 329,* 537–539.

Dunham, I., Shimizu, N., Roe, B. A., & Chissoe, S. (1999). The DNA sequence of human chromosome 22. *Nature, 402,* 489–495.

Fagerheim, T., Raeymaekers, P., Tonnessen, F. E., Pedersen, M., Tranebjaerg, L., & Lubs, H. A. (1999). A new gene (DYX3) for dyslexia is located on chromosome 2. *Journal of Medical Genetics, 36,* 664–669.

Fenson, L., Dale, P. S., Reznick, J. S., Bates, E., Thal, D. J., & Pethick, S. J. (1994). Variability in early communicative development. *Monographs of the Society for Research on Child Development, 59*, 1–173.

Field, L. L., & Kaplan, B. J. (1998). Absence of linkage of phonological coding dyslexia to chromosome 6p23–p21.3 in a large family data set. *American Journal of Human Genetics, 63*, 1448–1456.

Finucci, J. M., Guthrie, J. T., Childs, A. L., Abbey, H., & Childs, B. (1976). The genetics of specific reading disability. *Annual Review of Human Genetics, 40*, 1–23.

Fisher, S. E., Vargha-Khadem, F., Watkins, K. E., Monaco, A. P., & Pembrey, M. E. (1998). Localisation of a gene implicated in a severe speech and language disorder. *Nature Genetics, 18*, 168–170.

Fisher, S. E., Marlow, A. J., Lamb, J., Maestrini, E., Williams, D. F., Richardson, A. J., Weeks, D. E., Stein, J. F., & Monaco, A. P. (1999). A quantitative trait locus on chromosome 6p influences aspects of developmental dyslexia. *American Journal of Human Genetics, 64*, 146–156.

Froster, U., Schulte-Korne, G., Hebebrand, J., & Remschmidt, H. (1993). Cosegregation of balanced translocation (1:2) with retarded speech development and dyslexia. *Lancet*, No. 8864, 178–179.

Fundudis, T., Kolvin, I., & Garside, R. (1979). *Speech retarded and deaf children: Their psychological development*. New York: Academic Press.

Gayan, J., Forsberg, H., & Olson, R. K. (1994). Genetic influences on subtypes of dyslexia. *Behavioral Genetics, 24*, 513.

Gayan, J., Datta, H. E., Castles, A. E., & Olson, R. K. (1997). *The aetiology of group deficits in word decoding across levels of phonological decoding and orthographic decoding*. Paper presented at the annual meeting of the Society for the Scientific Study of Reading.

Gayan, J., Smith, S. D., Cherny, S. S., Cardon, L. R., Fulker, D. W., Brower, A. M., Olson, R. K., Pennington, B. F., & DeFries, J. D. (1999). Quantitative-trait locus for specific language and reading deficits on chromosome 6. *American Journal of Human Genetics, 64*, 157–164.

Gilger, J. W., Pennington, B. F., & DeFries, J. C. (1991). Risk for reading disability as a function of parental history in 3 family studies. *Reading and Writing, 3*, 205–217.

Gopnik, M. (1990). Feature-blind grammar and dysphasia. *Nature, 344*, 715.

Gopnik, M., & Crago, M. B. (1991). Familial aggregation of a developmental language disorder. *Cognition, 39*, 1–50.

Grigorenko, E. L., Wood, F. B., Meyer, M. S., Hart, L. A., Speed, W. C., Shuster, A., & Pauls, D. L. (1997). Susceptibility loci for distinct components of developmental dyslexia on chromosomes 6 and 15. *American Journal of Human Genetics, 60*, 27–39.

Grigorenko, E. L., Wood, F. B., Meyer, M. S., & Pauls, D. L. (2000). Chromosome 6p influences on different dyslexia-related cognitive processes: Further confirmation. *American Journal of Human Genetics, 66*, 715–723.

Hallgren, B. (1950). Specific dyslexia: A clinical and genetic study. *Acta Psychiatrica et Neurologica Scandinavia*, Suppl. 65.

Hardy-Brown, K. (1983). Universals and individual differences: Disentangling two approaches to the study of language acquisition. *Developmental Psychology, 19*, 610–624.

Hardy-Brown, K., & Plomin, R. (1985). Infant communicative development: Evidence from adoptive and biological families for genetic and environmental influences on rate differences. *Developmental Psychology, 21*, 378–385.

Hardy-Brown, K., Plomin, R., & DeFries, J. C. (1981). Genetic and environmental influences on the rate of communicative development in the first year of life. *Developmental Psychology, 17*, 704–717.

Hay, D. A., Prior, M., Collett, S., & Williams, M. (1987). Speech and language development of twins. *Acta Geneticae Medicae et Gemellologiae, 36*, 213–223.

Hier, D. B., & Rosenberger, P. B. (1980). Focal left temporal lobe lesions and delayed speech acquisition. *Journal of Developmental and Behavioral Pediatrics, 1*, 54–57.

Hugdahl, K., Synnevag, B., & Satz, P. (1990). Immune and autoimmune disorders in dyslexic children. *Neuropsychologia, 28,* 673–679.

Hurst, J. A., Baraitser, M., Auger, E., Grahm, F., & Norell, S. (1990). An extended family with a dominantly inherited speech disorder. *Developmental Medicine and Child Neurology, 32,* 352–355.

Ingram, T. T. S. (1959). Specific developmental disorders of speech in childhood. *Brain, 82,* 450–454.

Lewis, B. A. (1992). Pedigree analysis of children with phonology disorders. *Journal of Learning Disability, 25,* 586–597.

Lewis, B. A., & Thompson, L. A. (1992). A study of developmental speech and language disorders in twins. *Journal of Speech and Hearing Research, 35,* 1086–1094.

Lewis, B. A., Cox, N. J., & Byard, P. J. (1993). Segregation analysis of speech and language disorders. *Behavior Genetics, 23,* 291–297.

Locke, J. L., & Mather, P. L. (1989). Genetic factors in the ontogeny of spoken language: Evidence from monozygotic and dizygotic twins. *Journal of Child Language, 16,* 553–559.

Luchsinger, R. (1970). Inheritance of speech deficits. *Folia Phoniatrica, 22,* 216–230.

Matheny, A. P., & Bruggemann, C. E. (1973). Children's speech: Hereditary components and sex differences. *Folia Phoniatrica, 25,* 442–449.

Mather, P. L., & Black, K. N. (1984). Hereditary and environmental influences on preschool twins' language skills. *Developmental Psychology, 20,* 303–308.

Maynard-Smith, J., & Szathmary, E. (1995). *The major transitions in evolution.* Oxford: Freeman.

McReady, E. B. (1926). Defects in the zone of language (word-deafness and word-blindness) and their influence in education and behavior. *American Journal of Psychiatry, 6,* 267–277.

Morris, D. W., Robinson, L., Turic, D., Duke, M., Webb, V., Milham, C., Hopkin, E., Pound, K., Fernando, S., Easton, M., Hamshere, M., Williams, N., McGuffin, P., Stevenson, J., Krawczak, M., Owen, M. J., O'Donovan, M. C., & Williams, J. (2000). Family-based association mapping provides evidence for a gene for reading disability on chromosome 15q. *Human Molecular Genetics, 9,* 855–860.

Munsinger, H., & Douglass, A. (1976). The syntactic abilities of identical twins, fraternal twins, and their siblings. *Child Development, 47,* 40–50.

Neils, J., & Aram, D. (1986). Family history of children with developmental language disorders. *Perceptual and Motor Skills, 63,* 655–658.

Olson, R. K., Forsberg, H., & Wise, B. (1994). Genes, environment, and the development of ortho-graphic skills. In V. W. Berninger (Ed.), *The varieties of orthographic knowledge.* Vol. 1: *Theoretical developmental issues* (pp. 1–31). Dordrecht: Kluwer.

Osborne, R. T., Gregor, A. J., & Miele, F. (1968). Heritability of factor V: Verbal comprehension. *Perceptual and Motor Skills, 26,* 191–202.

Owen, F., Adams, P., Forrest, T., Stolz, L., & Fisher, S. (1971). Learning disorders in children: Sibling studies. *Monographs of the Society for Research in Child Development, 36,* No. 4.

Pennington, B. F. (1990). Annotation: The genetics of dyslexia. *Journal of Child Psychiatry and Psychology, 31,* 193–201.

Pennington, B. F., Smith, S., Kimberling, W., Green, P., & Haith, M. (1987). Left-handedness and immune disorders in familial dyslexics. *Archives of Neurology, 44,* 634–639.

Pennington, B. F., Gilger, J. W., Pauls, D., Smith, S. A., Smith, S. D., & DeFries, J. C. (1991). Evidence for major gene transmission of developmental dyslexia. *Journal of the American Medical Association, 266,* 1527–1534.

Pennington, B. F., Gilger, J. W., Olson, R. K., & DeFries, J. C. (1992). The external validity of age-discrepancy versus IQ-discrepancy definitions of reading disability: Lessons from a twin study. *Journal of Learning Disabilities, 25,* 562–573.

Petryshen, T. L., Kaplan, B. J., Hughes, M. L., & Field, L. L. (2000a). Evidence for the chromosome 2p15–p16 dyslexia susceptibility locus (DXY3) in a large Canadian data set. *American Journal of Medical Genetics (Neuropsychiatric Genetics)*, 96, 473.

Petryshen, T. L., Kaplan, B. J., Liu, M. F., & Field, L. L. (2000b). Absence of significant linkage between phonological decoding dyslexia and chromosome 6p23–21.3, as determined by use of quantitative-trait methods: Confirmation of qualitative analyses. *American Journal of Human Genetics*, 66, 708–714.

Pinker, S. (1994). *The language instinct: The new science of language and mind*. London: Penguin.

Plomin, R. (1986). *Development, genetics, and psychology*. Hillsdale, NJ: Erlbaum.

Plomin, R., DeFries, J. C., & Fulker, D. W. (1988). *Nature and nurture during infancy and early childhood*. New York: Cambridge University Press.

Rabin, M., Wen, X. L., Hepburn, M., Lubs, H. A., Feldman, E., & Duara, R. (1993). Suggestive linkage of developmental dyslexia to chromosome 1p34–p36. *Lancet*, 342, 178.

Randall, D., Reynell, J., & Curwen, M. (1974). A study of language development in a sample of 3–year-old children. *British Journal of Disorders of Communication*, 9, 3–16.

Rice, M. L. (1997). Specific language impairments: In search of diagnostic markers and genetic contributions. *Mental Retardation and Developmental Disabilities Research Reviews*, 3, 350–357.

Robinson, L., Morris, D. W., Turic, D., Duke, M., Webb, V., Milham, C., Hopkin, E., Pound, K., Fernando, S., Easton, M., Hamshere, M., Williams, N., McGuffin, P., Stevenson, J., Krawczak, M., Owen, M. J., O'Donovan, M. C., & Williams, J. (2000). *Dimensions of reading disability*. Unpublished paper.

Rutter, M., Tizard, J., & Whitmore, K. (1970). *Education, health, and behaviour*. London: Longmans.

Samples, J. M., & Lane, V. W. (1985). Genetic possibilities in six siblings with specific language learning disorders. *Asha*, 27, 27–32.

Scarr, S., & Carter-Saltzman, L. (1983). Genetics and intelligence. In J. Fuller & E. Simmel (Eds.), *Behavior genetics: Principles and applications* (pp. 217–335). Hillsdale, NJ: Erlbaum.

Schulte-Korne, G., Grimm, T., Nothen, N. M., Muller-Myshok, B., Cichon, S., Vogt, I. R., Propping, P., & Remschmidt, H. (1998). Evidence for linkage of spelling disability to chromosome 15. *American Journal of Human Genetics*, 63, 279–282.

Shankweiler, D., Liberman, I. Y., Mark, L. S., Fowler, C. A., & Fischer, F. W. (1979). The speech code and learning to read. *Journal of Experimental Psychology: Human Learning and Memory*, 5, 531–545.

Shaywitz, S. E., Shaywitz, B. A., Fletcher, J. M., & Escobar, M. D. (1990). Prevalence of reading disability in boys and girls. *Journal of the American Medical Association*, 264, 998–1002.

Smith, S. D., Kimberling, W. J., Pennington, B. F., & Lubs, H. A. (1983). Specific reading disability: Identification of an inherited form through linkage analysis. *Science*, 219, 1345.

Smith, S. D., Pennington, B. F., Kimberling, W. J., Fain, P. R., Ing, P. S., & Lubs, H. A. (1986). Genetic heterogeneity in specific reading disabilities. *American Journal of Human Genetics*, 39, 169a.

Smith, S. D., Pennington, B. F., Kimberling, B. F., & Ing, P. S. (1990). Genetic linkage analysis with specific dyslexia: Use of multiple markers to include and exclude possible loci. In G. T. Pavlidis (Ed.), *Perspectives on dyslexia*, Vol. 1: *Neurology, neuropsychology, and genetics* (pp. 77–89). West Sussex: Wiley.

Spitz, R. V., Tallal, P., Flax, J., & Benasich, A. A. (1997). Look who's talking: A prospective study of familial transmission of language impairments. *Journal of Speech and Hearing Research*, 40, 990–1001.

Stein, J. F. (1993). Visuospatial perception in disabled readers. In D. M. Willows, R. S. Kruk, & E. Corcos (Eds.), *Visual processes in reading and reading disabilities* (pp. 331–346). Hillsdale, NJ: Erlbaum.

Stein, J. F., & Walsh, V. (1997). To see but not to read: The magnocellular theory of dyslexia. *Trends in Neuroscience, 20,* 147–152.

Stevenson, J. (1991). Which aspects of processing text mediate genetic effects? *Reading and Writing, 3,* 249–269.

Stevenson, J., & Richman, N. (1976). The prevalence of language delay in a population of 3-year-old children and its association with general retardation. *Developmental Medicine and Child Neurology, 18,* 431–441.

Stevenson, J., Graham, P., Fredman, G., & McLoughlin, V. (1987). A twin study of genetic influences on reading and spelling ability and disability. *Journal of Child Psychiatry and Psychology, 28,* 229–247.

Stromswold, K. (1994). *The nature of children's early grammar: Evidence from inversion errors.* Paper presented at the Linguistic Society of America.

Tallal, P., Ross, R., & Curtiss, S. (1989). Familial aggregation in specific language impairment. *Journal of Speech and Hearing Disorders, 54,* 167–173.

Terwilliger, J. D., & Ott, J. (1994). *Handbook of human genetic language.* Baltimore: Johns Hopkins.

Tomblin, J. B. (1989). Familial concentration of developmental language impairment. *Journal of Speech and Hearing Disorders, 54,* 287–295.

Tomblin, J. B. (1996). Genetic and environmental contributions to the risk for specific language impairment. In M. L. Rice (Ed.), *Towards a genetics of language* (pp. 191–210). Mahwah, NJ: Erlbaum.

Tomblin, J. B., & Buckwalter, P. R. (1998). Heritability of poor language achievement among twins. *Journal of Speech and Hearing Research, 41,* 188–199.

Tomblin, J. B., Freese, P. R., & Records, N. L. (1992). Diagnosing specific language impairment in adults for the purpose of pedigree analysis. *Journal of Speech and Hearing Research, 35,* 832–843.

Turic, D., Robinson, L., Duke, M., Morris, D. W., Webb, V., Hamshere, M., Milham, C., *et al.* (2000). Linkage disequilibrium mapping provides evidence for a gene for reading disability on chromosome 6p21.3-22. *American Journal of Human Genetics.* Submitted manuscript.

Van der Lely, H. K., & Stollwerck, L. (1996). A grammatical specific language impairment in children: An autosomal dominant inheritance? *Brain and Language, 52,* 484–504.

Vargha-Khadem, F., & Passingham, R. E. (1990). Speech and language defects. *Nature, 346,* 226.

Vargha-Khadem, F., Watkins, K., Alcock, K., Fletcher, P., & Passingham, R. E. (1995). Praxic and nonverbal cognitive deficits in a large family with a genetically transmitted speech and language disorder. *Proceedings of the National Academy of Sciences, 92,* 930–933.

Vogler, G. P., DeFries, J. C., & Decker, S. N. (1985). Family history as an indicator of risk for reading disability. *Journal of Learning Disabilities, 18,* 419–421.

Wadsworth, S. J., DeFries, J. C., Stevenson, J., Gilger, J. W., & Pennington, B. F. (1992). Gender ratios among reading-disabled children and their siblings. *Journal of Child Psychiatry and Psychology, 33,* 1229–1239.

Walker, L., & Cole, E. (1965). Familial patterns of expression of specific reading disability in a population sample. *Bulletin of the Orton Society, 15,* 12–24.

Watkins, K. E., Gadian, D. G., & Vargha-Khadem, F. (1999). Functional and structural brain abnormalities associated with a genetic disorder of speech and language. *American Journal of Human Genetics, 65,* 1215–1221.

Wolf, M., & Bowers, P. G. (1999). The double-deficit hypothesis for the developmental dyslexias. *Journal of Educational Psychology, 91,* 415–438.

Yule, W., & Rutter, M. (1975). The concept of specific reading retardation. *Journal of Child Psychiatry and Psychology, 16,* 181–197.

Zerbin-Rudin, E. (1967). Congenital word-blindness. *Bulletin of the Orton Society, 17,* 47–54.

7

GENETICS IN CRANIOFACIAL DISORDERS AND CLEFTING

THEN AND NOW

ROBERT J. SHPRINTZEN

Department of Otolaryngology and Communicative Science
State University of New York
Upstate Medical University
Syracuse, New York

The past twenty years have brought a revolution to the study of human disease that has encompassed the large majority of the subspecialties in health care. The study of human genetics is a relatively new science that has gained enormous momentum from the Human Genome Project, a multinational and well-funded effort to completely describe and understand the human genome (and all other species' genomes) within the first few years of the twenty-first century. The burst of activity in genetics has allowed clinicians to understand the basis of human disease in areas as diverse as cancer and psychosis. Genes that cause both common and rare human abnormalities are rapidly being discovered and mapped to specific chromosomal locations nearly every day. Just prior to the year 2000, the genetic sequence for one entire human chromosome, chromosome 22, was fully ascertained. This is truly remarkable when one considers that the basic structure of DNA was not understood until the latter half of the twentieth century.

Unfortunately, there is a sizeable gap in the knowledge of genetics among scientists who study communicative disorders. There are several reasons for the failure of practitioners in the communicative sciences to latch onto the study of either molecular or clinical genetics. One reason is that genetics is a fairly new discipline in the health sciences and it may not have been included in the curricula of current practitioners. A second reason is that scientists studying molecular genetics were largely recruited from the academic fields of molecular and cellular biology and were basic scientists, unlike the majority of speech–language pathologists and audiologists, who are clinicians without extensive laboratory experience. Finally, the behavioral fields of health care, such as speech–language pathology and psychology, have been traditionally steeped in learning and environmental influence (nurture) rather than biology (nature), making the notion that genetics can influence behavior novel, at best. The "nurture" approach to communication impairments has often led researchers to seek explanations for communication disorders that relate to factors that may influence the individual, rather than factors that come from within the child. Because behavioral genetics is a relatively new addition to the study of humans, it is likely that many studies that previously reported the etiology of speech or language impairments in children may require some reconsideration.

It is the purpose of this chapter to discuss the role of genetics in the communicative disorders expressed by people with craniofacial anomalies. The impact on patient care and how clinicians might best cope with the integration of the state of the art in genetics into their management strategies are also discussed. The predictive power of understanding the causation of communicative impairment in children with clefts and the manner in which genetics influences treatment outcomes is also explored.

I. THE GENETICS OF CLEFTING: ITS EVOLUTION OVER THE PAST 30 YEARS

Attention to the issue of the genetics of clefting began to develop in the late 1960s and early 1970s as craniofacial scientists and clinicians began to develop a new field of expertise initially known as *syndromology*, a discipline that today is typically referred to as *dysmorphology*. F. Clarke Fraser, Robert J. Gorlin, David

Smith, John Opitz, and David Bixler were among the true pioneers in the early development of clinical genetics. They subsequently trained many students who have expanded the field, such as M. Michael Cohen Jr., who has developed a systematic method for categorizing children with multiple anomalies (Cohen, 1997). These scientists and others delineated many multiple anomaly disorders— referred to as *syndromes*, *sequences*, and *associations*—serving as an impetus to understand the basic causes of clefts.

An *anomaly* is what was formerly called a birth defect. Anomalies are simply deviations from normal structure or function that are considered to be abnormal. Normality can often be defined in terms of some type of normative data. For example, normal height may be defined as all measurements that fall within two standard deviations of the population mean for height. For 5-year-old American males, average height is approximately 110 centimeters. Two standard deviations below the mean are 99 cm and two standard deviations above the mean are 118 cm. Therefore, short stature for 5-year-old boys, which is an anomaly, is defined as being under 99 cm in height. Similar norms are available for head circumference, interocular measurements, ear length, and many other anthropometric measurements. Human behavioral abnormalities can also be considered to be anomalies (see Chapter 9). Because there are standardized tests for many human behaviors— such as IQ scores, language and articulation tests, audiograms, and other aspects of cognition and/or perception—the interpretation of abnormalities is not particularly difficult, and behavioral anomalies can be determined. Therefore, an IQ score of 65 is also an anomaly, as are aberrant articulation, delayed language, and hypernasal speech.

In the early years of studying the genetics of clefting, it was thought that the majority of clefts occurred as isolated anomalies. In an early article that was cited very frequently for many years following its publication, Fraser (1970) reported that the very large majority of children with clefts, 97%, did not have other anomalies or syndromes in association with their clefts. The implication of Fraser's report, which was based on birth records, is that nearly all children with clefts are otherwise normal. Many clinicians had observed that clefting did not follow a typical dominant or recessive inheritance pattern in most cases. Therefore, an alternative explanation was sought for presence of some familial cases among the large number of sporadic cases. The genetic model was also based on the assumption that nearly all cases of clefting were nonsyndromic. A *multifactorial* model was proposed (Fraser, 1970) postulating that clefting was usually caused by multiple factors for each affected person, including the contribution of multiple genes (or a *polygenic* contribution) plus nongenetic factors such as environmental agents, intrauterine environment, and the timing of embryonic development in relation to these nongenetic factors. Because there were multiple factors involved, with genetics playing only a partial role, *recurrence risks* (the probability that parents with a child who had a cleft would have another, or the risk that the child would have a child with a cleft) were calculated to be quite low, such as 2 to 4%.

The multifactorial theory of cleft causation was accepted widely as fact for over a decade, and today many genetic counselors still estimate recurrence risk based on the multifactorial model. It should be noted that prior to 1970 there were very few specialists who focused on clinical genetics, and genetic counseling was in its infancy. Toward the end of that decade, however, genetic counselors and a new generation of clinical geneticists began to filter into more hospital settings, many of which had well-established cleft palate/craniofacial centers. As these clinicians saw larger numbers of patients with cleft palates, they began to recognize that many of their patients had other anomalies in addition to their clefts.

In 1981, Rollnick and Pruzansky reported that the majority of the 2512 patients seen at their center in Chicago had anomalies in addition to their clefts, and that 44% of their patients had multiple anomaly syndromes. This landmark study was a retrospective review of all patient charts at the Center for Craniofacial Anomalies, but all of the patients had been seen by clinicians with expertise in dysmorphology. Four years later, Shprintzen et al. (1985a) found that over 60% of 1000 consecutive patients seen in New York had associated anomalies and that 53% had syndromes. Although this study was a chart review, the 1000 consecutive patients were all seen prospectively by the same dysmorphologist and genetic counselor. In a follow-up study, Shprintzen et al. (1985b) reported that over 9% of their diagnoses were made retrospectively after syndromic identification had been missed at the time of the first patient contact. There are several reasons for missing the diagnosis of multiple anomaly syndromes in many cases, including:

1. Many structural anomalies are not obvious or present at birth and may not become expressed until later in life. For example, many children who have postnatal growth deficiency may have normal birth weight and length, but then develop postnatal growth deficiency and short stature, as is the case in some skeletal dysplasias. Other examples include the development of myopia in Stickler syndrome or ectodermal dysplasia involving the hair and teeth in Rapp–Hodgkin syndrome that may not be evident at birth. Clefting is a common feature in both Stickler syndrome and Rapp–Hodgkin syndrome. In studies reporting percentages of anomalies from birth records, such as that of Fraser (1970), the frequency of anomalies must be lower than the actual number of associated abnormalities for two reasons: the already mentioned late expression of some structural anomalies and the person who examines newborns for anomalies is rarely an experienced clinical geneticist. Newborn examinations are typically brief and cursory, and only the most obvious problems are detected. If other anomalies are detected later in life, even within days of birth (following discharge from the hospital), the anomalies will not be added to birth records.

2. Some anomalies are behavioral in nature and thus cannot be expressed at birth and therefore cannot be detected until later in childhood. For example, essentially all children with velocardiofacial syndrome develop

learning disabilities and temperament disorders. Because the behavioral components may not become evident until 4 or 5 years of age, a very high percentage of children with this syndrome escape detection until school years.

3. The process of syndrome delineation is an ongoing one, and new syndromes are discovered continuously. First contact with a patient may precede the delineation of a particular syndrome so that the diagnosis cannot be applied. In the 1970s, only about 70 multiple anomaly syndromes with clefting as a clinical finding had been delineated. Today, over 400 are known.

As new molecular genetics technologies have become available, scientists have discovered genes that directly or indirectly cause anomalies of the craniofacial complex, as well as genes that are associated with other developmental effects. The absence of familial cases of clefting does not rule out a genetic causation. For example, although velocardiofacial syndrome (VCFS) has an established genetic cause (deletion of a small portion of 22q11.2), the large majority of new cases are spontaneous rearrangements of chromosome 22. Over 90% of cases of VCFS are sporadic, but caused by the same genetic deletion as familial cases.

II. HOW MIGHT MUTANT GENES CAUSE CLEFT LIP, CLEFT PALATE, AND CRANIOFACIAL ANOMALIES?

Genes may impact on the formation of the lip, palate, face, and head in a number of ways, although the end result of a cleft or craniofacial anomaly may be difficult to distinguish according to the primary molecular mutation. For example, Stickler syndrome involves a mutation in a gene on the long arm of chromosome 12. The gene affected in Stickler syndrome (COL2A1) is involved in the formation of collagen 2, a type of collagen involved in the formation of connective tissue, cartilage, and bone. The resulting effect of the mutation is to cause cleft palate, myopia, retinal detachments, and joint laxity. However, cleft palate is also caused by mutations in genes not involved in collagen formation, including a gene on the long arm of chromosome 5 known as the TREACLE gene (Jabs et al., 1991) that causes Treacher Collins syndrome or the fibroblast growth receptor gene 2 (FGFR2) located on the long arm of chromosome 10 that causes Apert syndrome. Many more genetic mutations have been found to cause clefting, including those for van der Woude syndrome on the long arm of chromosome 1 (Murray et al., 1990) and the gene for otopalatodigital syndrome type I on the long arm of the X chromosome (Biancalana et al., 1991), to name a few. The mechanisms by which these genes cause the clefts is variable. Some affect the embryonic fusion process by impairing cell-to-cell reactions, some cause hypoplasia of tissues, and some interfere with migration patterns from the branchial arches. In other words, there are many possible interruptions in the process of palate and/or lip formation that will result in clefts, and the mechanisms by which the genes cause the clefts is different for each one. Therefore, clefting is not a specific disease, but rather a symptom of many possible disease processes, and those processes may be affected by many genes. Clefting is therefore heterogenous in etiology and is often only a single symptom in a broader pattern of anomalies.

III. SYNDROMES OF CLEFTING

A syndrome is defined as multiple anomalies in a single individual with all of the anomalies having a single cause. The cause might be a chromosomal aneu-ploidy, a genetic mutation, a teratogen (an environmental agent), or some extrinsic factor impinging on the developing embryo. Clefting of the palate and/or lip may be caused by any of these types of causes. For example, there are many chromo-somal abnormalities that cause clefts associated with other anomalies, including trisomy 13 (an extra chromosome 13), trisomy 18 (an extra chromosome 18), trisomy 21 (Down syndrome), Turner syndrome (a female missing one X chro-mosome), del(18p) (a deletion from the short arm of chromosome 18), del(4p) (also known as Wolf–Hirschhorn syndrome, a deletion from the short arm of chromosome 4), del(5p) (also known as cri-du-chat syndrome, a deletion from the short arm of chromosome 5), and del(6q) (deletion from the long arm of chromo-some 6). Although clefting is a feature of all of these syndromes, the other anomalies are not the same because the genetic contributions of the various chromosomes are different. Trisomy 13 has polydactyly (extra digits) and severe brain malformations, and early death occurs in essentially all cases. Turner syn-drome is characterized by webbing of the neck, heart anomalies, short stature, and lack of secondary sexual characteristics, but is not often fatal, unlike trisomy 13. Therefore, in these various chromosomal syndromes, clefting is only one of many severe anomalies, but the pattern, or phenotype, is different and distinctive for each syndrome.

Genetic disorders of clefting outnumber all other syndromic etiologies. Genetic syndromes are caused by DNA rearrangements that include deletions of some DNA, additions of DNA, or substitutions of DNA sequences that cannot typically be seen under a microscope. Genetic disorders may be single gene or contiguous gene. Single-gene disorders are those where there is a mutation in one gene that alters its function. Single-gene disorders of clefting may be inherited as autoso-mal-dominant, autosomal-recessive, X-linked-dominant, or X-linked-recessive traits, although the majority are autosomal dominant.

There are hundreds of single-gene disorders that have clefting as a feature, and many of the genes for these disorders have been mapped. These include Stickler syndrome (autosomal dominant, long arm of chromosome 12), van der Woude syndrome (autosomal dominant, long arm of chromosome 1), Freeman–Sheldon syndrome (autosomal dominant, short arm of chromosome 11), and Smith–Lemli–Opitz syndrome (autosomal recessive, long arm of chromosome 7).

Contiguous-gene disorders are those where a very small piece of DNA is deleted from one of the chromosomes. The deletion is usually too small to be detected with even a high-resolution karyotype, but it is detectable using molecular genetic techniques, such as FISH (fluorescent *in-situ* hybridization). There are several contiguous-gene disorders that have very interesting speech and language phenotypes, including velocardiofacial syndrome (Figure 7.1) and Prader–Willi syndrome (Figure 7.2). Velocardiofacial syndrome is the most common syndrome associated with clefting, accounting for approximately 8% of all patients with clefts of the palate (including submucous cleft) without cleft lip (although cleft lip does occur in a small percentage of cases). Velocardiofacial syndrome is caused by a deletion of a small segment of the long arm of chromosome 22, and is inherited as an autosomal dominant disorder. The syndrome is characterized by language impairment, learning disabilities, mental illness, immune deficiency, heart malformations, and over 180 other anomalies (VCFSEF website, 2000). The deleted region contains approximately 30 genes. Prader–Willi syndrome is not typically associated with cleft palate, but hypernasal speech is common in young

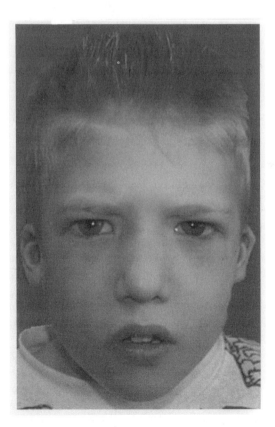

FIGURE 7.1   A child with velocardiofacial syndrome.

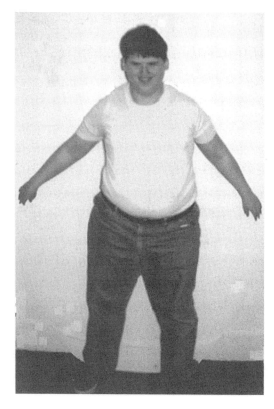

FIGURE 7.2   A child with Prader–Willi syndrome.

children with this disorder because of hypotonia. Other findings include obesity due to excessive and uncontrollable overeating (hyperphagia), small genitals in males, and small hands and feet. The hypernasality tends to resolve with age as muscle tone improves. Prader–Willi syndrome is caused by a deletion of the long arm of chromosome 15 when inherited from the father (i.e., absence of the paternal 15q11). However, when the deletion is inherited from the maternal chromosome 15 (absence of the maternal 15q11), a syndrome with a completely different phenotype is expressed in the child, Angelman syndrome. Angelman syndrome is characterized by severe cognitive impairment, absent speech development, and severe ataxia with essentially no resemblance to Prader–Willi syndrome. This difference in expression depending on the source of the deletion is known as *imprinting*.

Teratogens, agents external to the developing embryo that will cause abnormalities in the developmental process resulting in congenital anomalies, may be drugs (both legal and illegal), viruses and bacteria, environmental substances (such as heavy metals like mercury), and even disturbances in the maternal intrauterine environment caused by very high temperature elevations in the mother (maternal hyperthermia). Teratogenic syndromes are relatively rare, but there is a number of teratogens that do cause clefts and craniofacial disorders. The most common is ethyl alcohol, and fetal alcohol effects can result in cleft lip, cleft palate, and other craniofacial malformations, along with developmental delay and cognitive impairments. Anticonvulsant medications, such as phenytoins, may cause similar anomalies. Some viruses such as rubella and cytomegalovirus are also potent teratogens.

Factors extrinsic to the developing embryo can result in clefts. Perhaps the most common extrinsic cause of clefts is amniotic adhesions (Figure 7.3). If the mother's amnion ruptures or tears during early embryogenesis, as it begins to heal, strands of amniotic tissue may adhere onto the developing embryo with resulting disruption of fusing facial parts. If amniotic adhesions attach to the limbs, amputations or ring-like constrictions may occur (Figure 7.4). The anomalies caused by amniotic adhesions are known as the amnion rupture sequence (see Section IV). Because external factors are not genetic in etiology and typically represent random accidents, there is essentially negligible recurrence risk.

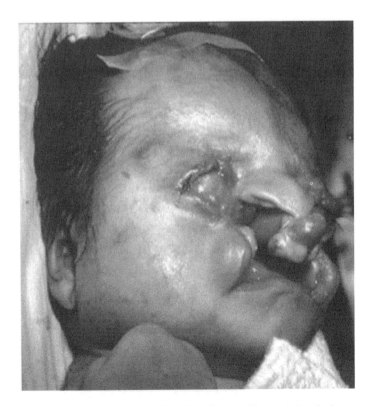

FIGURE 7.3   A newborn with facial clefts caused by amniotic adhesions.

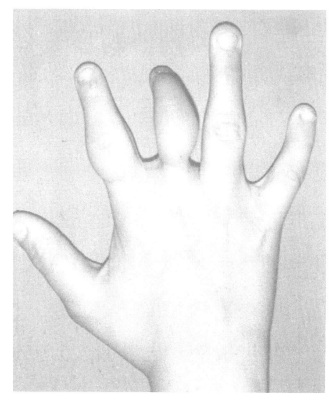

FIGURE 7.4   Ring-like constrictions in a patient with amnion rupture sequence.

IV. SEQUENCES AND ASSOCIATIONS

Sequences and *associations* are two additional categories of multiple anomaly disorders differentiated from syndromes because all of the anomalies cannot be traced back to a common etiological factor such as an abnormal chromosome, mutant gene, or teratogen. A sequence is the presence of multiple anomalies that can all be traced back to a single structural anomaly that interferes with subsequent development. In other words, a chromosomal, genetic, teratogenic, or extrinsic factor will cause some type of structural anomaly. The presence of that anomaly then has an adverse effect on the development of other structures or functions occurring from that time onward. The best known sequence is the Robin sequence, which was formerly known as Pierre Robin syndrome. In the case of Robin sequence, the one anomaly that gives rise to the others is micrognathia. The classical symptom triad associated with Robin sequence includes micrognathia, a wide U-shaped palatal cleft, and upper airway obstruction. In the developmental process of the palate, the palatal shelves are originally in a vertical position with the embryonic tongue sitting between them. As the mandible begins to grow, the tongue is free to descend from between the palatal shelves that then move into a horizontal position and begin to grow toward the midline for eventual fusion. If the tongue does not descend, the palatal shelves are prevented from migrating medially resulting in a cleft, most often U-shaped, because it reflects the shape of the intervening tongue. After birth, babies are obligate nose breathers and keep their mouths closed. With the mouth closed the tongue often drops back into the pharyngeal airway because it cannot move forward (glossoptosis), resulting in upper airway obstruction. Neither the cleft nor the airway obstruction would have occurred without the presence of the micrognathia. However, micrognathia has many possible causes. Micrognathia is a feature of many genetic syndromes, such as Stickler syndrome, spondiloepiphyseal dysplasia congenita, Treacher Collins syndrome, otopalatodigital syndrome, and diaphyseal dysplasia syndrome, to name only a few. Because micrognathia can also occur in chromosomal and teratogenic syndromes, it becomes obvious that micrognathia is etiologically heterogeneous. It should also be obvious that it is possible to have a syndrome and a sequence in the same patient. In other words, the syndromic feature of micrognathia can lead to Robin sequence. In fact, over a third of all Robin sequence cases are patients with Stickler syndrome, and 11% have velocardiofacial syndrome (Shprintzen, 1988; Shprintzen & Singer, 1992).

Associations are groupings of anomalies that have not been demonstrated to be a syndrome or sequence, but the patterns of anomalies are consistent even though the etiology is not known. A relatively common association that has clefting as a feature is CHARGE (coloboma, heart anomalies, atresia choanae, retarded growth and development, genital hypoplasia, and ear anomalies). VATER (vertebral defects, anal atresia, tracheoesophageal fistula, esophageal atresia, radial dysplasia) and VACTERL (vertebral anomalies, anal atresia, cardiac malformations, tracheoesophageal fistula, renal anomalies, and limb anomalies) are other well-recognized associations.

V. WHEN TO BE SUSPICIOUS

If multiple-anomaly syndromes are so common in patients with clefts, when should a clinician become suspicious? It is important to recognize that a child who has more than one major anomaly probably has a syndrome. The reason for this conclusion relates to the mathematical probability of two major anomalies occurring together in the same child by chance. For example, cleft lip and palate have been estimated to occur with a frequency of 1:750 live births. Congenital heart anomalies occur with a frequency of approximately 1:100 live births. What would be the expected frequency of a child being born with the combination of a congenital heart anomaly and cleft lip and palate? The probability is 1:75,000, which is 1:750×100. However, in actuality, children with clefts have a rather high frequency of having a heart anomaly. Several reports have placed the frequency of heart anomalies in patients with clefts at approximately 7% (Geis *et al.*, 1981; Shprintzen *et al.*, 1985a). This would place the actual frequency of clefting and heart anomalies at a minimum of 1:10,800. The discrepancy between an expected random association of 1:75,000 and the actual observation of 1:10,800 can be explained only if heart anomalies and clefting are usually related to a common cause. Furthermore, children who have clefts with heart anomalies also tend to have other malformations, which is additional evidence of the presence of multiple anomaly syndromes.

Clinicians should be aware that not all anomalies are easily detected, or even present at birth. For example, approximately 21% of children with velocardio-facial syndrome have a small or missing kidney on one side. Because people can function perfectly well on one kidney, unless specific tests, such as a renal ultrasound, are done, the anomaly may never be detected. Also, a feature of velocardiofacial syndrome is mental illness, which cannot be diagnosed until late childhood or early adult life. Therefore, the opportunity to observe syndromic effects may not be present at all times.

VI. THE PREDICTIVE POWER OF UNDERSTANDING CAUSATION

Does it make a difference if a cause for the presence of the cleft can be established? There are many benefits to establishing the primary etiology. Three factors that are of ultimate importance and that become evident with diagnosis are the *phenotypic spectrum*, the *natural history*, and the *prognosis* (Cohen, 1997). Diagnosis also leads to counseling for recurrence risk, some degree of predict-ability with regard to treatment outcomes, and a degree of comfort for the patient's family that the treating professionals are knowledgeable about the disorder that they are treating.

A syndrome's phenotypic spectrum refers to the anomalies that are known to occur in a particular disorder. Because not all anomalies are necessarily visible or detectable on physical examination, understanding the phenotypic spectrum allows the clinician to know where to search for possible problems and also how to triage the patient for comprehensive evaluation. For example, patients with Stickler syndrome frequently have a cleft palate, and high-frequency sensorineural hearing loss is found in 10 to 15%. The phenotypic spectrum also includes myopia and abnormalities of the epiphyses (the growth plates of the long bones) that may cause symptoms similar to arthritis. Although micrognathia and mild microstomia are common, most children with Stickler syndrome are attractive and develop-mentally normal (Figure 7.5). Therefore, the primary presentation of a child with Stickler syndrome is that of an otherwise normal child. However, knowing that

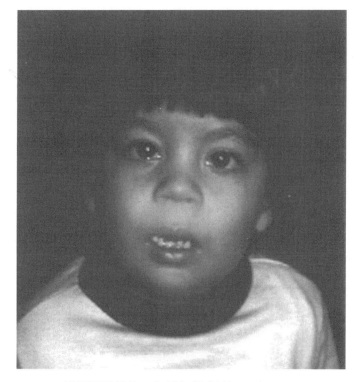

FIGURE 7.5   A child with Stickler syndrome.

both visual problems and joint abnormalities may be a part of the syndrome, the astute clinician will refer patients for ophthalmologic examination and radiographs of the ankles and knees to check for associated anomalies that might be a source of discomfort or dysfunction. Furthermore, because approximately a third of children with Robin sequence have Stickler syndrome, the diagnosis of Robin sequence in an infant should immediately alert the clinician to the strong likelihood that the baby may have Stickler syndrome, especially if there is no evidence of other major structural anomalies.

The natural history of a syndrome refers to the course of the disorder over time. There are many syndromes that have late-onset findings or distinctive growth patterns. Returning to Stickler syndrome, although babies with Stickler syndrome and Robin sequence often have severe micrognathia, they also have deficient maxillary growth. As a result, as they get older, the maxilla and mandible often become proportionate to each other even though both are deficient. Clinicians and researchers in the past, therefore, have often thought that the mandible shows "catch-up growth" in Robin sequence, even though the reality is that there is not so much "catch-up" of the mandible as there is "left behind" of the maxilla.

Another example of the power of understanding the natural history of the syndrome is the occurrence of both learning disabilities and mental illness in velocardiofacial syndrome. Learning disabilities occur with nearly 100% frequency in VCFS (Shprintzen & Goldberg, 1985) and bipolar disorder occurs with a greater than 80% frequency (Papolos *et al.*, 1996). Therefore, if a child with VCFS is seen prior to school age, the parents can be properly counseled about the probability of learning disabilities and the need to get special attention for the child before a pattern of school failure develops.

The final predictive component relates to a long-term prognosis. Understanding the certainty of outcome of some syndromes helps to guide treatment plans and make the expenditure of resources efficient. For example, though the early course of Beckwith–Wiedemann syndrome may be very precarious with omphalocele (herniation of the gut through the abdominal wall), severe hypotonia, macroglossia, possible upper airway obstruction, and hypoglycemia, the long-term prognosis is not as negative as the early presentation. Children with Beckwith–Wiedemann syndrome definitely benefit from all forms of therapy, including speech, physical, and occupational therapies. Their muscle tone tends to improve with age, and functioning is often normal or close to normal. Conversely, the prognosis in craniodiaphyseal dysplasia, a syndrome with severe bony overgrowth of the craniofacial structures, is that the disorder is progressive and irreversible, resulting in early death from cranial nerve compression and airway obstruction. The application of heroic craniofacial operations is futile because of the rapid progression of the disorder. There is a number of genetic syndromes with similar poor outcomes, including some of the lysosomal storage diseases (e.g., the mucopolysaccharidoses such as Hunter and Hurler syndromes), syndromes of premature aging (progeria and Werner syndrome), and syndromes with neurologic degeneration (Cockayne syndrome).

VII. INTEGRATION OF GENETICS INTO THE INTERDISCIPLINARY TEAM

Most interdisciplinary cleft palate and craniofacial teams are headed by individuals actively involved in the treatment of patients—such as surgeons, orthodontists, and speech pathologists—who may know little about genetics and the associated syndromes found in children with malformations of the head and neck. I have found that in most teams that involve geneticists in the evaluation of patients there is selective referral of cases, usually when there is a strong suspicion of the presence of a syndrome. In cases where the syndromic association is so obvious, the geneticist is probably needed the least. In other words, recognizing obvious syndromes with striking phenotypes, such as Treacher Collins syndrome or Apert syndrome, does not necessarily require the skill of a geneticist or dysmorphologist. However, there are hundreds of syndromes associated with clefting that have more subtle phenotypes that will not be recognized without careful pedigree analysis, physical examination, and knowledge of specific tests that can be applied when necessary. It is therefore suggested that geneticists should be the entry point for all patients into craniofacial and cleft palate centers.

As cited earlier, studies have shown that a very high percentage of children with clefts have associated malformations and syndromes (Rollnick & Pruzansky, 1981; Shprintzen et al., 1985a). With studies of major U.S. cleft palate centers showing that approximately 50% of patients have multiple anomaly disorders, what specialty is more relevant to the evaluation of patients with clefts than genetics?

In a discussion of the function of cleft and craniofacial teams, Shprintzen (1994) suggested that there are some inherent problems with the director of a team coming from a treatment-oriented discipline, such as plastic surgery or orthodontics. Specialists from treating disciplines may often steer the team toward biases that are discipline specific, but that may not necessarily be in the best interest of the patient. Proper patient management may benefit from having a "generalist," such as a geneticist, act as the team director (perhaps "referee" might be the best title), in order to take all possible diagnoses into account, as well as the natural history and prognosis. Therefore, it is suggested that perhaps the best person to make first and last contact with the patient is a geneticist: first contact for proper triage; last contact for proper counseling.

It is important for a clinical geneticist to be involved in assessing all patients seen at cleft centers. Because many anomalies are not necessarily present at birth or early in life, and because the natural history of many syndromes may reveal late onset findings, it is important that clinical geneticists have more than a single contact with a patient.

VIII. SYNDROMES COMMONLY SEEN IN CLEFT PALATE CENTERS

In studies of large populations at cleft palate centers where genetic services were applied to every patient, there have been some consistent findings that have major implications in terms of patient management. Rollnick and Pruzansky (1981) reviewed 2512 cases with clefts, Shprintzen et al. (1985a) examined 1000 consecutive cases with clefts, and Jones (1988) examined 428 consecutive cases with clefts. In all three studies, it was found that the highest rate of associated syndromes was found with cleft palate in the absence of cleft lip. In fact, patients with submucous clefts had the most frequent association with other anomalies and syndromes. The lowest frequency of associated anomalies was found for patients with cleft lip without cleft palate. Cleft palate without cleft lip was the most frequent cleft type seen in all three studies

According to Shprintzen et al. (1985a), several syndromes accounted for a high percentage of all cases seen in their study. Velocardiofacial syndrome, Stickler syndrome, and van der Woude syndrome accounted for approximately 13% of the total patient population at their center. Velocardiofacial syndrome accounted for 4.7% of the entire patient population and 8.1% of all patients with cleft palate without cleft lip (including submucous clefts). This finding was confirmed by Lipson *et al.* (1991), who reported that velocardiofacial syndrome accounted for approximately 5% of the patient population at their center in Sydney.

Robin sequence is a common diagnosis in many centers, and this should immediately prompt clinicians to suspect the probability that any of a number of common multiple anomaly syndromes may be at the root of the diagnosis. Shprintzen and Singer (1992) found that Stickler syndrome and velocardiofacial syndrome accounted for 45% of all Robin sequence cases (34 and 11%, respectively). Because of these common associations with Robin sequence, a handful of syndromes should be suspected immediately (Table 7.1).

TABLE 7.1   The Most Common Syndromes Associated with Robin Sequence in Descending Order of Frequency of Occurrence, with Indication of the Cause of Mandibular Abnormality, Excluding Chromosomal Syndromes

Syndrome	Reason for mandibular anomaly
Stickler syndrome	Micrognathia with shortening of ramus
Velocardiofacial syndrome	Retrognathia secondary to platybasia
Nonsyndromic Robin sequence	Positional deformation of mandible
Treacher Collins syndrome	Micrognathia with generalized mandibular hypoplasia of both body and ramus
Fetal alcohol syndrome	Micrognathia secondary to growth deficiency of mandibular body
Distal arthrogryposis	Retrognathia secondary to inability to manipulate mandible anteriorly
Freeman–Sheldon syndrome	Retrognathia secondary to inability to manipulate the mandible anteriorly
Spondyloepiphyseal dysplasia	Micrognathia with short ramus congenita syndrome
Diastrophic dysplasia syndrome	Micrognathia with short ramus
Popliteal pterygium syndrome	Retrognathia secondary to inability to manipulate the mandible anteriorly
Beckwith–Wiedemann syndrome	Mandible large, but macroglossia causes sequence
Amnion rupture sequence	Amniotic adhesions
Femoral dysgenesis syndrome	Micrognathia secondary to short ramus
Nager syndrome	Severe generalized mandibular hypoplasia

Sometimes, key anomalies can narrow the search for associated syndromes. For example, the presence of conotruncal heart anomalies provides a strong suspicion of the diagnosis of velocardiofacial syndrome, whereas severe myopia would strongly indicate Stickler syndrome. Limb anomalies—such as contractures, webbing of the neck, pigmentary anomalies, and other key findings—may help to provide necessary cues to the astute clinician so that proper triage and diagnosis can proceed. Table 7.2 lists some of the more common syndromes seen in cleft palate centers, including the associated anomalies that would be solid clues.

IX. DOES IT REALLY MAKE A DIFFERENCE?

Clinicians have been searching consistently for mechanisms to maximize treatment for their patients. To date, the emphasis has clearly been on the treatments themselves, with less emphasis on the amount of diagnostic rigor applied to the decision-making process. This is why the literature is filled with reports of success rates with operations like pharyngeal flaps or sphincter pharyngoplasties, or the effects of a particular operation on facial growth or dental occlusion. Very few investigations of this type have accounted for variations in anatomy or physiology that might be caused by syndromic effects. For example, among syndromes that have cleft lip and palate as a common feature, there is a number that essentially always shows maxillary growth deficiency, including Binder syndrome, popliteal pterygium syndrome, Bixler syndrome, and Rapp–Hodgkin syndrome. With or without repair of the cleft, patients with these syndromes will always have hypoplasia of the maxilla.

A single syndromic example will illustrate the importance of correct diagnosis. One of the most common manifestations of velocardiofacial syndrome is velopharyngeal insufficiency (VPI). There are multiple contributions to VPI in VCFS, including cleft palate (overt, submucous, or occult submucous cleft), congenital hypoplasia or aplasia of the adenoid, obtuse cranial base angle which increases pharyngeal volume), and pharyngeal hypotonia (Arvystas & Shprintzen, 1984; Shprintzen, 1982; Shprintzen et al., 1978). Because the VPI in this common syndrome is not as simple as the anatomic anomaly caused by the cleft, the treatment issues become much more complicated. Due to the unusual anatomic and physiologic problems associated with VCFS, the degree of hypernasality is almost always severe, even if the velopharyngeal gap tends to be relatively small. Experience has shown that the velopharyngeal valve must be nearly obstructed by a pharyngeal flap or surgical outcomes are almost always poor in VCFS. However, complicating matters is the medial deviation of the internal carotid arteries with ectopic placement (Mitnick et al., 1996). Depending on the placement of incisions in the posterior pharyngeal wall, there is a risk of severing the internal carotid artery, which would result in a potentially fatal surgical complication (MacKenzie-Stepner et al., 1987; Mitnick et al., 1996). Without the knowl-

TABLE 7.2   Some of the More Common Syndromes Seen in Cleft Palate Centers along with the Most Common Associated Features and Etiology

Amnion rupture sequence (amniotic adhesions)
Facial clefts, digit amputations, ring-like constrictions on limbs, possible cranial defects

Apert syndrome (autosomal dominant, mutation in FGFR2 gene at 10q26)
Craniosynostosis, syndactyly, hydrocephalus, cognitive impairment, airway obstruction, cleft palate

Beckwith–Wiedemann syndrome (autosomal dominant, IGF2 gene at 11p15.5)
Large at birth, mandibular prognathism, omphalocele or umbilical hernias, hypotonia, possible cognitive impairment, accelerated growth, macroglossia, creases in ear lobes, inguinal hernias, occasional heart anomalies, occasional hypoglycemia

Cleidocranial dysplasia syndrome (autosomal dominant, deletion at 6p21)
Absent or hypoplastic clavicles, delayed closure of cranial sutures, broad forehead, late dental eruption, finger anomalies, delayed mineralization of pubic symphysis, occasional osteosclerosis, hearing loss, cleft palate

de Lange syndrome (3q25.1–26.2 trisomy)
Short stature, cognitive impairment, limb reduction (arms), digital anomalies, coarse facies, synophrys, microcephaly, irritability, seizures, hypertonia, lack of facial expression, cleft palate, low anterior hairline, long eye lashes, anomalous auricles, hirsute ears, short neck, somatic hirsutism, renal anomalies, multiple hernias, pyloric stenosis, intestinal anomalies, cardiac malformations, micrognathia, Robin sequence possible

EEC syndrome (autosomal dominant, gene mapped to 7q11.2–q21.3)
Cleft palate, cleft lip, ectrodactyly, absent or hypoplastic nails, syndactyly, sparse hair, decreased pigmentation of the hair and skin, absent punctae in lower eye lids, missing or abnormal teeth, enamel hypoplasia, photophobia, occasional cognitive impairment, occasional kidney anomalies

Fetal alcohol syndrome (maternal ingestion of alcohol during pregnancy)
Cognitive impairment, low birth weight, microcephaly, short palpebral fissures, heart anomalies, short nose, flat philtrum, cleft palate, cleft lip, digital anomalies, joint abnormalities

Fetal hydantoin syndrome (maternal exposure to hydantoin)
Cognitive impairment, growth deficiency, cleft palate, cleft lip, short nose, flat philtrum, hypoplastic distal phalanges and nails of hands and feet, low anterior hair line, cardiac anomalies, genital anomalies

Freeman–Sheldon syndrome (autosomal dominant, gene mapped to 11p15.5)
"Whistling face" appearance, keel-shaped forehead, micrognathia, limited oral opening, ulnar deviation of fingers, multiple joint contractures, relatively short stature, cleft palate, Robin sequence, occasional cognitive impairment

Hay-Wells syndrome (autosomal dominant)
Attachment of upper and lower eyelids at the lateral margins, hypodontia or anodontia, absent or severely hypoplastic finger nails, sparse or absent scalp hair, midface deficiency, cleft palate, hypohidrotic ectodermal dysplasia

Holoprosencephaly (etiologically heterogenous)
Brain anomalies ranging from incomplete septation of the brain, absence of olfactory bulbs and tracts, hypotelorism (cyclopia in most severe form), microcephaly, anosmia, cognitive impairment, nasal anomalies, heart anomalies, single central incisor, cleft lip, cleft palate

Kabuki make-up syndrome, or Niikawa–Kuroki syndrome (unknown etiology)
Cognitive impairment, wide palpebral fissures showing some conjunctiva at outer canthus, protuberant large ears, positioned eyebrows, short stature, cleft lip, cleft palate, scoliosis, short fifth fingers, heart anomalies, hip dislocation

Kallmann syndrome (etiologically heterogenous)
Hypogonadism, anosmia, cleft lip, cleft palate, hearing loss

continued

TABLE 7.2 CONTINUED

Nager syndrome (autosomal recessive)
Severe micrognathia, cleft or absent palate, absent or hypoplastic thumbs, radial anomalies, external and middle ear anomalies

Noonan syndrome (autosomal dominant, mapped to 12q22)
Small stature, cognitive impairment, low posterior hair line, webbed neck, pectus excavatum or carinatum, pulmonary stenosis, vertebral anomalies, hypoplastic male genitals, ptosis, down-slanting eyes, vertical maxillary excess, occasional cleft palate (often submucous), hearing loss

Oculo-auriculo-vertebral sequence (etiologically heterogenous)
Facial asymmetry, spine anomalies, microtia, asymmetry of tongue motion, ocular anomalies, dermoid cysts, hearing loss, cleft palate, cleft lip, facial paresis, occasional cognitive deficiency, occasional kidney anomalies, occasional heart anomalies; sensorineural loss of hearing, occasional limb anomalies

Opitz syndrome (X-linked recessive, mapped to Xp22)
Hypertelorism, hypospadias, cryptorchidism, cognitive impairment, hernias, cleft larynx, heart anomalies, cleft palate and/or cleft lip, anal anomalies, renal anomalies

Otopalatodigital syndrome (X-linked recessive, mapped to Xq28)
Prominent superior orbital ridge, hypertelorism, downslanting eyes, cognitive deficiency, small stature, abnormal digits with curvature, cleft palate, Robin sequence, micrognathia

Popliteal pterygium syndrome (autosomal dominant)
Cleft palate and/or cleft lip, webbing of the space behind the knees (popliteal space), dysplastic toenails, external genital anomalies, lower lip pits

Rapp–Hodgkin syndrome (autosomal dominant)
Ectodermal dysplasia, cleft lip, cleft palate, hypohidrosis, sparse hair, hypoplastic or absent nails, missing and abnormal teeth, maxillary deficiency, hypospadias

Robinow syndrome (autosomal dominant)
Frontal bossing, hypertelorism, wide palpebral fissures, short nose, macrocephaly, cleft palate, cleft lip, progressive osteosclerosis of skull, shortening of the arms, brachydactyly, clinodactyly, vertebral anomalies, skeletal anomalies, small penis, cryptorchidism, minor female genital anomalies

Stickler syndrome (autosomal dominant, collagen 2 gene, long arm of chromosome 12)
Round face, micrognathia, maxillary deficiency, cleft palate, Robin sequence, myopia, vitreoretinal degeneration, joint laxity, epiphyseal dysplasia, talipes equinovarus

Townes–Brocks syndrome (autosomal dominant, deletion at 16q12.1–16q13)
Facial asymmetry, ear tags and pits, microtia, severe commissural cleft, digital anomalies, radial anomalies, anal anomalies, renal anomalies, hearing loss

Treacher Collins syndrome (autosomal dominant, Treacle gene, long arm of chromosome 5)
Micrognathia, absent or hypoplastic zygomas, defects of lower eye lids, absent lashes of inner two-thirds of lower eye lids, malar clefts, cleft palate, Robin sequence, cleft lip (uncommon), microtia, ossicular malformation, airway obstruction, choanal atresia, conductive hearing loss

Turner syndrome (deletion of one entire X chromosome)
Short stature, webbed neck, short neck, low posterior hair line, lack of sexual development, shield-shaped chest, heart anomalies, renal anomalies, small nails, osteoporosis, pigmented nevi, occasional cleft palate, occasional cognitive impairment

Van der Woude syndrome (autosomal dominant, gene on long arm of chromosome 1)
Cleft palate, cleft lip, pits or mounds of the lower lip, congenitally missing teeth

Velocardiofacial syndrome (autosomal dominant, 22q11 deletion)
Cleft palate, heart anomalies, facies characterized by a long nose with bulbous or dimpled tip and prominent root, puffy upper eyelids, allergic shiners, small ears with attached lobules and overfolded helices, learning disabilities, ADHD, eventual mental illness, scoliosis, hypocalcemia, immune deficiency, vascular anomalies, kidney anomalies, feeding difficulties, hypotonia

edge of the special circumstances associated with VCFS that cause VPI, treatment might not only be unsuccessful but may be potentially dangerous. Because VCFS was found to constitute 8.1% of the clinical population with cleft palate without cleft lip (Shprintzen *et al.*, 1985a), this "special" consideration is hardly very special.

X. HAS THERE BEEN AN EFFECT ON RESEARCH?

There has been an enormous amount of clinical research done over the past five decades in the area of cleft palate and craniofacial disorders focusing on language impairment, intellect, social skills, academic achievement, and many other components of human behavior. The large majority of these studies has admitted patients based on the presence of a cleft, but it is the rare study (prior to the past few years) that has excluded subjects based on the presence of a genetic or syndromic diagnosis. As stated above, velocardiofacial syndrome constitutes over 8% of patients with clefting of the secondary palate. In any study assessing behavioral parameters of children with cleft palate (such as language, intellect, and social skills), if 8% of the sample is children with VCFS, then the study data will be skewed sufficiently away from the norm to provide data that will show a significant difference. However, the lower scores in the "cleft" sample may have nothing to do with the cleft, but may have everything to do with VCFS. Many other syndromes that constitute the population of children with cleft palate also show cognitive or language impairments and may represent over half of all children with cleft palate. One of the key problems with clinical research is the need to keep study populations as homogenous as possible (Shprintzen, 1991). Otherwise, the source of variability of obtained data must be suspect.

XI. CONCLUSION

In summary, cleft palate or cleft lip and palate are not always isolated anomalies. In fact, more often than not, clefting represents a symptom of a more complicated disorder of maldevelopment. Ignoring this fact does not enhance patient care and may severely impair it.

REFERENCES

Arvystas, M., & Shprintzen, R. J. (1984). Craniofacial morphology in the velo-cardio-facial syndrome. *Journal of Craniofacial Genetics and Developmental Biology*, *4*, 39–45.
Biancalana, V., Le Marec, B., Odent, S., van den Hurk, J. A. M. J., & Hanauer, A. (1991). Oto-palato-digital syndrome type I: Further evidence for assignment of the locus to Xq28. *Human Genetics*, *88*, 228–230.

Cohen Jr., M. M. (1997). *The child with multiple birth defects*. New York: Oxford University Press.

Fraser F. C. (1970). The genetics of cleft lip and cleft palate. *American Journal of Human Genetics, 22*, 336–352.

Geis, N., Seto. B., Bartoshesky. L., Lewis, M. B., & Pashayan, H. M. (1981). The prevalence of congenital heart disease among the population of a metropolitan cleft lip and palate clinic. *Cleft Palate Journal, 18*, 19–23.

Jabs, E. W., Li, X., Coss, C. A., Taylor, E. W., Meyers, D. A., & Weber, J. L. (1991). Mapping the Treacher Collins syndrome locus to 5q31.3–q33.3. *Genomics, 11*, 193–198.

Jones, M. C. (1988). Etiology of facial clefts: Prospective evaluation of 428 patients. *Cleft Palate Journal, 25*, 16–20.

Lipson, A. H., Yuille, D., Angel, M., Thompson, P. G., Vanderwoord, J. G., & Beckenham, E. J. (1991). Velo-cardio-facial syndrome: An important syndrome for the dysmorphologist to recognize. *Journal of Medical Genetics, 28*, 596–604.

MacKenzie-Stepner, K., Witzel, M. A., Stringer, D. A., Lindsay, W. K., Munro, I. R., & Hughes, H. (1987). Abnormal carotid arteries in Velocardiofacial syndrome: A report of three cases. *Plastic and Reconstructive Surgery, 80*, 347–351.

Mitnick, R. J., Bello, J. A., Golding-Kushner, K. J., Argamaso, R. V., & Shprintzen, R. J. (1996). The use of magnetic resonance angiography prior to pharyngeal flap surgery in patients with velo-cardio-facial syndrome. *Plastic and Reconstructive Surgery, 97*, 908–919.

Murray, J. C., Nishimura, D. Y., Buetow, K. H., Ardinger, H. H., Spence, M. A., Sparkes, R. S., Falk, R. E., Falk, P. M., Gardner, R. J. M., Harkness, E. M., Glinski, L. P., Pauli, R. M., Nakamura, Y., Green, P. P., & Schinzel, A. (1990). Linkage of an autosomal dominant clefting syndrome (van der Woude) to loci on chromosome 1q. *American Journal of Human Genetics, 46*, 486–491.

Papolos, D. F., Faedda, G. L., Veit, S., Goldberg, R., Morrow, B., Kucherlapati, R., & Shprintzen, R. J. (1996). Bipolar spectrum disorders in patients diagnosed with velo-cardio-facial syndrome: Does a hemizygous deletion of chromosome 22q11 result in bipolar affective disorder? *American Journal of Psychiatry, 153*, 1541–1547.

Rollnick, B. R., & Pruzansky, S. (1981). Genetic services at a center for craniofacial anomalies. *Cleft Palate Journal, 18*, 304–313.

Shprintzen, R. J. (1982). Palatal and pharyngeal anomalies in craniofacial syndromes. *Birth Defects Original Articles Series, 18*(1), 53–78.

Shprintzen, R. J. (1988). Pierre Robin, micrognathia, and airway obstruction: The dependency of treatment on accurate diagnosis. *International Anesthesiology Clinics, 26*, 84–91.

Shprintzen, R. J. (1991). The fallibility of clinical research. *Cleft Palate Journal, 28*, 136–140.

Shprintzen, R. J. (1994). A new perspective on clefting. In R. J. Shprintzen & J. Bardach (Eds.), *Cleft palate speech management: A multidisciplinary approach* (pp. 1–15). St. Louis: Mosby.

Shprintzen, R. J., & Goldberg, R. B. (1985). Multiple anomaly syndromes and learning disabilities. In S. Smith (Ed.), *Genetics and learning disabilities* (pp. 153–174). San Diego: College Hill Press.

Shprintzen, R. J., & Singer, L. (1992). Upper airway obstruction and the Robin sequence. *International Anesthesiology Clinics, 30*, 109–114.

Shprintzen, R. J., Goldberg, R. B., Lewin, M. L., Sidoti, E. J., Berkman, M. D., Argamaso, R. V., & Young, D. (1978). A new syndrome involving cleft palate, cardiac anomalies, typical facies, and learning disabilities: Velo-cardio-facial syndrome. *Cleft Palate Journal, 15*, 56–62.

Shprintzen, R. J., Siegel-Sadewitz, V. L., Amato, J., & Goldberg, R. B. (1985a). Anomalies associated with cleft lip, cleft palate, or both. *American Journal of Medical Genetics, 20*, 585–596.

Shprintzen, R. J., Siegel-Sadewitz, V. L., Amato, J., & Goldberg, R. B. (1985b). Retrospective diagnoses of previously missed syndromic disorders amongst 1,000 patients with cleft lip, cleft palate, or both. *Birth Defects Original Article Series, 21*(2), 85–92.

8

STUTTERING AND GENETICS

OUR PAST AND OUR FUTURE

SUSAN FELSENFELD

Department of Speech–Language Pathology
Duquesne University
Pittsburgh, Pennsylvania

DENNIS DRAYNA

National Institute on Deafness
and Other Communicative Disorders
Rockville, Maryland

The Handbook of Genetic Communicative
Disorders

I. INTRODUCTION

When we consider the future for research investigating the genetics of stutter-ing, one thing is certain: there is no turning back. Molecular genetic technology will continue to grow, potentially at an exponential rate, and these advances will soon be brought to bear on the disorder of stuttering. The descriptive work that is the essential foundation for molecular genetics research has been in process for over 70 years. In the present chapter, we begin by summarizing this descriptive (behavioral) genetics research, beginning with some of the very early twin and family studies of stuttering. Rather than attempting to review this literature com-prehensively, we have chosen to highlight representative and/or particularly in-fluential behavioral genetics papers that have been published during the twentieth century. (For more comprehensive reviews of this literature, both current and historical, the reader is directed to Felsenfeld, 1996, 1997; Kidd, 1984; Ludlow, 1999; Pauls, 1990; Sheehan & Costley, 1977; Yairi et al., 1996.) Following this, we discuss current approaches to studying the role of genetics in the pathogenesis of stuttering. Our particular focus in this section is to provide a brief overview of the research methodologies of gene linkage and gene association, complex and elegant procedures that are at the forefront of stuttering genetics work at the present time. Finally, we end the chapter with a discussion of the ethical and social questions that our field will be required to address if and when "major stuttering genes" are found. Although the technology of gene finding is truly dazzling and can easily garner all of our attention, it is important that we begin to address the complex issues that will ensue when genetic science comes face to face with stuttering-affected families.

II. STUTTERING AND GENETICS: AN ABRIDGED HISTORICAL TIMELINE

A. 1930 TO 1950

Astute observers of the disorder of stuttering recognized its familial nature well before the birth of behavioral and molecular genetics as formal disciplines. Al-though it is not clear who is to be credited with the "first ever" published mention of the familial nature of stuttering, there are several empirical reports of this phenomenon in the American speech pathology literature beginning in the 1930s (e.g., Nelson, 1939), which is where our timeline begins.

In 1939, West, Nelson, and Berry published a large family study of stuttering. In it, they reported on the "family lines" of 204 stuttering probands (*propositi*) and compared these extended family pedigrees with those of 204 age- and gen-der-matched nonstuttering individuals, a sample size that is robust even by modern standards. Informant interviews were used to determine if any relatives had ever had problems with stuttering. When the number of affected relatives found in the pedigrees of the propositi were compared with those found in the control pedigrees, it became apparent that the relatives of stuttering propositi was considerably more likely to stutter, by a ratio of about 6 to 1. While favoring a biological (genetic) interpretation of their findings, West and his colleagues were careful to note that "strong precipitating factors" in the environment could theoretically cause stuttering to appear in cases where hereditary liability was minimal. Interestingly, West and colleagues expressed concern about the appropriate way to classify certain relatives in the pedigree, such as those who were reported to have "recovered" from stuttering. These same classification issues continue to plague genetics researchers today.

Wepman, also in 1939, published a family study that essentially replicated the principal findings of the West *et al.* (1939) investigation. Wepman identified 250 "stammerers" from clinics and schools in Chicago and Indiana, and paired these cases with "a like group of (250) nonstammerers" (p. 207). Wepman personally interviewed a key informant from each of these 500 families, and from these he constructed pedigrees showing the "position, age, and sex of each stammerer" (p. 207). The results of this investigation were remarkably similar to those reported in the West *et al.* study; once again, the proportion of stutterers found in the families of stuttering cases exceeded those found in the control families by a ratio of 6:1. In further describing the extent of familial aggregation of this disorder, Wepman observed that 69% (172/250) of the proband families had at least one stuttering-affected family member in addition to the proband subject (in modern parlance, they were family history positive). This was compared with the rather low percentage of control families who reported "some incidence of stammering" in the family background (39/250 or 16%). Like West and his colleagues, Wepman concluded that stuttering appeared to be inherited (biologically) in some families, although he too declined to take a "dogmatic stand" (p. 209) on the biological versus social origin of the observed familial aggregation for this disorder.

In 1945, Nelson, Hunter, and Walter completed a twin study of stuttering that was quite sophisticated in method for its day. Unlike earlier twin studies that had failed to differentiate clearly between identical (monozygotic, MZ) and fraternal (dizygotic, DZ) twins, these investigators understood that this distinction—specifically, the difference in concordance between these twin types—was critical for determining a trait's heritability. In this study, 200 complete twin pairs (69 MZ and 131 DZ pairs) between the ages of 4 and 40 years of age were evaluated. The twins were recruited without reference to speech status, that is, they were not selected because one or both members were known to stutter. Each twin was examined in the home to obtain evidence of their "similarities and speech habits" (p. 337). Although, by modern standards, the methods used to establish zygosity (twin type) in this study were crude, a serious attempt was made to classify twins appropriately. Somewhat unexpectedly, the prevalence of stuttering in this "unselected" twin sample was quite high: 20% of the 200 twin pairs were found to contain at least one stuttering member. This high rate of occurrence suggests either that the frequency of stuttering is significantly higher among twins than among singletons or, more likely, that the ascertainment of twins in fact was biased in favor of those who were speech-affected.

Concordance for stuttering was found to differ considerably as a function of zygosity. Of the 10 monozygotic pairs containing at least one stutterer, 9 were found to be concordant for the disorder (90%). In contrast, of the 30 dizygotic pairs containing a stuttering member, only 2 were judged to be concordant for stuttering (7%). Because appropriate methodological safeguards were not employed in the Nelson *et al.* (1945) study, these concordance values should be viewed with caution.

This large MZ–DZ difference was interpreted as evidence that heredity (or "germ plasm," to use their term) was important in conferring risk for stuttering. However, as was the case for the family studies of this period, alternative (social) explanations for the findings were explored by Nelson and her colleagues. Among the more creative such attempts was their suggestion that the higher concordance rates found for the MZ twins might be due to a form of "telepathic identity" that identical twins were thought to share (p. 342). Thus, as with previous inheritance studies of this era, these investigators were willing to consider both biological and social transmission hypotheses to explain their results, with clear bias in favor of biological explanations.

Also published during this time was a pedigree study that came to symbolize the growing anti-biological movement within the stuttering research community. Performed in 1940 by Marcella Gray, under the direction of Wendell Johnson, the pedigree study of the "X family" remains the most widely cited genetic study of the era. In contrast to the larger genetic studies being performed at the time, the study by Gray focused on a single, large (five-generation) pedigree that tracked two branches of the descendants of a female stutterer. One branch (the "Iowa" branch) was studied in more detail. This branch was significantly larger in size than the "Kansas" branch to which it was compared. There were 31 direct descendants about whom speech data were available in Generations 4 and 5 of the Iowa branch, in comparison to 17 descendants in the Kansas branch, a ratio of nearly 2:1. This size disparity appeared to arise from two sources: a smaller family size among the Kansas families and what appears to be a significant amount of missing or unknown data in this group. In comparison to the Iowans, many of whom were interviewed directly, speech information about the Kansas branch was obtained "in the course of interviews with members of the Iowa branch and by correspondence with members of the family who live(d) in Kansas" (p. 343).

When speech outcomes in these two branches were compared, the larger Iowa branch was found to contain a higher proportion of current or former stutterers in Generations 4 and 5 (11/31 direct descendants) than was found in the Kansas branch (1/17 direct descendants). What remains most notable about this study is its strong and somewhat unorthodox interpretation. In discussing her finding, Gray rejected a "sheer hereditarian hypothesis" (p. 345) to account for the differences in stuttering frequency found between the branches. Instead, relying on retrospective and anecdotal reports from the Iowa branch, she concluded that it was likely that the two branches had developed a different "semantic environment" with respect to speech and stuttering. Specifically, she concluded that members of the stuttering-dense Iowa branch were particularly "stuttering conscious," perhaps as the result of the strong influence of one powerful Iowan in Generation 4 who was himself a severe stutterer.

By modern standards, the incomplete and unsystematic ascertainment of descendants and the uncertain diagnostic procedures used in Gray's study render it little more than anecdotal. In this regard, it is like another infamous pedigree study—referred to as the Kallikak study—that was published by Goddard in 1914 (cited in Garrett, 1961). This investigation tracked the numerous descendants of Martin Kallikak, a busy gentleman who sired children with two women. One line was descended from "the dalliance of Martin Kallikak and a feeble minded tavern girl." This union was reported to have resulted in "hundreds of descendants of the lowest types of human beings." As a group, they represented a "dreary picture of shiftlessness, depravity, crime, and social worthlessness" (Garrett, p. 55). In contrast, the descendants of his wife ("a worthy Quakeress") produced "hundreds of the highest types of human beings," including "governors, college presidents, lawyers, physicians, teachers, and business men."

What is particularly amusing in the present context is Goddard's interpretation of his results. Being a hereditarian, he naturally concluded that the outcome differences between the two branches of this family were the result of differences in inheritance that could be traced back to Kallikak's two genetically dissimilar paramours! Apparently, it did not occur to Goddard that the descendants of the "feeble-minded tavern girl" were likely to experience economic and social disadvantage that would almost certainly have impeded their educational and vocational opportunities. Of course, such a simplistic interpretation for a complex phenomenon—whether social or biological in its bias—is currently considered quaint at best. In like manner, our field's "X family" study should be viewed as having historical interest but limited scientific credibility by professionals in the modern era.

B. 1950 TO 1970

In comparison to the previous two decades, the 1950s and 1960s may be considered the "quiet" era for studies examining the genetics of stuttering. Although the reasons for this are not entirely clear, it is likely that biologically oriented research, in general, fell out of favor during this period, because it was philosophically incompatible with Wendell Johnson's very influential environmentalist (diagnosogenic) theory of stuttering etiology. It is ironic, therefore, that one of the few notable family studies of stuttering to be performed during this era was completed by Johnson himself (Johnson et al., 1959). As part of a larger descriptive study investigating the onset of stuttering, Johnson and his colleagues obtained information about speech history from 150 families with "allegedly stuttering children" and 150 matched control families with "allegedly nonstuttering children." Results revealed that about 6% of the control parents reported a positive family history of stuttering, in comparison to 23% of the parents of the "allegedly stuttering children" (nearly a fourfold increase in the latter group). Although Johnson and his colleagues did not dispute this finding—they acknowledged that stuttering indeed appeared more often among the relatives of the "allegedly stuttering children"—the interpretation of this finding reflected their anti-hereditarian beliefs, as illustrated in the following quote:

> There are two main reasons, of course, why characteristics run in families. One is biological, genetic, hereditary in a physical sense of the word. . . . The other reason is social— customs, tradition, training. . . . The reason why stuttering tends to run in families seems to be rather definitely a matter of tradition rather than genes. . . . What runs in families (in those cases in which something seems to) appears to be a background of experience with stuttering and therefore a kind of concern, a set of attitudes and a tendency to deal in certain ways with children who are just learning to talk, and with the normal imperfections in their speech (p. 70).

During this same time, Gavin Andrews and Mary Harris were performing a seminal epidemiological investigation of stuttering in Newcastle-upon-Tyne, England (Andrews & Harris, 1964). As part of this investigation, family history information was obtained via interviews and questionnaires from the families of 213 stuttering cases (probands) derived from three nonoverlapping samples, a school-based sample of 9- to 11-year-old stuttering children ($N = 78$) and two clinic-based groups, Group A and Group B. Clinic Group A consisted of 83 children (mean age of 6 years) who were seen for stuttering therapy at a university clinic during a 3-year period. Clinic Group B had 52 cases (mean age of 20 years) that consisted of "all of the adolescent and adult stutterers under treatment at the [university] Clinic during 1963" (p. 133).

In comparison to earlier family studies of stuttering, the Newcastle study was considerably more sophisticated. Rather than simply reporting the proportion of families that had stuttering members other than the proband case, this investigation reported stuttering risk separately (by relative type) for first-degree family members (e.g., the differential risk to brothers versus sisters of stuttering probands). In addition, this study included an analysis of risk to relatives as a function of proband gender; indeed, the observation that stuttering rates are slightly elevated in families containing a *female* proband was first reported here. Collapsing across subject samples and proband gender, the results of the Newcastle study indicated that approximately 13% of the first-degree relatives of a proband case were also stuttering-affected (13% of parents and 14% of siblings). Comparable data from control families were not reported; instead, these values were compared with previously published population prevalence rates for stuttering in childhood and adolescence (about 3%). Stuttering liability was not equivalent for the two sexes in the Newcastle samples. Not surprisingly, more male relatives (fathers and brothers) than female relatives (mothers and sisters) were found to stutter (19 versus 7%, respectively). Perhaps more interestingly, as noted earlier, there was a slight but significant differential risk to family members as a function of the gender of the proband. The risk of stuttering among the relatives (parents and siblings) of female probands was significantly higher than the risk among relatives of male probands (20 versus 12%, respectively). (This particular finding has not been replicated universally; cf. Ambrose *et al.*, 1993.)

Unlike prior family studies, the Newcastle investigators engaged in frank genetic hypothesis testing, speculating about modes of genetic transmission that appeared to be most compatible with their data. After examining the pattern of transmission across families, they concluded "transmission by a common dominant gene with a multifactorial background appear(ed) to be a reasonable hypothesis" (p. 143). The potential importance of nongenetic factors was also acknowledged by these investigators, who wrote, quite reasonably, "Genetic inheritance, whether single gene or polygenic, does not by any means rule out the possibility that other, nongenetic, causes may also be at work; indeed, a complex and varying disorder of function, such as stuttering, is *a priori* likely to be the result of a number of converging forces" (p. 139).

C. 1970 TO 1990

Compared to the previous two decades, genetics research experienced a renaissance during the 1970s and 1980s, in large part due to the efforts of one human geneticist from Yale University and his colleagues. The Yale group, led by Kenneth Kidd, published thirteen papers on the topic of stuttering and genetics between 1977 and 1984. (These are collectively referred to as the Yale Family Study series.) Building upon the methodological progress begun by Andrews and Harris in the Newcastle Study, the Yale Family Study brought genetics research into the modern era regarding stuttering. One important advance was the study team itself, which included quantitative (behavioral) geneticists, molecular biologists, and speech–language pathologists. It is now well understood that genetics research investigating complex phenotypes requires the expertise of scientists in many disciplines. For stuttering, the Yale series represents the birth of this collaborative effort.

By the time the final review papers summarizing the study results were published (Kidd, 1983, 1984), the Yale project had obtained speech history information from approximately 600 adolescent and adult stutterers of European descent and slightly more than 2000 of their first-degree relatives. Most of the proband subjects were referred to the investigators by speech–language pathologists, who were responsible for diagnosing the cases as stuttering-affected. Approximately half of the proband subjects were interviewed to confirm the diagnosis, and half completed self-report questionnaires. Unlike the proband cases, a diagnosis of stuttering among the first-degree relatives did not require verification by a speech–language pathologist. Instead, relatives were classified as "stuttering-affected" through a variety of mechanisms, most typically via informant (proband) report.

While recognizing that direct interview of relatives would have been a preferable diagnostic strategy, the Yale investigators defended their decision by noting that "any error in incidence figures introduced because of failure to directly interview all relatives is considered small and, if present, would only elevate the frequency of stuttering in the relatives" (Kidd, 1983, p. 199). (See Pauls [1990] for a critique of this aspect of the Yale Family Study design.)

The stuttering frequencies found among the relatives of the proband cases in the Yale Family Study were quite similar to those reported for relatives in the earlier Newcastle investigation performed by Andrews and Harris in 1964. Collapsing across proband gender, the results of the Yale study revealed that approximately 16% of the first-degree relatives of a proband case were also stuttering-affected: 13% of parents, 14% of siblings, and 21% of offspring (Kidd, 1983). In addition, as had Andrews and Harris, Kidd (1983) found the risk of stuttering among the first-degree relatives of female probands to be higher than the risk among relatives of male probands (20 versus 13%, respectively). Compared to population prevalence rates for stuttering, Kidd concluded that the stuttering frequencies found among the proband relatives in his studies were significantly elevated, providing additional support for the observation that stuttering aggregates within biological families.

More than any previous genetic study of stuttering, the Yale series illustrated the power and breadth of the family study design, and this is arguably one of its greatest achievements. One example of this attention to phenotypic detail is reflected in two papers published in 1983 that addressed the phenomenon of stuttering recovery (Cox & Kidd, 1983; Seider et al., 1983). In most prior genetic studies of stuttering, persistent and recovered cases were not well differentiated, although, as noted earlier, the problem of classifying recovered cases was recognized for some time. Kidd and colleagues used their rich data set to study this phenomenon, and, in so doing, provided future researchers with a model for including epidemiological questions into a behavioral genetics design for this disorder. What emerged from their analysis of recovery continues to intrigue researchers today. Among the first-degree relatives of persistent adult probands, the investigators found that between 45 and 51% of those who had "ever stuttered" had reportedly recovered. Female relatives were significantly more likely to report recovery (66%) than were male relatives (46%), and they were also more likely to report that they began stuttering at an earlier age and recovered at an earlier age, on average (12;0 years for males and 9;3 years for females).

One of the primary objectives of the Yale Family Study was to test competing hypotheses about the transmission of stuttering using state-of-the-art segregation analyses programs. A complementary objective appeared to be to provide readers with basic information about genetic modeling. Over a 10-year period, Kidd and his colleagues authored six tutorial papers that discussed model-fitting and its interpretation (Cox, 1988; Kidd, 1977, 1980, 1983, 1984; Kidd et al., 1978). In 1984, Cox, Kramer, and Kidd published the first, and still largest, segregation analysis of this disorder (Cox *et al.*, 1984a). Compared to previous family studies that (by necessity) had merely speculated about the most likely mode of transmission for stuttering, the Cox *et al.* investigation used specialized segregation programs to actually test competing transmission models. To do so, the pedigree data from 386 adult probands and their first-degree relatives from the Yale Study were entered into two segregation programs (POINTER and PAP). Results from both programs were consistent and indicated that the best-fitting model was one in which stuttering was transmitted as a multifactorial-polygenic condition (i.e., a condition in which multiple genetic loci and/or environmental factors influence the liability to stutter). Although the multifactorial model fit their obtained data most closely, Cox and colleagues noted that segregation at one or more major loci could not be rejected for a subset of families.

In addition to testing alternative transmission models, Kidd and his colleagues presented a cogent explanation for the observed gender effects for stuttering. Their sex-specific (also called sex-modified or sex-limited) threshold model, described in varying detail in several papers (Kidd, 1980, 1983, 1984; Kidd, Kidd, & Records, 1978), essentially proposed that stuttering genotype(s) are expressed as different susceptibilities depending on sex. Because the "stuttering threshold" is hypothesized to be higher for females, it is assumed that more precipitating (genetic or environmental) factors that contribute to stuttering would have to be present for females to cross the threshold and manifest the disorder. This model of stuttering makes two predictions, both of which fit the observed stuttering data well: (1) more males than females in the population ought to stutter, and (2) a female stutterer, who carries more deleterious predisposing factors, should have more affected relatives. Although these gender effects had been recognized for some time, Kidd and colleagues were the first to offer a sophisticated and potentially testable model to explain their occurrence.

Finally, the Yale Family Study should be credited with being the first behavioral genetic investigation of stuttering to include an assessment of environmental variables as a project objective. Using a rather "shotgun" assessment strategy, Cox, Seider, & Kidd (Cox *et al.*, 1984b) interviewed 14 stuttering-dense and 10 control families to determine if any of the 124 prenatal, medical, developmental, social, educational, or parental variables they sampled distinguished persons who stuttered from their nonstuttering relatives and from control cases. Interestingly, despite the large number of variables tested, few significant group differences were found. Because the study was flawed methodologically—for example, the investigators relied heavily on retrospective recall, and many of the assessment items lacked sensitivity—the results do not provide a definitive test of environmental (etiologic) hypotheses for this disorder. However, its limitations notwithstanding, this final empirical paper in the Yale series did make an important statement: nongenetic factors, though inherently difficult to identify, are worthy of study. It is slightly ironic, but somehow fitting that, in bringing to a close their extraordinarily productive program of research, the team that became known as the pioneers of genetics research for stuttering provided the field with a nascent (albeit imperfect) model for conceptualizing and assessing nongenetic factors within stuttering and nonstuttering families.

Although the Yale team dominated stuttering genetics research in the 1970s and 1980s, one influential twin study not associated with the Yale Family Project was published during this time. In 1981, Pauline Howie reported her findings from 29 same-sex twin pairs (6–27 years of age) who had been selected for study because at least one member had reported a history of stuttering. When the age-corrected pairwise concordance rates found among the 16 monozygotic pairs were compared with the rates found among the 13 dizygotic pairs, the results suggested a strong genetic effect for stuttering. Specifically, 63% of the monozygotic twins in this study (10/16 pairs) were concordant-affected pairs, in comparison to only 19% (3/13) of the dizygotic pairs. Although these differences suggest an important role for genetics, Howie herself noted that a large subgroup of her identical twins (about 40%) were stuttering-discordant. She reasoned that the existence of these discordant MZ pairs highlighted the "importance of the interaction of genetic and environmental factors in the etiology of this disorder" (p. 317), a sensible conclusion that had been reached by virtually all of her predecessors.

Although limited, including a rather modest sample size and the heterogeneous age range of the participating twins, the results of Howie's (1981) study are actually more interpretable than the results reported in the much larger twin study performed by Nelson *et al.* in 1945. Howie was able to take advantage of improvements in statistical analysis and zygosity testing that were not available in previous decades. In addition, by the time this study was performed, there was more knowledge extant about the necessary safeguards required in twin designs. For example, Howie understood the importance of ensuring diagnostic independence (i.e., making sure that speech diagnoses were made blindly with respect to both zygosity and co-twin speech status) and the necessity of using a standard and precisely described definition for classifying twins as stuttering-affected or unaffected.

D. 1990 AND BEYOND

The 1990s continued to be a productive period for research investigating the genetics of stuttering. Two multidisciplinary teams emerged to build on the work of their predecessors in behavioral genetics. One of these teams (the Illinois group) published data from their prospective family study of stuttering in young children (Ambrose *et al.*, 1993, 1997), while the other (the Australian group) reported results from two quasi-population-based twin studies (Andrews *et al.*, 1991; Felsenfeld *et al.*, 2000). In addition to these behavioral genetics studies, the 1990s witnessed the beginning of several independent molecular genetic (linkage) studies of stuttering, including a genetic linkage study of stuttering supported by the National Institutes of Health described later. Indeed, the 1990s may well be remembered as the "decade of maturity" for research in stuttering genetics, reflecting, in large part, the addition of molecular science to the field's behavioral genetic research portfolio.

The principal genetic objectives of the University of Illinois's Early Childhood Stuttering Project were similar to those of prior family studies of stuttering, and included verifying familial aggregation, examining rates of disorder across relative types, investigating gender effects, and testing alternative models of transmission using segregation analysis. By and large, the results of these analyses complemented and replicated the findings reported in earlier investigations. What most clearly distinguishes this project from its predecessors is the age of the proband cases. Unlike most prior genetic studies of stuttering, the 69 proband cases in the Illinois project were all preschool-aged children who were "close to the onset of stuttering." Ambrose, Yairi, and Cox (1993) reported a proband sample of 69 children, aged two and six years, and Ambrose, Cox, and Yairi (1997) reported a sample of 66 children, aged two to eight years. It was not made clear if these samples were independent or if there was subject overlap between the two studies. This difference in case selection was considered significant by the Illinois researchers for two primary reasons: (1) it reduced the sampling bias that may have been present in family studies that ascertained only chronic adult stuttering cases, and (2) the pedigree information that was gathered about the family members of the incipient proband subjects was assumed to be "fresher" and hence more reliable.

One finding of particular interest emerged from the Illinois project. Revisiting an issue that had interested the Yale group 20 years earlier, Ambrose *et al.* (1997) divided their proband subjects into those who were persistent stutterers and those who appeared to have recovered from stuttering by 36 months post-onset. When the pedigrees of these groups were compared, a significant tendency for recovery status to "breed true" within families was observed; in other words, families tended to express either primarily persistent or primarily recovered stuttering profiles. Ambrose and her colleagues put forth an interesting biological hypothesis to explain this effect, arguing that perhaps "persistent stuttering may be the expression of underlying stuttering, with the same major [genetic] locus component as recovered stuttering, but with other genes promoting a tendency to persist" (1997, p. 577).

Two twin studies of stuttering were also performed during the 1990s, both of which identified their stuttering cases from the Australian Twin Project (ATP). In the first of these investigations, Andrews *et al.* (1991) examined the questionnaire responses of 3810 adult twin pairs to identify individuals who had responded affirmatively to an item about stuttering. From this large sample, 135 complete pairs were identified that contained at least one self-reported stuttering member (50 MZ and 85 DZ pairs). Of the 50 MZ pairs, 10 (20%) were concordant for stuttering, in comparison to only 3% of the DZ pairs. When genetic models were fitted to these data, the best-fitting model was one in which 71% of the variance in liability was attributed to genetic variance, with the remaining 29% attributed to the individual's unique environment.

At the end of the decade, researchers in the United States and Australia combined forces to complete a second twin study of stuttering, this time sampling a younger cohort from the ATP (Felsenfeld *et al.*, 2000). The proband subjects in this study were drawn from a sample of 4269 pairs of twins aged 21–28 years. These twins were mailed health questionnaires in 1990–1992, and responses were received from 1567 pairs and 634 individual twins (a total of 3768 respondents). Two items about stuttering were included on the questionnaire, and these were used to identify positive stuttering cases ("positive screens"). Once identified, these positive screens ($n = 331$), their co-twin, and a sample of control cases were interviewed by phone to confirm the diagnosis. Ultimately, 91 complete twin pairs (38 MZ and 53 DZ pairs) containing at least one stuttering member were identified in the interview phase of the study. Of these, 17/38 MZ and 8/53 DZ pairs were concordant for presence of the disorder, corresponding to pairwise concordance rates of 45 and 15% for MZ and DZ twins, respectively. Multivariate structural equation modeling of these data revealed that approximately 70% of the variance in liability to stuttering in both men and women was attributable to genetic effects, with the remainder due to nonshared environmental effects. Prior to this analysis, the data were corrected for ascertainment bias using a bivariate analysis procedure. This procedure is described in greater detail by Felsenfeld *et al.* (2000). It is worth noting that this modeling result, which attributes a very substantial amount of variance in stuttering liability to genetics, is virtually identical to the modeling result reported for the older twin cohort examined by Andrews and colleagues in 1991.

III. GENE FINDING: THE "TODAY" AND "TOMORROW" OF STUTTERING RESEARCH

The advances in behavioral genetics just described, impressive as they are, pale in comparison to the astronomical scientific growth that has occurred over the last two decades in molecular genetic laboratories around the world. Genetic maps of humans have been constructed and refined, most of the human genes have been enumerated, and large regions of the human genome have had their DNA sequence completely determined (Hunt *et al.*, 1999). The tools and techniques of the Human Genome Project have also provided a tremendous impetus to the study of genes that cause disease in humans. These advances have been used to elucidate the defects that underlie hundreds of different genetic diseases, encompassing all of the common genetic diseases of humans, plus scores of rare ones. The purpose of this section is to introduce the concepts of disease gene identification and to describe how modern molecular genetics methods are used to accomplish this task (see Chapter 2).

A. GENETIC LINKAGE STUDIES

Most of the human disease genes identified to date have made use of genetic linkage information. Briefly stated, genetic linkage is the observance of co-inheritance between two traits as they are passed from parent to offspring. Genetic linkage is a relative rarity. For any two simple traits taken at random, co-inheritance can be observed roughly 1% of the time or less. It is so rare, in fact, that Gregor Mendel formulated one of his Laws of Inheritance (sometimes called the Law of Independent Assortment) to state this fact. However, if one searches hard enough, one can eventually find traits that violate Mendel's law, and are inherited together. The reason traits are inherited together is that the genes that cause those two traits reside immediately adjacent to each other on the same chromosome. When closely arranged, these genes are rarely or not at all subject to the normal mixing processes that all chromosomes undergo as they are passed from parent to offspring.

An example of how linkage information is useful is the study of nail-patella syndrome, a very rare genetic disease in which the affected individuals have disorders of their fingernails, toenails, and kneecaps (Aschner, 1934). Nail-patella syndrome is inherited as a simple trait, indicating it is caused by the action of a single mutant gene. More than 50 years ago, it was discovered that in families with nail-patella syndrome the disease was always co-inherited with the blood type that the affected parent passed to their affected offspring (McKusick, 1991). In other words, the gene specifying ABO blood group was linked to the gene that caused nail-patella syndrome. Subsequently, it became known that the ABO blood group gene resides on human chromosome 9, and by the principle of linkage, the nail-patella syndrome gene was thus assigned to chromosome 9 (Ferguson-Smith et al., 1976). Although the nature of the nail-patella syndrome gene was completely obscure, the knowledge of its position on chromosome 9 ultimately allowed this gene to be identified. This general approach to finding genes has come to be known as positional cloning, that is, the cloning of a gene based solely on its position in the genome.

Genetic linkage studies received a tremendous boost from the development of a large array of simple genetic markers for the human (Weissenbach et al., 1992). These markers are variants in the DNA sequence that occur naturally among individuals at specific places distributed throughout the genome. Through molecular biological laboratory methods, it is possible to assay the variation present at a single site. Since the chromosomal location of each of these markers is known, the observance of linkage between one of these markers and an inherited disease tells us where the gene causing that disease is located. In practice, some 350 such markers, spaced evenly down the length of each chromosome, are typed on the DNA of each individual in the family. This genotypic information is then subjected to computerized linkage analysis to measure the precise degree of statistical support for linkage at each of these 350 positions. This type of statistical information is typically reported as LOD scores, which give the logarithm of the odds that the disease is linked to a marker divided by the odds of it being unlinked. A LOD score of 3, representing 1000 to 1 odds in favor of linkage, is generally accepted as proof of linkage for a single gene trait.

This general approach has been applied with spectacular success to a wide range of human diseases. By the year 2000, we had already learned the location of almost a thousand disease genes, including genes that cause neurological disease, metabolic disease, endocrine disease, digestive disease, pulmonary disease, psychiatric disease, and diseases of many other systems within the body (Collins, 1995). The great strength of positional cloning is that no information about the gene or the product of the gene is required. No information about the biochemistry, pathology, physiology, or normal function of the gene is necessary; only that it causes disease in a way that can be traced in families.

B. GENE-FINDING AND CANDIDATE EVALUATION

A good genetic linkage study can provide a tremendous amount of positional information. With sufficient families available for study, a linkage study can narrow the location of a single gene down to a region of 1/1000th the length of the entire genome. Thus, while there are roughly 100,000 genes within the human genome, linkage studies can narrow the number of genes under consideration by a thousand-fold, to roughly a hundred. However, these 100 candidate genes still present a formidable task: each one must be examined in detail, in both normal and affected individuals. Even before this, however, one must be certain one knows all the genes that exist within the region of the genome identified in the linkage studies.

Although gene identification was a major laboratory undertaking in past positional cloning efforts, this part of the process has been greatly simplified by the Human Genome Project. The Human Genome Project has made several important resources freely available to the research community. First, continuously overlapping sets of clones of human genomic DNA have been isolated and mapped, so that the DNA of any region identified in a linkage study is available in isolated pure form. This DNA is required in cloned form for all subsequent genetic analyses of the disease gene region, and its ready availability saves tremendous time and effort. Second, a large fraction of all human genes has been identified, sequenced, and stored in easily searchable databases, notably the Expressed Sequence Tag (EST) database at the National Center for Biotechnology Information (NCBI) at the National Institutes of Health. (dbEST can be accessed at: http://www.ncbi.nlm.nih.gov/dbEST/index.html.) The comprehensive nature of these databases, and their ease of use, have substantially changed the process by which all genes within a genomic region are identified.

C. GENE IDENTIFICATION

Current methods of gene discovery within a genomic region rely on the availability of DNA clones covering that region, the use of high-throughput DNA sequencing, and EST databases. In brief, the current method of choice is to use automated DNA sequencing methods to obtain a random sampling of the genomic DNA sequence across the region. This sequence is then used to search EST databases to find which genes, as represented by their expressed sequences, reside within that region of the genome. The random sample sequencing strategies typically result in a survey of roughly two-thirds of the DNA sequence. With this approach, it is possible or even likely that some expressed sequences will be missed. However, because genes are arranged in exons (coding sequences) spread across larger stretches of noncoding DNA within the genome, it is unlikely that any gene will go completely undetected. Other databases, such as the Unigene database, can be used to piece together disparate EST sequences and help provide a view of the complete expressed gene as it resides within the genomic region of interest. (Unigene can be accessed at: http://www.ncbi.nlm.nih.gov/UniGene/index.html.) A so-called "rough draft" of the complete sequence of the human genome will soon be available, and this will be followed by the completely finished sequence shortly thereafter. The availability of this DNA sequence, together with publicly available annotation that will precisely point out the likely genes within this sequence, will have a tremendous effect on this task. These resources will eliminate the necessity of laboratory work to identify all the genes within a genomic region, as this information will be available in convenient form in electronic databases, such as GenBank. (GenBank can be accessed at: http://www2.ncbi.nlm.nih.gov/genbank/query form.html.)

D. GENE EVALUATION

Once all the genes within the candidate region have been identified, each one must be evaluated. Many times, the apparent biological function of a candidate gene will make it of particular interest for evaluation. This strategy is sometimes referred to as the positional candidate gene approach. It should be borne in mind that many apparently attractive candidates have ultimately turned out to not be the gene responsible for the disease. Since these failures are typically not published, the overall success rate of the positional candidate approach may well be exaggerated. Nevertheless, as our understanding of biology increases, this approach is likely to become more useful.

The evaluation of candidate genes is essentially an association study, in which researchers attempt to correlate the presence of mutation(s) in a gene with the presence of disease in humans. Many genes have a number of natural variations in their DNA sequence. Most of these differences have little or no functional consequence, so any apparent mutation in a candidate gene must be carefully evaluated to prove if it indeed causes the disease. This remains the most labor-intensive part of the positional cloning process. It makes large use of DNA sequencing, and requires DNA of individuals affected with the disease from many different families. Ultimately, proof that a particular gene is responsible for a particular disease comes from several lines of evidence. Critically, however, the gene must contain mutation(s) in affected individuals that are not observed in normal individuals. Other types of evidence contributing to proof of causality include the nature of the gene product and the tissues in which the gene is expressed.

E. COMPLEX DISEASES

The traditional positional cloning process outlined above has been spectacularly successful in the studies of single-gene Mendelian disorders. However, such disorders are rare in the population. Much more common are diseases that, although they have a clear genetic component, also have nongenetic causes and are not inherited in any simple fashion. Many speech and language disorders fall into this category, including stuttering. How will this affect the efforts to locate and isolate the genes involved in these disorders?

In the absence of simple inheritance patterns, the methods used to search for linkage in complex diseases must be modified. For example, the traditional LOD score method is based on the assumption that a single gene underlies the disease, and that the disease shows some approximation of Mendelian inheritance in families. Since neither of these conditions is true for complex disorders, other methods have been developed. In particular, allele-sharing methods have become popular (Blackwelder & Elston, 1985). These methods make no assumptions about the mode of inheritance, but simply measure the number of alleles shared among affected individuals in a family. For example, if a marker is unlinked to the gene that causes the disease in two affected siblings, those two siblings should share zero alleles at that locus 25% of the time, they should share one allele 50% of the time, and they should share two alleles 25% of the time. In such nonparametric linkage strategies, the data at marker loci are analyzed to look for distortions of this 25:50:25 percent ratio. If, for example, affected siblings share alleles much more often than expected, then linkage is probable, and that marker is likely to be close to a gene that contributes to that disease.

A number of other strategies can also be used to aid linkage studies of complex diseases. One popular choice is to employ a genetically isolated population. Such populations frequently have a much more limited number of genes that cause a particular disease. Working in such a population effectively raises the signal-to-noise ratio, since it increases the possibility that a single major locus is at work, and reduces the likelihood that other minor loci will be contributing to the disease (Wright et al., 1999). Although such a strategy has been employed in numerous instances to simplify linkage studies of single gene traits, its use in the study of complex traits has produced a mixed track record to date. For example, studies of schizophrenia using isolated populations have frequently failed to refine or even confirm the localizations obtained in previous studies using outbred populations. Nevertheless, the theoretical power of such populations argues strongly for their continued use, and it is likely that some of these will come to fruition.

F. CANDIDATE GENE EVALUATION IN COMPLEX DISEASES

Evaluation of candidate genes in complex diseases (such as stuttering) is more difficult than in Mendelian diseases. In Mendelian diseases, having a particular genotype is necessary and sufficient to cause the disease. In complex diseases, this is not the case. Thus, an individual can have the disease gene and not have the disease, for example, which makes candidate gene evaluation difficult. A number of strategies have been used to address this problem, including most of the strategies used for evaluation of genes in Mendelian disorders, with some modifications.

A common strategy to confirm or refute a particular candidate gene is to employ an association study, like that used in Mendelian disorders. Association studies for complex diseases often measure the occurrence of DNA sequence differences in a particular gene in a large group of people with the disease, and compare this frequency to that in a large group of people without the disease or in the general population. These associations, which are evaluated statistically, can provide strong evidence that the candidate gene has an involvement in the disease process, but this evidence is essentially indirect (Saunders *et al.*, 1993). No matter how strong the statistical association, it does not provide information on how the gene product contributes to the disease, or even prove the gene is causative. Especially in the current era, which is focused on reductionist approaches in the biological and medical sciences, additional information about the role of the candidate gene in the disease is required.

While the discovery of genes underlying complex diseases is in its infancy, it is clear that proof of the involvement of any gene here will require a broader array of evidence than that so far accepted for Mendelian diseases. Since many cases of complex disease are certain to be phenocopies (that is, the same disease caused by different genes, or even nongenetic causes), the study populations will necessarily be very large. However, this is a surmountable hurdle, given the many thousands or even millions of individuals in the population who are diagnosed with these disorders.

G. THE NIH STUTTERING STUDY

The National Institute on Deafness and Other Communication Disorders at the National Institutes of Health (NIH) is currently undertaking a genetic linkage study of stuttering. The genetic epidemiology of stuttering has many similarities to that of other disorders that have been successfully studied by this approach (Drayna, 1997). The study design focuses on affected relative pairs, predominantly affected siblings, and uses nonparametric analysis methods, including the allele-sharing methods described above. Enrollment will necessarily be large (several hundred affected relative pairs) to identify linkage in the face of the significantly non-Mendelian inheritance observed for this disorder.

If predisposing genes for stuttering are identified, there are several steps that can be taken to improve the diagnosis and treatment of this condition. For example, we may one day be able to identify subgroups of affected cases on the basis of their differing "genetic profiles." This information may be useful in "matching" clients to particular treatments that will be most effective for their profile, and in predicting long-term outcomes (such as the likelihood that recovery or relapse will occur).

IV. THE HUMAN FACE OF THE MOLECULAR GENETICS REVOLUTION

The general public is becoming increasingly informed about, and interested in, advances in medical genetics, such as those just described. Attention to this topic is undoubtedly particularly strong among families who have an aggregating disorder. To illustrate the human complexities of this situation, imagine a hypothetical family with multiple stuttering members who is told by a speech–language pathologist that genes "play a significant role" in conferring a risk for this disorder. How might this information be received? Can we anticipate the questions or concerns that may arise as a consequence of this information? For example, will this family assume that we can identify the specific relatives who are at greatest risk? Will they believe that, because their family's stuttering is "genetic" in origin, it is immutable and therefore untreatable? If major genes for stuttering are identified and publicized in the media, will there be an expectation that a drug or surgical cure for the disorder is just around the corner? Will the family inquire about a screening test for their presymptomatic children? Will they worry that speech therapy will no longer be covered by insurance? Will family members blame one another for "passing along" the stuttering genes?

To respond to these and other sensitive issues arising from the new genetics, a growing research alliance has developed between geneticists and scholars in the fields of law, sociology and medical ethics (see Chapter 10). The Human Genome Project has actively promoted this effort by creating a multidisciplinary division to address the ethical, legal, and social implications (ELSI) of human genetics research. Approximately 5% of the Human Genome Project's budget is devoted to funding ELSI grants and educational programs, and, although some would argue that this expenditure is too modest, it nonetheless represents an attempt on the part of Genome Project scientists to be proactive about the potential societal impact of the technical information they will disseminate (see Chapter 10). It is now clearly recognized, for example, that public and professional education programs about genetics must be developed to ensure that the populace has a reasonable level of "genetic literacy." (The ELSI Division of the Human Genome Project can be accessed at http://www.ornl.gov/hgmis/resource/elsi.html.)

The American Speech–Language–Hearing Association (ASHA) has also begun formal efforts to address this and other ELSI needs for the profession. In 1998, ASHA coordinated the development and distribution of a questionnaire about genetics that was mailed to 600 randomly selected ASHA members (Willig *et al.*, 2000). Of the 364 ASHA members who responded to this survey, fewer than 20% reported that they had had any formal course work in genetics. When asked how they had acquired knowledge about recent genetic advances, a large majority indicated that most or all of their knowledge came from the popular media. Several possible mechanisms to enhance the genetic literacy of the professional membership were proposed by Willig and her colleagues, including developing university courses, integrating consumer panels into curricula, and increasing educational opportunities for ASHA members and consumers.

GENETIC LITERACY AND LAY BELIEFS ABOUT INHERITANCE

As information about genetics continues to filter into our daily lives, three observations have become increasingly clear. First, there is substantial public interest in topics relating to gene-finding, genetic testing, gene therapies, and the Human Genome Project. Second, the public is generally ill-equipped to interpret this highly complex information and apply it to their own health management. And, third, it is unclear who should assume primary responsibility for ensuring that new genetic information does more "good than harm," is culturally sensitive, and is nondiscriminatory (Nelkin, 1992; Richards, 1996; Wexler, 1992). To further complicate matters, we now recognize that genetic disorders have a particular potency for those who are affected and their families, perhaps because they are seen as transmitted directly by a parent or through a parental line. As Richards (1996) has observed, the issue of who is "responsible" for a familial condition may become a topic for overt discussion and, in the worst case, may result in a situation in which "accusations of blighted inheritance will fly between family members" (p. 265). The very act of pedigree construction can sometimes become emotionally charged, even for a disorder as seemingly benign as stuttering. There may be a reluctance to admit that other family members had the disorder; this is particularly true for certain age cohorts or cultural groups where an admission that a disorder has existed is perceived as a personal failing or a source of shame (Richards, 1996). To return to our example, grandmother may not want to talk about the fact that her brother stuttered and may minimize or even suppress this information in an attempt to preserve his privacy and dignity.

How do we effectively assess and then enhance the genetic sophistication of the population? This is a complex task, particularly given the variety of constituent groups whom we might want to investigate, including clinicians who treat clients with familial disorders, the clients and families themselves, and journalists who are charged with reporting the latest genetic breakthroughs to the public (Durant *et al.*, 1996). At the present time, there is limited published information about the current level of genetic literacy within our specific constituent groups (e.g., speech–language pathologists, audiologists, and clients with communicative disorders). There are, however, a few qualitative studies that have examined lay beliefs about inheritance in families affected with other familial conditions, such as breast and ovarian cancer (Richards, 1997) and Huntington disease (Richards, 1997; Wexler, 1992). Though preliminary, these investigations have provided insights about common beliefs and misconceptions about inheritance that may serve as models for developing similar studies within our own profession.

One interesting finding to emerge from this research is that most adults, even those with limited scientific sophistication, have opinions about inheritance. These lay beliefs may be very strongly held in some families, and people may be very resistant to "scientific" explanations that challenge their longstanding ways of thinking. Thus, when faced with probability-based explanations of heredity provided by health practitioners that conflict with their personal experiences, the lay beliefs will often prevail (Richards, 1996; Richards & Ponder, 1996). Although frequently innocuous, this dissonance can compromise the integrity of genetic counseling sessions. In some cases, less than optimal management decisions may be made as families are put in a position to choose between their longstanding lay beliefs about inheritance and the scientific data they are being presented (Ponder *et al.*, 1996; Richards, 1996).

A second finding of interest is that people's (mistaken) beliefs about inheritance are generally not idiosyncratic; rather, they can generally be sorted into a small number of recurring categories of misperception (Ponder *et al.*, 1996; Richards, 1996, 1997; Wexler, 1992). These categories will undoubtedly change and expand as research on this topic continues. However, at present, the following five categories appear to capture many of the beliefs about inheritance that are expressed by the lay populace:

1. *Genetic connections ought to somehow mirror kinship closeness.* Even though people intellectually realize that biological kinship and emotional kinship are distinct, these boundaries sometimes become blurred when people view their own family. Statements such as "My brother and I share nothing in common; we must not share many genes," or "I'm much closer to my mother than to my father; my mother and I must have more genes in common" are typical of this kind of reasoning. Although factually erroneous—you share, on average, 50% of your genes with your brother, regardless of how much you like him—it is still difficult for some people to accept that they share substantial genetic material with individuals towards whom they do not feel warmly.

2. *There must be a pattern to explain who becomes affected within a family.* When specific "rules" to explain familial transmission are lacking, as they always will be for complex disorders such as stuttering, some families simply invent their own transmission rules. So, for example, a family might explain to you that their daughter won't be a stutterer like her father, because in their family "stuttering always skips a generation." Other families create different rule systems: "It only happens to the firstborns," "It only happens to the boys," and so forth. Once families decide upon a set of rules, they are often very resistant to change, even

in the face of contradictory evidence within the family itself. (Exceptions to the rule tend to be minimized.) As in many aspects of life, rules about inheritance seem to bring a semblance of order to a situation that might otherwise be disturbingly unpredictable.

3. *Reproductive outcomes cannot really be governed by chance and probability.* With each pregnancy, the genetic dice are rolled again; put simply, each pregnancy is a completely independent event. Families who have one speech-affected child might reason that they have already had their "special child," and surely the odds of producing another special child are minimal. Unfortunately, for multifactorial-polygenic genetic disorders such as stuttering, there is likely to be an uncertain but elevated risk for each pregnancy. Thus, having already had one affected child will not reduce the risk for future conceptions.

4. *Traits are inherited in clusters.* Many people mistakenly believe that independent traits are actually inherited in clusters. As such, if an individual does not "take after" the affected relative in their family—in appearance, for instance—it is assumed that they won't inherit the disorder from that person either. For example, a mother might say about her son, "He won't stutter like my husband because he doesn't 'take after' him." The mistake many people make is to assume that traits such as facial or personality resemblance and stuttering are linked, when, in fact, they are biologically unrelated.

5. *Healthy lifestyle choices can counterbalance any inherited susceptibility.* People may acknowledge that there is some inherited tendency for a particular disorder within their family, but may believe that they can prevent or minimize its effects by making "good lifestyle choices." For example, a family with multiple stuttering members in its extended branches may indicate that their children are not at particular risk for stuttering because they have made a conscious decision to adopt a "relaxed" family style. This statement reflects an implicit belief that a sensible lifestyle choice can serve a protective function that has the potential to eliminate or counterbalance any genetic liability that may exist.

V. CONCLUDING REMARKS

Twin and family studies of stuttering have appeared in the literature since the 1930s, and most have reached the same conclusion: genes are important for determining who will and will not ever stutter. This body of descriptive work, though not extensive, has laid the necessary foundation for the molecular genetic (linkage and association) projects that are currently being performed or planned. At the time of this writing, major genes that predispose to stuttering have not yet been located. However, it is reasonable to predict that such genes, if they exist, will be identified and the studies replicated within the coming decade. Once this occurs, it will set off a chain of scientific events that may culminate in very promising improvements for those who stutter. In the meantime, important psychosocial and educational issues relating to the "new genetics" must be considered. Most persons who stutter, and their speech–language clinicians, do not have the requisite scientific sophistication they will need to interpret the molecular genetic findings that may emerge in the near future. It would therefore seem prudent to make interdisciplinary research in these areas an immediate priority.

Finally, we end with a quotation from Susan Wexler, a neuropsychologist at Columbia University who has been tracking down the gene for Huntington disease for more than a decade. By her own admission, it has been a long and frustrating road, a journey made particularly poignant because Huntington disease runs in her family, and she herself is at considerable risk. She reflected on the importance of moving forward with genetic linkage studies of disorders by arguing the following:

> It may be true that knowing the cause of a disease at a molecular level may do nothing toward advancing palliation or cure. But it makes intellectual sense to go after the gene, the cause of the disease, as one possible avenue of interdiction. . . . If you want to stop the damage of the Nile constantly overflowing its banks, you could either build protections along the length of the river shore or go to the source of the Nile and try to control the flow before damage occurs. (1992, p. 241)

For stuttering, we have been building protections along the shore for some time, trying to contain the problem therapeutically as best we know how. As we begin a new century, it is time to see how much can be accomplished by searching for the source of the Nile.

REFERENCES

Ambrose, N. G., Cox, N., & Yairi, E. (1997). The genetic basis of persistence and recovery in stuttering. *Journal of Speech, Language, and Hearing Research, 40,* 567–580.

Ambrose, N. G., Yairi, E., & Cox, N. (1993). Genetic aspects of early childhood stuttering. *Journal of Speech and Hearing Research, 36,* 701–706.

Andrews, G., & Harris, M. (1964). The syndrome of stuttering. *Clinics in Developmental Medicine,* No. 17. London: Spastic Society Medical Education and Information Unit.

Andrews, G., Morris-Yates, A., Howie, P., & Martin, N. (1991). Genetic factors in stuttering confirmed. *Archives of General Psychiatry, 48,* 1034–1035.

Aschner, B. (1934). A typical hereditary syndrome: Dystrophy of the nails, congenital defect of the patella and congenital defect of the head of the radius. *Journal of the American Medical Association, 102,* 2017–2020.

Blackwelder, W., & Elston, R. (1985). A comparison of sib-pair linkage tests for disease susceptibility loci. *Genetic Epidemiology, 2,* 85–97.

Collins, F. S. (1995). Positional cloning moves from perditional to traditional. *Nature Genetics, 9,* 347–350.

Cox, N. (1988, April). Molecular genetics: The key to the puzzle of stuttering? *Asha,* 36–40.

Cox, N., & Kidd, K. (1983). Can recovery from stuttering be considered a genetically milder subtype of stuttering? *Behavior Genetics, 13,* 129–139.

Cox, N., Kramer, P., & Kidd, K. (1984a). Segregation analyses of stuttering. *Genetic Epidemiology, 1,* 245–253.

Cox, N., Seider, R., & Kidd, K. (1984b). Some environmental factors and hypotheses for stuttering in families with several stutterers. *Journal of Speech and Hearing Research, 27,* 543–548.

Drayna, D. (1997). Genetic linkage studies of stuttering: Ready for prime time? *Journal of Fluency Disorders, 22,* 237–241.

Durant, J., Hansen, A., & Bauer, M. (1996). Public understanding of the new genetics. In T. Marteau & M. Richards (Eds.), *The troubled helix: Social and psychological implications of the new human genetics* (pp. 235–248). Cambridge: Cambridge University Press.

Felsenfeld, S. (1996). Progress and needs in the genetics of stuttering. *Journal of Fluency Disorders, 21,* 77–103.

Felsenfeld, S. (1997). Epidemiology and genetics of stuttering. In R. F. Curlee & G. M. Siegel (Eds.), *Nature and treatment of stuttering: New directions* (pp. 3–23). Boston: Allyn and Bacon.

Felsenfeld, S., Kirk, K., Zhu, G., Statham, D., Neale, M., & Martin, N. (2000). A study of the genetic and environmental etiology of stuttering in a selected twin sample. *Behavior Genetics.* Submitted manuscript.

Ferguson-Smith, M, Aitken, D., Turleau, C., & de Grouchy, J. (1976). Localisation of the human ABO: Np-1:AK-1 linkage group by regional assignment of AK-1 to 9q34. *Human Genetics, 34,* 35–43.

Garrett, H. E. (1961). *General psychology* (2nd ed.). New York: American Book Company.

Gray, M. (1940). The X Family: A clinical and laboratory study of a "stuttering" family. *Journal of Speech Disorders, 5,* 343–348.

Howie, P. (1981). Concordance for stuttering in monozygotic and dizygotic twin pairs. *Journal of Speech and Hearing Research, 24,* 317–321.

Hunt, A. R., Collins, J. E., Bruskiewich, R., *et al.* (1999). The DNA sequence of human chromosome 22. *Nature, 402,* 489–495.

Johnson, W., *et al.* (1959). *The onset of stuttering.* Minneapolis: University of Minnesota Press.

Kidd, K. (1977). A genetic perspective on stuttering. *Journal of Fluency Disorders, 2,* 259–269.

Kidd, K. (1980). Genetic models of stuttering. *Journal of Fluency Disorders, 5,* 187–201.

Kidd, K. (1983). Recent progress on the genetics of stuttering. In C. Ludlow & J. Cooper (Eds.), *Genetic aspects of speech and language disorders* (pp. 197–213). New York: Academic Press.

Kidd, K. (1984). Stuttering as a genetic disorder. In R. F. Curlee & W. H. Perkins (Eds.), *Nature and treatment of stuttering: New directions* (pp. 149–169). Boston: Allyn and Bacon.

Kidd, K., Kidd, J., & Records, M. A. (1978). The possible causes of the sex ratio in stuttering and its implications. *Journal of Fluency Disorders, 3,* 13–23.

Ludlow, C. (1999). A conceptual framework for investigating the neurobiology of stuttering. In N. B. Ratner & E. C. Healey (Eds.), *Stuttering research and practice: Bridging the gap* (pp. 63–84). Mahwah, NJ: Erlbaum.

McKusick, V. (1991). *Mendelian inheritance in man* (9th ed.). Baltimore: Johns Hopkins University Press.

Nelkin, D. (1992). The social power of genetic information. In D. J. Kevles & L. Hood (Eds.), *Scientific and social issues in the Human Genome Project* (pp. 177–190). Cambridge: Harvard University Press.

Nelson, S. (1939). The role of heredity in stuttering. *Journal of Pediatrics, 14,* 642–654.

Nelson, S., Hunter, N., & Walter, M. (1945). Stuttering in twin types. *Journal of Speech Disorders, 10,* 335–343.

Pauls, D. L. (1990). A review of the evidence for genetic factors in stuttering. In *Research needs in stuttering. ASHA reports 18* (pp. 34–38). Rockville, MD: American Speech–Language–Hearing Association.

Ponder, M., Lee, J., Green, J., & Richards, M. (1996). Family history and perceived vulnerability to some common diseases: A study of young people and their parents. *Journal of Medical Genetics, 33,* 485–492.

Richards, M. (1996). Families, kinship, and genetics. In T. Marteau & M. Richards (Eds.), *The troubled helix: Social and psychological implications of the new human genetics* (pp. 249–273). Cambridge: Cambridge University Press.

Richards, M. (1997). It runs in the family: Lay knowledge about inheritance. In A. Clarke & E. Parsons (Eds.), *Culture, kinship, and genes: Towards cross–cultural genetics* (pp. 175-194). New York: St Martin's.

Richards, M., & Ponder, M. (1996). Lay understanding of genetics: A test of a hypothesis. *Journal of Medical Genetics, 33*, 1032–1036.

Saunders, A. M., Strittmatter, W. J., & Schmechel, D. (1993). Association of apolipoprotein E allele epsilon4 with late-onset familial and sporadic Alzheimer's disease. *Neurology, 43*, 1467–1472.

Seider, R., Gladstein, K., & Kidd, K. (1983). Recovery and persistence of stuttering among relatives of stutterers. *Journal of Speech and Hearing Disorders, 48*, 402–409.

Sheehan, J., & Costley, M. (1977). A reexamination of the role of heredity in stuttering. *Journal of Speech and Hearing Disorders, 42*, 47–59.

Weissenbach, J., Gyapay, G., Dib, C., Vignal, A., Morissette, J., Millasseau, P., Vaysseix, G., & Lathrop, M. (1992). A second-generation linkage map of the human genome. *Nature, 359(6398)*, 794–801.

Wepman, J. (1939). Familial incidence of stammering. *Journal of Heredity, 30*, 207–210.

West, R., Nelson, S., & Berry, M. (1939). The heredity of stuttering. *Quarterly Journal of Speech, 25*, 23–30.

Wexler, N. (1992). Clairvoyance and caution: Repercussions from the Human Genome Project. In D. J. Kevles & L. Hood (Eds.), *Scientific and social issues in the Human Genome Project* (pp. 211–243). Cambridge: Harvard University Press.

Willig, S., Moss, S., & Lapham, E.V. (2000). The new genetics: What does it mean to us? *The ASHA Leader, 5*, 4–5.

Wright, A., Carothers, A., & Pirastu, M. (1999). Population choice in mapping genes for complex diseases. *Nature Genetics, 23*, 397–404.

Yairi, E., Ambrose, N., & Cox, N. (1996). Genetics of stuttering: A critical review. *Journal of Speech and Hearing Research, 39*, 771–784.

9

CONCEPTS IN BEHAVIORAL

GENETICS AND THEIR

APPLICATION TO DEVELOPMENTAL

AND LEARNING DISORDERS

JEFFREY W. GILGER

Human Biology Program
University of Kansas
Lawrence, Kansas

Human behavioral genetics is an interdisciplinary mixture of the biological (genetic) and social sciences. Defining human behavioral genetics and its roots can be difficult. The definition depends somewhat on one's concept of behavior, whether there is a focus on quantitative versus molecular approaches, and if the consideration is typical or atypical variation or disease. Still, the defining question of the field is if and how genes affect human behavior.

The general principles behind the modern human behavioral genetic approaches began with the works of Charles Darwin, Francis Galton, and Gregor Mendel. Subsequent advances in mathematical and statistical approaches, as well as molecular genetics, have made the field what it is today (Bouchard & Propping, 1993; Neale & Cardon, 1992; Plomin et al., 1997; Sherman et al., 1997). Traditionally, the behaviors of interest in the field have been based in psychology, and included phenotypes like personality, speed of processing information, intelligence, and academic skills, among others (Fuller & Thompson, 1978; Minton & Schneider, 1985; Plomin et al., 1997). Over time, however, the field has expanded beyond these classic traits to include traits more commonly associated with other disciplines such as medicine and genetic epidemiology—for example, obesity, fragile X syndrome, Alzheimer disease, and addictive behaviors (Fuller & Simmel, 1983; Gilger & Hershberger, 1998; McGuffin et al., 1994; Plomin et al., 1994, 1997; Plomin & McClearn, 1993; Sherman et al., 1997).

In this chapter I endeavor to describe some of the concepts germane to the field and how these concepts apply to the area of developmental disorders and learning disabilities. The general purpose of this chapter is to provide the reader with a preliminary familiarization with the field as well as provide some concrete data regarding what we know about certain developmental disorders. Although there are many aspects of the field that I could discuss, I have chosen to focus on five within a logical framework of classical quantitative genetics: (1) the way in which behavioral genetic methods partition individual differences for a trait, like learning, into the proportion due to the *additive main effects* of genetic and nongenetic factors; (2) the manner in which human behavioral genetics examines the possibility that *nonadditive complexities* in development may contribute to disorders related to learning and development; (3) how human behavioral genetic methods have been used to detect and describe environmental influences independent of genetics; (4) how human behavioral genetic methods have helped us better define the characteristics of disorders and understand the basis for the correlations or associations among disorders within individuals; and (5) the way that human behavioral genetic methods have been used to describe the relationships between disorders and normal variation in learning or developmental skills.

It is not possible to cover all of these areas in great detail, and more in-depth reviews and examples of the specific problems addressed by behavioral genetics can be found in the references provided throughout this chapter. Although behavioral geneticists have studied many different behaviors, this chapter is aimed specifically at exemplary developmental, communicative, and learning disorders. There are many such disorders as listed in Table 9.1, and the etiology of each of these has been studied to some extent. The three disorders that are the focus of this paper are Developmental Reading Disorder (DRD or dyslexia), Attention Deficit Hyperactivity Disorder (ADHD), and autism, and general descriptions of these disorders are provided in Table 9.2. It is important to bear in mind that the

TABLE 9.1   Types of Learning Disorders or Primary Symptoms Associated With Commonly Recognized Developmental Learning Disabilities

Reading
Motor Coordination
Mathematics
Spelling
Attention
Writing
Activity
Memory
Social Skills
Nonverbal Abilities
Language

Note. These symptoms may occur separately or as a group (comorbidity) in a single individual.

TABLE 9.2   General Descriptions of the Primary Deficits in Developmental Reading Disorder (DRD), Autism, and Attention Deficit Hyperactivity Disorder (ADHD)

DRD
An unexplained inability to acquire normal reading skills[a]
Male-Female sex ratio = 1.5:1
Population prevalence = 5–10 per 100

Autism
Deficits in verbal and nonverbal skills, and imaginative activities; Impairments in social interactions; Restricted repertoire of activities and interests[b]
Male-Female sex ratio = 3:1
Population prevalence = 2–6 per 10,000

ADHD
Inattentiveness, impulsivity, over activity[c]
Male–female sex ratio = 2–9:1
Population prevalence = 4–10 per 100

Note: These symptoms lists are condensed from the Diagnostic and Statistical Manual of Mental Disorders (APA, 1994) and Pennington (1991).

[a]In addition to problems with reading, certain exclusionary criteria are typically applied as well to rule out various causes for the disorder such as mental retardation, psychiatric disturbance, inappropriate or inadequate learning experience, and gross brain abnormality.

[b]These are three general categories of deficits. Some or all of these deficits may exist in various degrees in any one person (see text for a discussion of symptom boundaries).

[c]These general symptoms are found in various combinations and degrees.

specific research reports reviewed in this chapter may have used variants of the
general definitions provided in Table 9.2. Nonetheless, the key criteria listed in
Table 9.2 are usually part of these research definitions.

I. INTRODUCTION TO THE BASIC MODEL OF
HUMAN BEHAVIORAL GENETICS

The basic approach of human behavioral genetics needs to be described at the
outset. It is essentially mathematical, with its basis in quantitative genetic theory
originating from work with plants and animals (Falconer, 1981; Fuller &
Thompson, 1978; Plomin *et al.*, 1997). While there is some variation in experimental approach, human behavioral geneticists are essentially interested in parti-
tioning phenotypic variance into its genetic and nongenetic components, or:

$$V_p = V_g + V_e \qquad (1)$$

where V_g is the genetic variance, V_e is the variance due to environment, and V_p
is the population phenotypic variance. Recall that the term "phenotype" refers to
the observable effects of genes, that is, phenotypes are analogous to the behaviors
or traits we are studying. Thus, at the first level of examination, the basic behavioral genetic model is additive in nature, and considers only the main effects of
genetic and nongenetic factors as they explain individual differences in phenotypes observed in the population of study.

An important assumption of quantitative genetics is implicit in Eq. (1), namely,
that the trait under study is a reflection of the additive and equal effects of many
genes along with environmental influences, or a multifactorial polygenic model
(MFP). The actual number of genes assumed in an MFP model is undefined in
actuality and may range from 2 or 3 in a multiple allelic system to 100 or more;
but, in either situation, the genetic and nongenetic effects combine to give a
relatively unimodal and smooth distribution of the phenotype as illustrated in
Figure 9.1 (Falconer, 1981; Fisher, 1918). An allele is an alternate form of a gene.
The locations of genes on chromosomes are called loci, although sometimes the
terms gene and locus are used synonymously. It is worth reiterating that complex
and continuously varying phenotypic distributions can be due to many genes or
even a very few given the right conditions (Fisher, 1918).

Classical human behavioral genetic methods rely on naturalistic experiments
with analogues in plant and animal research where various combinations of strains
or breeds can be manipulated in controlled conditions. In the case of humans,
the resemblance among relatives in naturally occurring experimental designs
is studied. These sets of relatives vary in the degree to which they share genes
and environments. Specifically, variations of twin, adoption, and family study
designs are used, where individual differences for human phenotypes can be
quantified in terms of heritability (h^2) and environmentality (e^2) (for a discussion

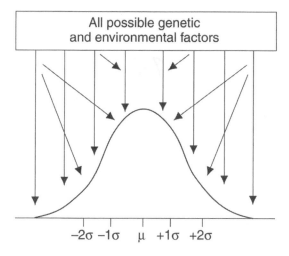

FIGURE 9.1 Many psychometrically assessed traits or complex phenotypes yield a continuous distribution from low to high. This continuum is often unimodal and fairly normal, with the fewest percentage of individuals scoring at the extreme ends.

of these designs see Fuller & Thompson, 1978; Neale & Cardon, 1992; Plomin *et al.*, 1997).

Heritability is a statistically standardized form of V_g, while environmentality is the standardized form of V_e, namely, h^2 is the proportion of variance in a trait attributable to genetic effects and e^2 is the proportion of trait variance attributable to nongenetic factors and error (Falconer, 1981). The sum of h^2 and e^2 must account for all the phenotypic variance, and, because they are standardized, estimates of h^2 and e^2 derived from the same sample and for the same trait will theoretically sum to 1.0 (Falconer, 1981). It is important to note that, like any statistic, h^2 and e^2 are estimates of hypothetical true values, and they will tend to vary from sample to sample in response to measurement error and genetic and environmental differences in the samples (Falconer, 1981). Therefore, when h^2 of a trait is mentioned, it is not necessarily indicating a static all-or-none quantity or quality for a trait.

A. ADDITIVE MAIN EFFECTS OF GENES AND ENVIRONMENTS ON DISORDERS OF READING, ATTENTION, OR ACTIVITY, AND AUTISM

The basic quantitative model (Eq. (1)) has been applied to many traits, and for the vast majority *both* genes and environments seem to be important (Gilger & Hershberger, 1998; Plomin *et al.*, 1997). This conclusion, based on decades of human research, should not be surprising. Yet, in the past, the social and scientific zeitgeist has swung between extremes, focusing either on genes and away from environment, or vice versa. Because of popular social and scientific paradigms that at times have favored environmental etiologies of behaviors, geneticists have had to carefully convince the professional and lay community that genes are, to some extent, important in the development and expression of nearly every human trait thus far examined. For some phenotypes, such as certain psychiatric disorders and adult intelligence, genetic effects typically equal or exceed environmental effects, while for other phenotypes, such as religiosity or adolescent antisocial personality, the reverse may be true (Eaves *et al.*, 1989; Lyons *et al.*, 1995; McGuffin *et al.*, 1994; Plomin *et al.*, 1994, 1997; Riggins-Caspers & Cadoret, 1999; Rowe, 1994; Truett *et al.*, 1992).

Heritability estimates across a number of cognitive and personality traits typically are statistically significant with values rarely below 0.20 or above 0.80, with a common average heritability of approximately 0.45–0.55 (Gilger & Hershberger, 1998; Plomin *et al.*, 1994, 1997; Rowe, 1994). Some phenotypes, however, such as autism, yield very high estimates of h^2. Autism, in fact, is considered to be one of the most heritable psychiatric conditions, with an h^2 in excess of 0.80–0.90 (Bailey *et al.*, 1996; Smalley *et al.*, 1988).

An h^2 for autism of this magnitude means that in situations where multiple family members are so affected the familial resemblance is primarily due to genes and not environments (e.g., parental treatment). In fact, the familial recurrence risk for autism (when there is already one child in a family with autism) is approximately 100 times that of the general population base rate of 4–6 per 10,000 people (Bolton *et al.*, 1994; Smalley *et al.*, 1988). Although this massive elevation in risk is due mainly to biological factors, bear in mind that the actual average risk to each additional offspring in such families is only approximately 100 times 0.0004 to 0.0006, or 0.04–0.06. Therefore, it is still unlikely that parents with one child who has autism will have another, assuming of course that they opt to have additional offspring (Jones & Szatmari, 1988).

It is noteworthy that for discontinuous phenotypes—such as the presence or absence of a psychiatric disorder like autism—quantitative genetic theory assumes that there are multiple genetic and environmental factors operating on an underlying trait continuity and that there is a threshold for trait diagnosis or expression that must be met (Falconer, 1981). Thus, human behavioral genetic studies address whether there is a significant h^2 for the *liability* of a disorder like autism (Gottesman, 1991; Heath & Madden, 1995) and, as noted previously, the h^2 for the liability of autism is quite high.

Similar to autism, most studies suggest that ADHD also has a high h^2. Across studies using a variety of diagnostic methods (e.g., questionnaire or standardized interview), the average h^2 is approximately 0.70 (Plomin *et al.*, 1997). This estimate applies to the liability of a qualitative diagnosis of ADHD as well as the variability of ADHD symptoms assessed as a continuously distributed trait.

ADHD also has a high familiality, and studies suggest elevated recurrence risks when there is already a first degree relative with the diagnosis. For example, a number of studies have shown that 25 to 40% of the first-degree relatives of probands (the proband is the person through whom we ascertain the family for study) with ADHD showing some or all of the cluster of ADHD symptoms, and this is significantly higher than the population base rate of 4–10% (Biederman *et al.*, 1986; Faraone *et al.*, 1991; Pauls *et al.*, 1993). That the h^2 for ADHD is so high again suggests that this familiality is primarily a reflection of genes shared among family members rather than experiences in common to family members.

In contrast to ADHD and autism, the heritability of DRD is in the moderate range. First, there is family resemblance for normal reading skills: family members are correlated for general reading ability and studies using standardized reading tests have estimated the h^2 of reading at approximately 0.30–0.50 (Plomin *et al.*, 1997). With regard to atypically low reading ability, both qualitative liability and quantitative scale models of DRD yield h^2 estimates approximating 0.40–0.50 (DeFries & Gillis, 1993; Olson *et al.*, 1994; Smith *et al.*, 1996).

Some reports on DRD (and ADHD as well) refer to a specialized form of heritability analysis, namely group heritability analysis, signified as h^2_g (DeFries & Fulker, 1988; DeFries & Gillis, 1993). The interpretation of h^2_g is different from that of h^2: in the case of reading ability or disability, h^2_g indicates the genetic proportion of the difference in average reading scores between groups of individuals with DRD and groups of individuals who are normal readers. Thus, an h^2_g for DRD of 0.50 (DeFries & Gillis, 1993) means that 50% of the difference in reading scores between normal and disordered groups of readers is due to genetics.

Similar to ADHD and autism, DRD is familial. The population base rate of DRD is 5–10%, and research indicates that relatives of people with DRD are at higher risk to also display the disorder than the population at large (Gilger *et al.*, 1991; Pennington & Gilger, 1996; Smith *et al.*, 1996). Specifically, across several studies, approximately 40–50% of the first degree relatives of a DRD proband have or had DRD themselves. Furthermore, risk varies depending on whether or not the offspring's parents have overcome (or compensated for) their reading problem (Gilger *et al.*, 1996a,b; Pennington & Gilger, 1996). For example, Table 9.3 shows that offspring are at greatest risk when a parent has not compensated (i.e., still displays DRD) and least at risk for a reading problem when a parent has compensated (i.e., no longer tests as having DRD). The basis of this parental compensation effect is unclear, and it may involve genetic or environmental factors that operate on brain systems that affect reading or general cognitive ability.

The heritability and recurrence rate data for autism, ADHD, and DRD can be used by the clinician to help with diagnostic, risk assessment, and early identification, as well as prognostic concerns. It is important to recognize, however, that the heritability and risk rates of these disorders are not 1.0 or 100%. Thus, it is clear that the environment makes a contribution to the liability or expression of these disorders. The precise nature of these environmental factors eludes us for the most part, although two generalizations can be made. First, save the rare exception, these disorders do not come about because of the way children are treated by their parents or because the symptoms or behaviors are learned from siblings or parents. This is not to say that the family atmosphere has no effect on

TABLE 9.3   Proportion of School-Aged Offspring Who
Had DRD as a Function of Parental Type[a]

Type of mating pair			
AA/AC	AU	CU	UU[b]
80%/60%	60%	30%	20%

Note: Modified from Gilger *et al.* (1996).

[a]Parents were diagnosed as Affected (A), Unaffected (U) or
Compensated (C) based on the presence or absence of reading problems in childhood and adulthood. A = had DRD while school-aged
and still do when tested as an adult; U = did not have DRD in
childhood and do not test as DRD in adulthood; C = had DRD in
childhood, but no longer test as DRD in adulthood. With three
parental types there are six mating types. There were too few of the
CC types of matings to include in this analysis. Number in each cell
represents the proportion (rounded) of offspring from these matings
that tested as DRD in childhood. Note that there is a linear decrease
in risk to offspring dependent on whether a child comes from a
family with an A type, C type, or U type parent.

[b]Theoretically, the proportion of affected offspring in this cell
should be close to the population base rate of 5–10%. The increased
magnitude realized is due to the manner in which families were
brought into the study: all were selected through a DRD proband,
thus artificially increasing the rates of DRD in the families even
when both parents are of the U type.

the expression or development of these disorders; it clearly can. But rather that
the resemblance among brothers, sisters, and parents for these disorders reflects
primarily genes and not shared experiences. This point is elaborated later on in
this chapter. Second, research suggests that much of the environmental variance
in these disorders represents effects on the brain that occurred prenatally or
perinatally (Filipek, 1995; Smith *et al.*, 1996). Thus, again, these developmental
disorders do not typically come about through childhood traumatic experiences,
bad parenting, or bad modeling by a disordered relative. Instead, given the normal
range of experiences, these disorders arise because of structural and functional
brain differences culminating from the interplay of genes and early adverse
environmental events that may vary child to child.

B. NONADDITIVE COMPLEXITIES IN THE DEVELOPMENT OF
DISORDERS OF READING, ATTENTION, OR ACTIVITY, AND AUTISM

The basic model of Eq. (1), in which the phenotypic variance in a population
is explained in terms of the main effects of genes and environments, can be

expanded to include additional terms, namely, it is recognized that V_p may also reflect nonadditive components or components that are not strictly genetic or nongenetic in their origin. Unless these components are explicitly considered in the statistical models, they are subsumed under the heritability and environmentality estimates (or error terms, which are typically subsumed under V_e).

Given what we know about neurophysiology, neurodevelopment, and human behavior, it is unlikely that genes and environments act in a simple additive and independent fashion to yield the structures and functions of the brain that ultimately give rise to thoughts, feeling, and actions. In fact, there is every reason to expect that genes interact with other genes and environments to form and operate the systems required for human behavior. Here, we are speaking of genotype–environment interactions as nonadditive effects beyond the main effects of genes or environments alone. We do not mean the same thing as what some have called "interactionism" or the situation where genes and environments act together to modify phenotypes (Anastasi, 1958; Riggins-Caspers & Cadoret, 1999; Whalsten, 1990). Here, we mean that different genotypes may react in different ways to the same environment.

One step toward recognizing this is an expansion of Eq. (1):

$$V_p = V_g + V_e + 2\text{cov}(g)(e) + V_{gxe} \tag{2}$$

where $2\text{cov}(g)(e)$ represents genotype–environment correlations, and V_{gxe} represents genotype–environment interactions. Also, V_g can be expanded to reveal what it contains:

$$V_g = V_I + V_A + V_D \tag{3}$$

where V_I represents epistasis, V_D dominance, and V_A additive effects of genes (Falconer, 1981). Dominance and epistasis are considered nonadditive in that the alleles at each locus contributing to trait variance or liability interact within loci (dominance) or across multiple loci (epistasis).

And, finally, some have suggested still other factors in the development of a phenotype, including the combinatorial emergenic properties of many genes and random epigenetic properties of biologic systems, both of which theoretically can contribute to phenotypic variability, but probably only in small and person-specific ways at a population level (Lykken, 1982).

1. Dominance and Epistasis

One form of nonadditive genetic variance, V_D, has been demonstrated to exist for a number of traits, among them personality, alcoholism, certain psychiatric disorders, IQ, and types of mental retardation (Alsobrook & Pauls, 1998; McGuffin et al., 1994; Plomin et al., 1994, 1997; Smith et al., 1996, 1998). Of particular relevance to this paper is the evidence that single genes with dominance effects may contribute to the liability for DRD, autism, and ADHD (McGuffin et al., 1994; Plomin et al., 1997). Thus, V_g for the disorder is not simply additive as expected under a classic MFP model. That single genes with significant effects may exist for these disorders also increases the likelihood that future molecular work will be able to identify and clone the key genes that predispose someone to develop ADHD, DRD, or autism (see later discussions in this chapter). On the other hand, clear and measurable evidence for genetic effects on learning-related behaviors due to the interaction across genes, or V_I, has been very difficult to find given the standard quantitative methods that rely solely on phenotypic data. Yet, it is theoretically likely that such effects occur. The actual identification of V_I for complex human behaviors like learning probably lies at first in future work using molecular genetic techniques in human and nonhuman models.

2. Genotype–Environment Correlations and Interactions

There are several methods for detecting genotype–environment correlations and interactions, including biometrical model fitting and correlational methods using adoption and/or twin data (Blangero, 1993; Neale & Cardon, 1992; Plomin *et al.*, 1997). Genotype–environment correlations are of three main types—active, reactive, and passive—each of which represents the situation in which particular genotypes are associated with particular environments (Plomin, 1986; Scarr & McCartney, 1983). There is some thinking that, for human behaviors, these three types of correlations to some extent are age dependent, with passive being more significant in the younger ages, and active and reactive becoming increasingly important as one grows older. Briefly, the active form pertains to the situation where environments are chosen or sought out by individuals that are conducive to or in alignment with their genetic propensities. Reactive pertains to the situation where a person's genetic make-up evokes or causes a response from, or change in, the environment; and the passive form occurs when a person (usually a child) passively receives genotypes that are correlated with their family experiences or environments. In contrast to correlations, genotype–environment interactions pertain to the differential response of certain genotypes to certain environments. Thus, particular genotypes may fare better in one environment, while other genotypes fare better in another environment.

Genotype–environment correlations and interactions for certain personality and cognitive traits have been found, but only a very few (Plomin *et al.*, 1997). Although genotype–environment interactions have not been thoroughly studied for DRD, autism, and ADHD, such complexities in their development may be identified in future work. For example, we may find that certain environments or experiences—for example, a virus in a pregnant woman, maternal immune response, a perinatal complication, a subtle brain injury, or a nonstimulating or deprived early infancy—interact with certain genotypes such that the risk to develop DRD, autism, or ADHD increases dramatically only when an individual with a specific genotype has these environmental experiences. In fact, there is some evidence that increased rates of prenatal or perinatal complications and minor congenital malformations are frequent in children with ADHD and autism

(Chandola *et al.*, 1992; Folstein & Rutter, 1977; Steffenberg *et al.*, 1989). Although the etiology and cause–effect relationships of these complications or malformations is debated, some (e.g., Folstein & Rutter, 1977) have suggested that they reflect a form of genotype–environment interaction where, without these environmental complications, full-blown expression of ADHD or autism would not come about.

Research looking specifically at genotype–environment correlations for DRD, autism, and ADHD is also rare, though significant genotype–environment correlations, primarily of the passive form, have been documented for related cognitive variables such as language (reading is a language-based disorder) and IQ (Plomin *et al.*, 1997). For example, passive genotype–environment correlations have been identified for language skills as early as 1 year of age (Hardy-Brown & Plomin, 1985; Hardy-Brown *et al.*, 1981). A preliminary study by Gilger *et al.* (in review) has also shown that reactive or active genotype–environment correlations seem particularly strong for children predisposed to a language disorder compared to their linguistically normal peers. According to this preliminary research, it appears that environments may adapt or respond differently to a child with atypical language skills compared to children with typical skills. This differential environmental response (e.g., over-attention by caregivers, solicitation of special education services) may be elicited by the child's atypical behavior. Thus, in some sense, genes may drive behavior as well as the environments in which behaviors develop. It is possible, if not likely, that such an effect is present for other atypical behaviors like ADHD, autism, and DRD.

C. ENVIRONMENT VERSUS GENETICS FOR DISORDERS OF READING, ATTENTION, OR ACTIVITY, AND AUTISM

The methods of human behavioral genetics can teach us about how genes influence behavior and how nongenetic factors operate as well. Variants of twin, family, and adoption designs are the only means by which genes and environments can be conjointly or independently studied, especially when data representing a number of different familial relationships are analyzed simultaneously (Plomin *et al.*, 1997; Rowe, 1994, 1997; Sherman *et al.*, 1997).

1. Intra- Versus Extrafamilial Environments

In quantitative theory, the environmental factors influencing a trait can be divided into two basic components (Falconer, 1981; Plomin *et al.*, 1997): those shared by relatives and those not shared by relatives. The V_e component of Eq. (1) can be expanded to show that

$$V_e = V_{es} + V_{ns} \tag{4}$$

where V_{es} represents shared or between-family environmental variance, and V_{ns} indicates nonshared or within-family environmental influences. Thus, in behavioral genetics the summary concept of e^2 is often separated into common or shared familial environmental influences (symbolized here as E_s) and nonshared familial environmental influences (symbolized here as E_{ns}). E_{ns} represents the standardized proportion of phenotypic variance that is unique and not commonly experienced by members of the same family. Thus, E_{ns} factors cause phenotypic differences among family members. This is in contrast to E_s, which represents the proportion of phenotypic variance due to environmental factors that are common to family members and that will tend to make family members alike (but that can cause between-family differences in the population). While the relative importance of E_s and E_{ns} can change with age, perhaps unexpectedly, it is not E_s, but E_{ns}, that seems to account for much of the nongenetic variance we find for many complex human traits (Eaves *et al.*, 1989; Plomin & Bergeman, 1991; Plomin *et al.*, 1997; Rowe, 1994).

For instance, if we consider the proportion of variance or liability for DRD, autism, and ADHD that is accounted for by nongenetic factors, most is explained by nonshared influences. In other words, although each of these disorders has a significant environmental component, this component seems to represent non-shared events such as pre- or perinatal accidents, trauma, infection, or some other unknown event not shared by members of the same family or, if shared, an event that affects family members in different ways.

Research indicating that E_{ns}, and not E_s, is typically a more important contributor to individual differences in many behaviors is contrary to the intuitive belief about the role of parental and sibling environments in behavioral development (Plomin *et al.*, 1997; Rowe, 1994). However, there has been some confusion over the implications of this general finding. This research does not mean that the family environment is unimportant. Children do learn a lot from parents and siblings, and there is little doubt that these familial experiences contribute significantly to behavioral development. The key point is that, even if family members are raised in the same home, all members will not necessarily perceive, react, or learn in identical ways even when given similar experiences. Thus, for example, the environment created by an aggressive or angry father does not necessarily teach aggressive behaviors in the same way to all of his sons and daughters. Similarly, two brothers with autism are not alike because of their cold and detached mother. If, in fact, E_s sorts of effects were practically and statistically significant, then we could theoretically identify the major environmental causes of these disorders and provide treatment or prevention (e.g., provide parents with parenting skills that would ameliorate ADHD or autism in their children). Unfortunately, the lack of success in identifying environmental factors that have major and consistent effects comes in part from their E_{ns} nature (Rowe, 1994).

2. Genotype–Environment Correlations Revisited

Human behavioral genetics also highlights the potential confounding of genes and environments in social science research, namely, human behavioral genetics has shown how passive genotype–environment correlations may underlie and confound many of the conclusions drawn from standard psychological research that has used family samples.

Behavioral genetics reminds us that, in families, the environment created by the parents and passed on to their offspring is partly a reflection of the parents' genes. Because genes (as well as environments) are passed on to and affect offspring family data can confound genetic and nongenetic effects. This confounding or correlation between parental genes and environments is the essence of a passive genotype–environment correlation (Hardy-Brown & Plomin, 1985; Plomin et al., 1997). Because of this potential correlation, an association between an apparent environmental factor in the home and a child's behavior may not be a phenomenon of learning or experience. Instead, it may be a consequence of the genes transmitted from the parent to the child, the effects of which will manifest themselves in the child's development as well as in the home environment the parent creates (Rowe, 1994).

So why is this concept important? It is important because it makes consumers of research more aware that experiments that do not unambiguously separate genetic from environmental effects transmitted in families may be drawing erroneous conclusions. We may assume, for instance, that the offspring of parents with DRD become poor readers because of an inadequate reading environment that the parents with DRD create (e.g., few books in the home, poor parental modeling of reading, disinterest in advancing literacy skills). But, in fact, research suggests that parent–child similarity for DRD is a reflection of shared genes and not a shared family environment.

Other good illustrations of this potential confound can be found in the language development literature (Gilger, 1995). For example, several environmental risk factors in families that are predictive of poor communication skills in young children have been identified (Molfese, 1989; Stromswold, 1998; Tomblin et al., 1991). Among these risk factors are low or poor values for parental educational achievement level, familial linguistic environment, socioeconomic status, and parental IQ. According to the literature, the worse a parent scores on these factors, the greater the risk that children in these families will develop a language or communication problem. Prior work in this area has traditionally interpreted these parent–offspring environmental correlations in terms of how the environment created by the parent can adversely affect the child's acquisition of communication skills, and there is little doubt that in some ways this is a valid conclusion. However, behavioral genetic studies strongly suggest that a large proportion of the variance shared between parental levels on these factors and offspring communicative competence may be due to the genes passed from parents to their children, rather than the environment the parents create (Gilger, 1995; Plomin et al., 1997; Rowe, 1994, 1997). These shared genes may influence IQ, general language competence, and educational attainment in both parents and their children. So the observed correlation between, say, a mother's verbal IQ test score and the verbal test score of her child do not necessarily tell us about the underlying

causal relations regardless of how plausible or intuitively appealing an environmental hypothesis may seem. Experimental designs other than simple family
studies are needed to better partition genetic and environmental effects, such as
twin and adoption projects.

D. THE BASIS OF THE ASSOCIATION AMONG VARIOUS DISORDERS, INCLUDING THOSE OF READING, ATTENTION, OR ACTIVITY, AND AUTISM

Up to this point, the major discussion has revolved around univariate analyses.
Advances in theory, statistics, and computer tools also allow for multivariate
analyses. Rather than simply considering the h^2 or e^2 of traits one by one,
multivariate analysis allows us to consider the basis for the covariance often
observed among traits, namely, it has allowed us to ask questions about the basis
for cognitive or personality profiles, and the basis of the comorbidity so often
reported in medicine and psychiatry (Gilger & Pennington, 1995; Nigg & Goldsmith, 1998; Plomin *et al.*, 1997).

Definitional Issues in Psychiatry

Questions pertaining to symptom or disease heterogeneity, symptom boundaries, and comorbidity for ADHD, DRD, and autism have been investigated (Gilger
& Pennington, 1995; McGuffin *et al.*, 1994; Nigg & Goldsmith, 1998; Plomin *et
al.*, 1997). By and large, these studies suggest that these associations are due to
some extent to significant shared genetic variance, that is, these disorders co-occur
more frequently in individuals than predicted by chance because they have genes
in common.

Still other research has helped refine symptom boundaries and may lead us
toward identifiable subtypes of psychiatric and learning disorders like schizophrenia and depression, as well as DRD, ADHD, and autism (Gottesman, 1991;
McGuffin *et al.*, 1994; Reus & Freimer, 1997). Interesting findings in this area
concern the symptom boundaries of autism and ADHD.

Studies of families ascertained through a proband with autism have suggested
that the disorder may lie on a continuum or a spectrum of autistic-like behaviors
or syndromes (McGuffin *et al.*, 1994). Often, these studies show that family
members may display autism or a variety of subtle, autistic-like behaviors such
as social deficits. Moreover, family members may show an even broader range of
cognitive and learning disabilities, especially in the speech–language domain
(Piven *et al.*, 1990).

Similarly, in studies looking at the families of probands with ADHD, a variety
of other behavioral or cognitive disorders often aggregate in addition to ADHD,
and it is common for relatives to display more than one problem (i.e., comorbidity). Family studies of various forms have found ADHD to be associated with
conduct, oppositional and antisocial behaviors, tic disorders (e.g., Tourette syndrome), and, of course, learning problems like DRD (DeFries & Gillis, 1993;

189

Faraone *et al.*, 1991; Gillis *et al.*, 1992; Nigg & Goldsmith, 1998; Pauls *et al.*, 1993; Pennington, 1991; Smith *et al.*, 1996).

Together, the family research on ADHD and autism suggests that these two disorders may have a broader phenotype than was once thought. One way to think of this is that there may be genes that predispose people toward the development of a number of cognitive or behavioral problems, sometimes culminating in ADHD or autism. However, the expression of these genes varies, probably depending on the effects of other genes and environmental factors. Family and genetic research may eventually lead us to an understanding of these complexities and identify what the underlying liability is as well as how and why it is expressed in different ways. This knowledge, in turn, may guide us to better diagnostic and treatment methods.

Before closing, one other interesting comorbidity finding deserves mention. Immune-related disorders such as allergies and autoimmune diseases may occur more frequently in persons with DRD, autism, and ADHD, as well as in their relatives (Bryden *et al.*, 1994; Gilger & Pennington, 1995). Again, the basis of this comorbidity is a complex issue, and some researchers debate if the comorbidity even exists. Still, it is an intriguing finding and may have some support based on neurodevelopmental theory (Bryden *et al.*, 1994). But for now, it is unclear if the comorbidity is due to shared genes that affect both the immune system and neurodevelopment, if it is a reflection of some unknown but shared environmental event, if the research suggesting significant comorbidity is flawed somehow, or some other explanation (Gilger & Pennington, 1995).

E. DISORDERS OF READING, ATTENTION, OR ACTIVITY, AND AUTISM VERSUS NORMAL VARIATION IN RELATED SKILLS

Many psychometrically assessed traits or complex phenotypes yield a continuous distribution from low to high. This continuum is often unimodal and fairly normal, with the fewest percentage of individuals scoring at the extreme ends (see Figure 9.1). Examples of such traits include intelligence and reading, as well as quantitatively measured levels of activity and personality (Eaves *et al.*, 1989; Matarazzo & Pankeratz, 1980; Minton & Schneider, 1985). Depending on the phenotype and scale, the higher or lower a person's score lies on these continua, the more likely a person is to have clinically significant problems. Indeed, an important part of the operational definition of many clinical disorders like DRD and ADHD is falling beyond an extreme threshold on some continuous trait distribution.

There is some controversy regarding whether the etiology of the extreme lower (or higher) tail of a trait continuum is distinct from the etiology of normal variation in the rest of the distribution. The resolution of this question has implications for our understanding of the nature of behavioral extremes as well as our nosological approaches to the definition of behavioral disorders or psychiatric disease.

As was mentioned previously, the quantitative MFP model assumes that many genes with small, equal, and additive effects act together with a variety of environmental factors to produce the range of phenotypes observed. In agreement with an MFP model, there are data to suggest that some disorders may simply represent the extreme values on a normal continuum, where all points on the scale are influenced by the same multifactorial etiologic agents (Eaves *et al.*, 1989; Plomin & Rende, 1991). On the other hand, there is also evidence that the etiology of extremes for other traits may be unique, for example, very low intelligence appears to differ in etiology from the rest of the continuum of intelligence in the population (Achenbach, 1982; Penrose, 1963). Specifically, unique etiologic agents (i.e., major disease genes or chromosomal abnormalities) seem to be more prevalent in individuals with IQs less than 50 compared to individuals with IQs in the rest of the range.

Researchers have begun to study empirically the common assumption that other communicative, psychological, or cognitive disorders are of unique etiology separate from the etiology of related phenotypes within the normal range. There are a number of methods available to test this assumption, including molecular genetics, and some or all of them have been applied to DRD and ADHD. Although the results are a bit ambiguous regarding ADHD, in large part they support that DRD is not of unique etiology and may represent part of the normal continuum of reading skills (Gilger *et al.*, 1996a,b; Plomin *et al.*, 1997; Smith *et al.*, 1996, 1998). An oligogenic or QTL model of susceptibility to DRD is currently favored (see the following section).

In contrast is a study by Dale *et al.* (1998). They applied the DeFries–Fulker twin method (DeFries & Fulker, 1988) to vocabulary test data obtained from a large sample of 3-year-old twins and found that the genetic and nongenetic factors operating on the vocabulary skills of toddlers at the very low end of the continuum were different from the factors influencing the vocabulary abilities of toddlers within the normal range. In other words, there were separate etiologic distributions subsumed under what was believed to be a single unimodal distribution of vocabulary skill. The situation suggested by the Dale *et al.* report is depicted in Figure 9.2 (Gilger, 1998).

II. MOLECULAR WORK AND HUMAN BEHAVIORAL GENETICS

Although traditional quantitative genetic approaches to the study of human behavior will continue to be important, the advent and success of the Human Genome Project point the way to a new type of behavioral genetic research: the ability to map, identify, and eventually clone the specific genes that affect complex human phenotypes. This has exciting potential.

Finding specific genes with significant effects at the molecular level for phenotypes like DRD, autism, and ADHD was generally unimaginable until fairly recently. One approach to gene searches is, in a sense, a compromise between the traditionally distinct schools of Mendelian (single gene) and MFP models. This approach looks for genes that additively increase susceptibility to a disorder but do not necessarily have major effects. These types of genes are called Quantitative

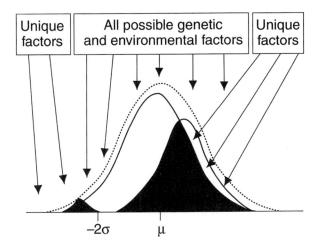

FIGURE 9.2   Separate etiologic distributions subsumed under what was believed to be a single unimodal distribution of vocabulary skill.

Trait Loci (QTL) (Gelderman, 1975; Plomin *et al.*, 1994). The key difference between a classic MFP or Mendelian system and QTL is that in the latter case genes of varying effect size are responsible for heritable aspects of the variance in a quantitative phenotype (or underlying liability for expression of a qualitative phenotype like autism). In other words, there may be an unknown number of genes underlying a trait like reading ability or disability, but there may be substantial variability in the proportion of trait variance each gene accounts for; some of the key loci can have large effects and some can have small effects, but all together these QTL add up in various combinations to produce a continuum of trait variability or liability.

Large-scale and international collaborations have begun to study a variety of human behaviors using QTL approaches motivated in part by the successful application of the approach to continuous traits in plants and nonhuman animals (Gelderman, 1975; Lander & Botstein, 1989). For instance, quantitative and molecular QTL methods have shown that reading disability is not governed by a classic MFP system. Rather, it appears that the disorder reflects the effects of a limited number of QTL and that the extreme low end of the reading ability distribution where dyslexia is diagnosed is an expression of the same etiologic factors, as is the rest of the distribution (Gilger *et al.*, 1996a,b; Smith *et al.*, 1998). With regard to the actual location of these QTL, the most reliable finding reported thus far for DRD is that at least one gene (or quantitative trait locus) is on chromosome 6 (Smith *et al.*, 1998). Although not as well replicated as the chromosome 6 results, other QTL for DRD may lie on chromosomes 15, 1, and 2, and perhaps others (Froster *et al.*, 1993; Grigorenko *et al.*, 1997; Lubs *et al.*, 1993; Smith *et al.*, 1998). These QTL, genes, or "susceptibility alleles," modify a person's liability for a reading disorder. While the general locations of DRD QTL may be known (although not precisely), we do not understand what the precise nature of these genes is or what protein they produce that affects brain growth or function.

Interestingly, QTL for autism, ADHD, and other disorders have also been tentatively located on chromosome 6 (Alsobrook & Pauls, 1998; Daniels *et al.*, 1998; Plomin *et al.*, 1994). That in at least one region on 6 is a major complex of genes that modify the human immune system may be of more than passing interest given the literature previously described where an association between immune system disorders and DRD, ADHD, and autism have been reported (Gilger & Pennington, 1995).[1]

The DRD molecular genetic QTL research has already been described, and similar searches for the locations of genes responsible for ADHD and autism have also been conducted or are in progress. Genetic research on ADHD and autism, more so than DRD, has also taken another approach to gene searches. Rather than searching blindly in hopes of hitting the correct chromosomal area containing a gene affecting the phenotype of interest, some studies of ADHD and autism have started with a known gene that affects brain development and function and looked to see if this gene is somehow defective or different in populations of individuals with autism or ADHD. This is sometimes called the candidate gene approach (Crowe, 1993).

Various candidate genes have been studied to see if they influence the liability to, or expression of, ADHD and autism (Alsobrook & Pauls, 1998; Blum & Noble, 1997). Although the results are not conclusive, some studies have reported associations between ADHD and dopamine receptor–transporter genes, monoamine oxidase A, serotonin receptor genes, dopamine conversion enzyme genes, among others. For autism, dopamine gene systems, c–Harvey–RAs oncogene (affects signal transduction pathways, but apparently not in the brain), and the DRB1 region of the human leukocyte antigen gene system (see Chapter 2) on chromosome 6 have all been implicated, yet none definitely so. Whether these candidate genes become confirmed contributors to these disorders awaits future research. However, it is clear that whatever contribution these genes make they do not explain all of the disorder liability or expression—there are definitely other genetic and nongenetic components that need to be identified.

III. TOWARD THE FUTURE

In this chapter, I have summarized five general areas in which human behavioral genetics has contributed significantly to our understanding of behavior in general and DRD, autism, and ADHD in particular. In closing, there are several

---

[1]At the time this manuscript is going to press, several genes thought to contribute to the liability for autism have been found. See <www.nichd.gov/autism/>.

issues perhaps worth considering as the field of human behavioral genetics moves into the twenty-first century.

First, quantitative genetic methods are not obsolete. Unfortunately, many researchers have jumped on the molecular genetics bandwagon and foregone the important information that can be gleaned from quantitative work. For example, because of the careful quantitative work on DRD, we are able to fully describe its inheritance, provide clinically useful data as to risk and prognosis, and think critically about how the genetics of the disorder act in neural development, phenotypic expression, and the development of reading skills in general (Gilger et al., 1996a,b; Olson et al., 1994; Pennington, 1997; Pennington & Gilger, 1996; Smith et al., 1996). We would have none of this important information if we skipped this quantitative work in favor of molecular gene searches. Traditional human behavioral genetics work should be used conjointly with molecular work in the future to tell us where we should be going and how the genes we find operate.

Second, in the future it must be remembered that behavioral genetics has shown us that the pathway from gene to human behavior is dynamic and complex (Gilger, 1995). Different genes turn on and off or change in relative effect at different times in our lives, genes interact with each other and with the environment, genes do not lead directly to behaviors, and so on. Understanding the complexities of this pathway as they influence expression of, or risk for, communicative disorders, DRD, autism, and ADHD is an essential although very difficult task facing us in the future.

Third, it is notable that collaborations between animal and human researchers are ongoing. Animal research is proving valuable to our discovery of genes for a range of phenotypes in humans including Alzheimer disease, hearing impairments, personality, alcoholism, epilepsy, and obesity among many others (Jones & Mormede, 1999; Pfaff et al., 1999). Animal models of human behavior are powerful means to ascertain candidate genes or loci because of the controls and experimental crosses that can be applied, including selection studies and knockout genetics (Capecchi, 1994). That animal and human genomes often have a great deal of homology is fortunate, and bridges between animal and human genetics will and should continue to grow.

Animal research will also be needed in the future to help us understand how we go from the molecular structure of genes to gene products, to neurological growth and function, and ultimately to behavior. Ironically, the excitement of the potential of the Human Genome Project is, in some ways, misleading: finding genes and loci will be relatively (not absolutely) easy with the automated techniques now available. As mentioned previously, the real problem will be ascribing the gene to behavior pathways for complex behaviors, especially how these pathways include environmental factors and gene–gene or genotype–environment interactions.

ACKNOWLEDGMENTS

During the preparation of this manuscript, the author was supported in part by a University of Kansas GRF Grant.

REFERENCES

Achenbach, T. M. (1982). *Developmental psychopathology* (2nd ed.). New York: Wiley.

Alsobrook, J. P., & Pauls, D. (1998). Molecular approaches to child psychopathology. *Human Biology, 70*, 413–432.

Anastasi, A. (1958). Hereditary, environment, and the question of "How?". *Psychological Review, 65*, 197–208.

Bailey, A., Phillips, W., & Rutter, M. (1996). Autism: Towards an integration of clinical, genetic, neuropsychological and neurobiological perspectives. *Journal of Child Psychology and Psychiatry, 37*, 89–126.

Biederman, J., Munir, K., Knee, D., Habelow, W., Armentano, M., Autor, S., Hoge, S. K., & Waternaux, C. (1986). A family study of patients with attention deficit disorder and normal controls. *Journal of Psychiatric Research, 20*, 263–274.

Blangero, J. (1993). Statistical genetic approaches to human adaptability. *Human Biology, 65*, 941–966.

Blum, K., & Noble, E. P. (1997). *Handbook of psychiatric genetics.* New York: CRC.

Bolton, P., MacDonald, H., Pickles, A., Rios, P., Goode, S., Crowson, M., Bailey, A., & Rutter, M. (1994). A case-control family history study of autism. *Journal of Child Psychology and Psychiatry, 35*, 877–900.

Bouchard, T. J., & Propping, P. (Eds.) (1993). *Twins as a tool of behavioral genetics.* New York: Wiley.

Bryden, M. P., McManus, I. C., & Bulman-Fleming, M. B. (1994). Evaluating the empirical support for the Geschwind–Behan–Galaburda model of cerebral localization. *Brain and Cognition, 26*, 103–167.

Capecchi, M. R. (1994, March). Targeted gene replacement. *Scientific American*, 52–59.

Chandola, C. A., Robling, M. R., Peters, T. J., Melvill-Thomas, G., & McGuffin, P. (1992). Pre- and peri-natal factors and the risk of subsequent referral for hyperactivity. *Journal of Child Psychology and Psychiatry, 33*, 1077–1090.

Crowe, R. R. (1993). Candidate genes in psychiatry: An epidemiological perspective. *American Journal of Medical Genetics, 48*, 74–77.

Dale, P. S., Simonoff, E., Bishop, D. V. M., Eley, T. C., Oliver, B., Price, T. S., Purcell, S., Stevenson, J., & Plomin, R. (1998). Genetic influence of language delay in two-year-old children. *Nature: Neuroscience, 1*, 324–328.

Daniels, J., McGuffin, P., Owen, M. J., & Plomin, R. (1998). Molecular genetic studies of cognitive ability. *Human Biology, 70*, 281–296.

DeFries, J. C., & Fulker, D. W. (1988). Multiple regression analysis of twin data: Etiology of deviant scores versus individual differences. *Acta Geneticae Medicae et Gemellologiae, 37*, 205–216.

DeFries, J. C., & Gillis, J. (1993). Genetics of reading disability. In R. Plomin & G. McClearn (Eds.), *Nature, nurture, and psychology* (pp. 59–76). Washington, DC: APA Press.

Eaves, L. J., Eysenck, H. J., & Martin, N. G. (1989). *Genes, culture, and personality: An empirical approach.* San Diego: Academic Press.

Falconer, D. S. (1981). *Introduction to quantitative genetics* (2nd ed.). London: Longman.

Faraone, S. V., Biederman, J., Keenan, K., & Tsuang, M. T. (1991). Separation of DSM-III attention deficit disorders and conduct disorder: Evidence from a family genetic study of American child psychiatric patients. *Psychological Medicine, 21*, 109–121.

Filipek, P. A. (1995). Neurobiological correlates of developmental dyslexia: How do dyslexics' brains differ from those of normal readers? *Journal of Child Neurology, 10*(Suppl. 1), S62–S67.

Fisher, R. A. (1918). The correlation between relatives on the supposition of Mendelian inheritance. *Transactions of the Royal Society of Edinburgh, 52,* 399–433.

Folstein, S., & Rutter, M. (1977). Infantile autism: A genetic study of 21 twin pairs. *Journal of Child Psychology and Psychiatry, 18,* 297–321.

Froster, U., Schultz-Korne, J., Hedebrand, J., & Remschmidt, H. (1993). Cosegregation of balanced translocation (1;2) with retarded speech development and dyslexia. *Lancet, 342,* 178–179.

Fuller, J. L., & Simmel, E. C. (Eds.) (1983). *Behavior genetics: Principles and applications.* Hillsdale, NJ: Erlbaum.

Fuller, J., & Thompson, W. (1978). *Foundations of behavior genetics.* St. Louis: Mosby.

Gelderman, H. (1975). Investigations on inheritance of quantitative characters in animals by gene markers, I: Methods. *Theoretical and applied genetics, 46,* 319–330.

Gilger, J. W. (1995). Behavioral genetics: Concepts for research in language and language disabilities. *Journal of Speech and Hearing Research, 38,* 1126–1142.

Gilger, J. W. (1998). Late talking toddlers may have special genes. *Nature (Medicine), 4,* 7–8.

Gilger, J. W., & Hershberger, S. (1998). Introduction to special issue on human behavioral genetics: Synthesis of quantitative and molecular approaches. *Human Biology, 70,* 155–157.

Gilger, J. W., & Pennington, B. F. (1995). Why associations among traits do not necessarily indicate their common etiology: A comment on the Geschwind–Behan–Galaburda model. *Brain & Cognition, 27,* 89–93.

Gilger, J. W., Pennington, B. F., & DeFries, J. C. (1991). Risk for reading disabilities as a function of parental history in three samples of families. *Reading and Writing, 3,* 205–217.

Gilger, J. W., Borecki, I., Smith, S. D., DeFries, J. C., & Pennington, B. F. (1996a). The etiology of extreme scores for complex phenotypes: An illustration using reading performance. In C. Chase, G. Rosen, & G. Sherman (Eds.), *Developmental dyslexia: Neural, cognitive and genetic mechanisms* (pp. 63–85). Baltimore: York.

Gilger, J. W., Hanebuth, E., Smith, S. D., & Pennington, B. F. (1996b). Differential risk for developmental reading disorders in the offspring of compensated versus noncompensated parents. *Reading and Writing: An Interdisciplinary Journal, 8,* 407–417.

Gilger, J. W., Ho, H-Z., Whipple, A., & Spitz, R. (in review). Gene–environment correlations for typically and atypically developing children aged 2–12 years.

Gillis, J., Gilger, J. W., Pennington, B. F., & DeFries, J. C. (1992). Attention deficit hyperactivity disorder in reading disabled twins: Evidence for a genetic etiology. *Journal of Abnormal Child Psychology, 20,* 303–316.

Gottesman, I. I. (1991). *Schizophrenia genesis: The origins of madness.* New York: Freeman.

Grigorenko, E. L., Wood, F. B., Meyer, M. S., Hart, L. A., Speed, W. C., Shuster, A., & Pauls, D. L. (1997). Susceptibility loci for distinct components of developmental dyslexia on chromosomes 6 and 15. *American Journal of Human Genetics, 60,* 27–39.

Hardy-Brown, K., & Plomin, R. (1985). Infant communicative development: Evidence from adoptive and biological families for genetic and environmental influences on rate differences. *Developmental Psychology, 21,* 378–385.

Hardy-Brown, K., Plomin, R., & DeFries, J. C. (1981). Genetic and environmental influences on the rate of communicative development in the first year of life. *Developmental Psychology, 17,* 704–717.

Heath, A., & Madden, P. F. (1995). Genetic influences on smoking behavior. In J. R. Turner, L. R. Cardon, & J. K. Hewitt (Eds.), *Behavior genetic approaches in behavioral medicine* (pp. 45–66). New York: Plenum.

Jones, B. C., & Mormede, P. (Eds.) (1999). *Neurobehavioral genetics: Methods and applications.* Boca Raton, FL: CRC.

Jones, M. B., & Szatmari, P. (1988). Stoppage rules and genetic studies of autism. *Journal of Autism and Developmental Disorders, 18,* 31–40.

Lander, E. S., & Botstein, D. (1989). Mapping Mendelian factors underlying quantitative traits using RFLP linkage maps. *Genetics, 121,* 185–199.

Lubs, H. A., Rabin, M., Feldman, E., Jallad, B. J., Kushch, A., & Gross-Glenn, K. (1993). Familial dyslexia: Genetic and medical findings in eleven three-generation families. *Annals of Dyslexia, 43,* 44–60.

Lykken, D. T. (1982). Research with twins: The concept of emergenesis. *Psychophysiology, 19,* 361–373.

Lyons, M. J., True, W., Eisen, S., Goldberg, J., Meyer, J. M., Faraone, S., Eaves, L. J., & Tsuang, M. T. (1995). Differential heritability of adult and juvenile antisocial traits. *Archives of General Psychiatry, 52,* 906–915.

Matarazzo, J. D., & Pankeratz, L. D. (1980). Intelligence. In R. H. Woody (Ed.), *Encyclopedia of clinical assessment* (pp. 697–713). San Francisco: Jossey-Bass.

McGuffin, P., Owen, M. J., O'Donovan, M. C., Thapar, A., & Gottesman, I. I. (1994). *Seminars in Psychiatric Genetics.* London: Royal College of Psychiatrists.

Minton, H., & Schneider, F. (1985). *Differential psychology.* Prospect Heights, IL: Waveland.

Molfese, V. J. (1989). *Perinatal risk and infant development: Assessment and prediction.* New York: Guilford.

Neale, M., & Cardon, L. (1992). *Methodology for genetic studies of twins and families.* Dordrecht, The Netherlands: Kluwer.

Nigg, J., & Goldsmith, H. H. (1998). Developmental psychopathology, personality, and temperament: Reflections on recent behavior. *Human Biology, 70,* 387–412.

Olson, R. L., Forsberg, H., & Wise, B. (1994). Genes, environment and the development of orthographic skills. In V. W. Berninger (Ed.), *The varieties of orthographic knowledge,* Vol. 1: *Theoretical and developmental issues* (pp. 27–71). Dordecht, The Netherlands: Kluwer Press.

Pauls, D., Leckman, J. F., & Cohen, D. J. (1993). Familial relationship between Gilles de la Tourette's syndrome, attention deficit disorder, learning disabilities, speech disorders and stuttering. *Journal of the American Academy of Child and Adolescent Psychiatry, 32,* 1044–1050.

Pennington, B. F. (1991). *Diagnosing learning disorders: A neuropsychological framework.* New York: Guilford.

Pennington, B. F. (1997). Using genetics to dissect cognition. *American Journal of Human Genetics, 60,* 13–16.

Pennington, B. F., & Gilger, J. W. (1996). How is dyslexia transmitted? In C. Chase, G. Rosen, & G. Sherman (Eds.), *Neural and cognitive mechanisms underlying speech, language and reading* (pp. 41–62). Baltimore: York.

Penrose, L. S. (1963). *The biology of mental defect* (3rd ed.). London: Sidgwick & Jackson.

Pfaff, D. W., Berrettini, W. H., Joh, T. H., & Maxson, S. C. (Eds.) (1999). *Genetic influences on neural and behavioral functions.* Boca Raton, FL: CRC.

Piven, J., Gayle, J., Chase, G., Fink, B., Landa, R., Wzorek, M. M., & Folstein, S. E. (1990). A family history of neuropsychiatric disorders in the adult siblings of autistic individuals. *Journal of the American Academy of Child and Adolescent Psychiatry, 29,* 177–184.

Plomin, R. (1986). *Development, genetics, and psychology.* Hillsdale, NJ: Erlbaum.

Plomin, R., & Bergeman, C. S. (1991). The nature of nurture: Genetic influence on "environmental" measures. *Behavioral and Brain Sciences, 14,* 373–427.

Plomin, R., & McClearn, G. (Eds.) (1993). *Nature, nurture and psychology.* Washington, DC: APA.

Plomin, R., & Rende, R. (1991). Human behavioral genetics. *Annual Review of Psychology, 42,* 1–66.

Plomin, R., Owen, M. J., & McGuffin, P. (1994). The genetic basis of complex behaviors. *Science, 264*, 1733–1739.

Plomin, R., DeFries, J. C., McClearn, G., & Rutter, M. (1997). *Behavioral genetics: A primer.* New York: Freeman.

Reus, V. L., & Freimer, N. B. (1997). Understanding the genetic basis of mood disorders: Where do we stand? *American Journal of Human Genetics, 60*, 1283–1288.

Riggins-Caspers, K., & Cadoret, R. J. (1999). Detecting and measuring gene–environment interaction in human temperament (aggressivity) and personality deviation (conduct disorder, antisocial personality). In B. Jones & P. Mormede (Eds.), *Neurobehavioral genetics: Methods and applications* (pp. 163–186). New York: CRC.

Rowe, D. C. (1994). *The limits of family influence: Genes, experience, and behavior.* New York: Guilford.

Rowe, D. C. (1997). A place at the policy table? Behavior genetics and estimates of family environmental effects on IQ. *Cognitive Science, 24*, 133–158.

Scarr, S., & McCartney, K. (1983). How people make their own environments: A theory of genotype–environment effects. *Child Development, 54*, 424–435.

Sherman, S. L., DeFries, J. C., Gottesman, I. I., Loehlin, J. C., Meyere, J. M., Pelias, M. Z., Rice, J., & Waldman, I. (1997). ASHG Statement: Recent developments in human behavioral genetics: Past accomplishments and future directions. *American Journal of Human Genetics, 60*, 1265–1275.

Smalley, S. L., Asarnow, R. F., & Spence, M. A. (1988). Autism and genetics: A decade of research. *Archives of General Psychiatry, 45*, 953–961.

Smith, S., Gilger, J., & Pennington, B. (1996). Genetics of learning disorders. In D. Rimoin, J. M. Connor, & R. Pyeritz (Eds.), *Emery and Rimoin's principles and practice of medical genetics* (pp. 1767–1790). New York: Churchill Livingstone,.

Smith, S. D., Kelley, P. M., & Brower, A. M. (1998). Molecular approaches to the genetic analysis of specific reading disability. *Human Biology, 70*, 239–256.

Steffenberg, S., Gillberg, C., Hellgren, L., Andersson, L., Gillberg, I. C., Jakobsson, G., & Bohman, M. (1989). A twin study of autism in Denmark, Finland, Iceland, Norway and Sweden. *Journal of Child Psychology and Psychiatry, 28*, 229–247.

Stromswold, K. (1998). Genetics of spoken language. *Human Biology, 70*, 297–324.

Tomblin, B., Hardy, J. C., & Hein, H. (1991). Predicting poor communication status in preschool children using risk factors present at birth. *Journal of Speech and Hearing Research, 34*, 1096–1105.

Truett, K. R., Eaves, L. J., Meyer, J. M., Heath, A. C., & Martin, N. G. (1992). Religion and education as mediators of attitudes: A multivariate analysis. *Behavior Genetics, 22*, 43–62.

Whalsten, D. (1990). Insensitivity of the analysis of variance to heredity–environment interaction. *Behavioral and Brain Sciences, 13*, 109–161.

10

GENETIC PRIVACY AND ETHICAL, LEGAL, AND SOCIAL ISSUES

SHARON DAVIS

Professional and Family Services
The Arc of the United States
Silver Spring, Maryland

Rapid advances are being made in learning the genetic basis of human disease and disability through Human Genome Project research. With the ability to pinpoint specific genes, scientists are designing diagnostic tests to detect genetic errors in people suspected of having a genetic condition or being at risk of developing one. They hope to be able to treat, cure, or even prevent genetic disorders (see Chapter 11). Unfortunately, many researchers, clinicians, and individuals who will be impacted are unaware of some of the implications of expanded genetic knowledge.

This chapter addresses some of these issues, including those regarding genetic testing, genetic discrimination, and protecting genetic privacy. When genetic information becomes known to third parties, it has implications for affected individuals. Fears of genetic discrimination may be real. Such fears and other social and psychological concerns about one's genetic status may make individuals reluctant to engage in genetic testing or participate in genetic research. Such reluctance may mean they do not receive the benefits of treatments or take precautions to prevent genetic diseases.

I. GENETIC TESTING

The joint National Institutes of Health–Department of Energy Task Force on Genetic Testing (1997) defines a genetic test as "the analysis of human DNA, RNA, chromosomes, proteins, and certain metabolites in order to detect heritable disease-related genotypes, mutations, phenotypes, or karyotypes for clinical purposes" (p. 7). Genetic tests are used to predict risk of disease, identify carriers, and establish prenatal and clinical diagnosis or prognosis. The definition also includes prenatal, newborn, and carrier screening and testing in families with a history of genetic disorders. It does not include genetic tests done solely for research.

One of the concerns of the Task Force on Genetic Testing is that the use of genetic testing is likely to expand rapidly without an accompanying increase in genetic specialists who can interpret tests and counsel individuals about the meaning of the tests. This means that providers with little formal training or experience in genetics will have the burden of interpreting test results and predicting future risks for their patients. These practitioners need to understand that genetic tests present unique problems.

Genetic tests will be used increasingly to predict future disease in healthy people. Yet, the predictions are not always certain, and often no independent test is available to confirm the prediction. The uncertainty of knowing what may happen in the future may cause psychological distress to individuals who learn they have a gene that may or may not result in future disease or disability. The situation is made worse by the fact that genetic tests are being rapidly developed for newly discovered genes, but no treatment is available. Getting positive test results means some people will be forced to make personal decisions about reproduction. Genetic tests are also unique in that they reveal information about risk of future disease in healthy relatives of the person tested. Providers need to know how to communicate genetic risks to relatives while keeping results confidential. Finally, some ethnic groups may be concerned about discrimination and stigmatization because of their heightened risk of certain genetic conditions. This needs to be taken into consideration when they are counseled (NIH–DOE Task Force on Genetic Testing, 1997).

In addition to not having enough genetic counselors who are knowledgeable about the implications of genetic testing, there are concerns about the tests themselves. They are not 100% accurate. Some tests have a large number of false positive results; others fail to detect the gene. The cost-effectiveness of the test is another issue. It may be too expensive for broad use. Furthermore, not all tests in use have been validated in broad populations. There are concerns that the demand for a test will be greater than effective delivery, and there may not be enough laboratories that are proficient in assuring accuracy and quality control. There are also problems with test interpretation, as many commercially available gene tests are still controversial. Many professionals are struggling with their interpretation and thus their usefulness as diagnostic tests (Welch & Burke, 1998).

Clearly, genetic knowledge has implications for practitioners, researchers, and families who deal with communicative disorders. They should know about the legal and social issues related to genetic discrimination and the potential effects on an individual's life. There are ethical issues related to maintaining confidentiality of genetic information and issues related to informed consent in testing and genetic research. Before consenting to testing or research participation, all involved should understand the implications of having genetic knowledge that is not kept confidential. These are topics that have arisen in the 1990s, instigated by the federal funding allocated to examining ethical, legal, and social issues related to the Human Genome Project.

II. GENETIC DISCRIMINATION

A major concern about having knowledge of one's genetic status is that of discrimination. Genetic discrimination describes the differential treatment of individuals or their relatives based on their actual or presumed genetic differences as distinguished from discrimination based on having symptoms of a genetic-based disease (Geller *et al.*, 1996). In other words, genetic discrimination is not based on having a disability, but based on having a gene that may (or may not) cause the person to show symptoms of a disability sometime in the future. It is aimed at people who appear healthy or whose symptoms are so mild that their functioning and health are not affected.

Discrimination based on genetic characteristics includes those individuals who have a gene or genes predisposing them or their offspring to developing disease, conditions, or late-onset disorders. Late-onset refers to disorders that may not show visible signs until late in the individual's life. One example is Huntington disease, a progressive genetic disorder characterized by late-onset neurological symptoms typically arising in the third to fourth decade of life. Men and women who are carriers for a genetic condition (who show no signs of disease) may also be discriminated against because of their potential to have children with genetic conditions. Errors in our genes are responsible for an estimated 4000 clearly hereditary diseases and conditions (U.S. Department of Energy and the Human Genome Project, 1996), many (or possibly most) affecting communication. For example, Frances S. Collins, Director of the National Institute for Human Genome Research (1995), estimates that each person carries "four to five really fouled-up genes and another couple of dozen that are not so great and place the person at risk for something" (p. 16).

A. EXAMPLES OF DISCRIMINATION

In a 1993 survey (Geller *et al.*, 1996), 455 people known to have defective genes, but who had no symptoms, reported having experienced genetic discrimination. Just over 200 of these respondents were interviewed. People contacted were individuals who had or were at risk to develop a genetic condition or were parents who had a child with a genetic condition. They reported discrimination by health and life insurance companies, clinical professionals, adoption agencies, armed services, employers, educational institutions, and blood banks.

One of the most common forms of discrimination is denial of health insurance based on a person's genes. Insurance companies gather and use medical information to predict a person's risk of illness and death. They use this risk information to determine which individuals and groups they will insure and at what price. That information plays a critical role for people in determining access to health care. In the Geller *et al.* study (1996), people who were asymptomatic were denied health insurance. Some individuals or families were treated differently once the genetic diagnosis was established. Some group insurance plans refused to provide coverage for qualified individuals with a genetic diagnosis, and in a few cases, relatives of an individual with a presumed genetic disease lost their insurance coverage. People were also denied life insurance because of their genes.

Employment is another area with reported cases of discrimination. Many individuals believe they were not hired or were fired because they were at risk for genetic conditions. In other cases, individuals who were employed were reluctant to change jobs because they feared losing health insurance coverage (Geller *et al.*, 1996). Their worries are well founded. Alpert (1993) reported that one employer study found that 50% of companies surveyed used medical records in making employment-related decisions. Another study (Office of Technology Assessment, 1991) found that many companies will not hire people with a preexisting medical condition.

Discrimination has also occurred when medical professionals counseled individuals about childbearing by urging prenatal diagnostic testing or telling them they should not have children. One HMO told a pregnant woman whose fetus tested positive for cystic fibrosis that it would cover the cost of an abortion, but would not cover the infant under the family's medical policy if she elected to carry the pregnancy to term (McGoodwin, 1996). Similarly, some adoption agencies have unfairly treated prospective parents with a genetic condition by refusing adoption or assuming they should adopt only children at risk of inheriting a disability. In other situations, one person with a 50% chance of developing Huntington disease was discharged from the armed services even though he was asymptomatic. A few children were denied opportunities in school because of a perceived genetic abnormality. Some people with hemochromatosis were rejected as blood donors when there was no medical reason to reject the blood (Geller *et al.*, 1996).

The possibility of being a victim of genetic discrimination is beginning to be recognized by the public. Articles have appeared in the popular press describing instances of discrimination. Congress has debated legislation governing privacy, as have state legislatures. As a result, people who fear potential genetic discrimination may be discouraged from obtaining genetic information that could bring health benefits to them and their families.

B. PROTECTION FROM DISCRIMINATION

The concern about possible genetic discrimination has led legislators in a number of states to pass laws banning genetic discrimination in health insurance and employment. The federal Health Insurance Portability and Accountability Act of 1996 (PL 104-191) offers protections to some people in health insurance by limiting preexisting condition exclusions. It also prohibits discrimination against individuals based on health status, including their genetic information.

The interest in regulating the uses of genetic information and offering special protections to guard its privacy is based on two arguments. One is that genetic tests may predict future risks for healthy persons, and the second is that these tests may infer risk about relatives (Reilly, 1997). Others also argue that genetic discrimination is wrong because we are powerless to change our hereditary characteristics. There is precedent in according a higher level of protection to some forms of medical records. Those currently regarded as requiring more privacy are psychiatric records and HIV test results. Reilly (1997) argued that, if genetic testing permeates medical care in the next 20 years, it will be very difficult to implement a law that requires separate treatment of a portion of many people's medical records. He points out that nearly everyone would benefit from enactment of a general medical privacy law covering access to and use of all health information. The draft rules, which go into effect in February 2002, apply only to computerized records, not those kept on paper. They would limit the release of information without the patient's consent, require health plans to tell patients how their information is being used, and give patients access to their records and the right to make corrections (Mohammed, 1999).

The Americans with Disabilities Act (ADA) offers protection from discrimination to individuals currently affected by a genetic condition or disease. It also applies to individuals who are regarded as having a disability. The Equal Employment Opportunity Commission (EEOC), which oversees enforcement of nondiscrimination in employment, has ruled (1995) that ADA applies specifically to individuals who are subjected to discrimination on the basis of genetic information relating to illness, disease, condition, or other disorders. This interpretation extends coverage to people who have genes making them predisposed to a disease that may cause disability or who have genes for a late-onset disorder. However, it may not protect carriers of genetic disorders who do not manifest symptoms of the disease (the unaffected carrier). They may be discriminated against based on concerns about health costs of future affected dependents.

The Americans with Disabilities Act does not cover the insurance industry. Insurance companies may deny health, life, disability, and other forms of insurance to people with defective genes if there is a sound basis for determining risks consistent with state law. Health maintenance organizations can also refuse to cover an individual with a genetic diagnosis even if the individual has no symptoms of the genetic disorder, provided there is a sound basis for the decision based on actual risk experience (Alper & Natowicz, 1993).

III. GENETIC PRIVACY

Genetic discrimination can be reduced if an individual's genetic status remains private. Genetic privacy means that individuals have the right to decide what genetic information others can know and what they want to know about themselves (The Arc, 1997). The importance of protecting privacy of medical records is not new, but protecting genetic privacy has its own set of issues.

A person's genes can tell a lot about that person. Employers, insurance companies, educational institutions, adoption agencies, and others can find out what conditions or diseases a person may have or be predisposed to getting. However, genetic test results can be misinterpreted by such organizations that are unfamiliar with genetics and the correct interpretation of the results of such tests. Having a gene for a certain condition does not necessarily mean the individual will ever show symptoms of the condition. This is a fact insurance companies and prospective employers may not know and thus incorrectly assume the presence of a condition (The Arc, 1997).

People who learn that they have a gene that places them at increased risk for certain diseases face the dilemma of whether to tell other family members about their potential susceptibility to disease. This information is relevant to their biological relatives, for other family members may also have the gene and be at increased risk. It also has implications for family members being at risk of genetic discrimination, since genetic information about an individual is also information about that person's family.

In addition to these problems, genetic testing provides highly sensitive health-related information that some individuals believe is important to know and others choose not to know. Genetic information is significantly different from other medical information since genetic testing often involves other family members who may or may not want to know or do not want to provide genetic information. When family members are tested, those who have negative test results may feel survivor guilt for knowing they do not carry the same risk as those family members who test positive. Parents who test positive and have passed a defective gene to their children may feel guilt and shame for their role.

A. SOURCES OF GENETIC INFORMATION AND CONCERNS ABOUT PRIVACY

Genetic information is obtained through the study of body cells. Genes are the basic units of heredity that are passed down from one generation to the next. Genes are made up of a body chemical called DNA (deoxyribonucleic acid). DNA can be obtained through several different ways, such as from saliva, hair, fingernails, blood, semen, skin, and nail clippings. Most gene testing uses blood as the method of obtaining a sample of DNA. Gene testing can also include biochemical tests for the presence or absence of key proteins that signal aberrant genes (National Cancer Institute, undated).

Genetic information is routinely stored within hospital databanks. It is collected with the goal of improving patient care or to reduce the likelihood of disease (Council for Responsible Genetics, 1995). Genetic information is stored for many other reasons. Researchers collect genetic information in hopes of preventing future disease and for discovering treatments and cures for genetic diseases and conditions. DNA is used to establish the identity of individuals suspected of committing crimes. It is used to prove paternity in order to determine who is responsible for child support. It can also be used to identify bodies that are damaged from fire or military combat. Scientists are collecting DNA samples from skeletons of humans who lived thousands of years ago in order to better understand the process of our evolution (Baker, 1997). DNA-based tests are also used for prenatal testing, identification of a carrier for a specific condition, diagnostic testing, presymptomatic testing, and risk-oriented or susceptibility testing such as determining susceptibility to inherited breast cancer (Kotval, 1994).

Genetic databanks (sometimes referred to as DNA databanks) are computerized databases that store records obtained through genetic testing. Gene databanks are used for several different purposes, but predominantly for forensic purposes when genetic information is obtained from blood, semen, hair, and other sources of DNA at a crime scene. Other databanks store actual biological samples from genetic tests and newborn blood samples taken to test for PKU and other genetic conditions. In addition to these databanks, researchers collect genetic material. A survey of informed consent documents collected from 104 research studies revealed that only 24% requested permission of participants for DNA banking or tissue storage. Most do not mention privacy or ownership of genetic material or possible secondary use by researchers or commercial companies (Wertz, 1997a).

There are many situations where people must provide personal information. Several include applying for a job, life or health insurance, credit or financial aid, and benefits from the government. As the use of genetic testing grows, insurers will want to obtain test results in order to determine the health status of the applicant or employee. Such information can be highly sensitive and personal. Once this information is provided, the companies or institutions or individuals are under no obligation by law to protect it. In fact, there is no law that says that a blood sample collected for one kind of DNA testing cannot be used for another purpose (Baker, 1997). Neither do individuals have the right to check their DNA file to see if the information is correct.

As already mentioned, an individual's genetic information may be used by people who are not health professionals. For example, insurance companies or employers may want to screen out applicants or possible new hires whose genetic information is considered undesirable. Although the definition of desirable or undesirable genetic information remains somewhat ambiguous, certainly genes related to communicative disorders may be labeled "undesirable." This could have negative impact on the individual and family members. Even if some types of medical information are kept in separate files so that fewer people can see it, if a "release of medical record" form is signed, insurers are entitled to see everything, including separate files (Wertz, 1997b).

Another concern is that, as medical records become more centralized and computerized, they will more easily be made available to corporations, social services agencies, and others, similar to the wide availability of credit histories (Alper & Natowicz, 1993). Anyone who has ever filled out an application for individual life, health, or disability insurance should have filled out an "MIB Notice" within their application. Through the Medical Information Bureau (MIB), insurance companies have access to the medical records of people who have applied for insurance. The MIB—a private, nonprofit corporation—manages a computerized databank of information to provide insurance companies with medical and certain nonmedical information about applicants for insurance. Originally created to prevent insurance fraud, the MIB holds medical information for 10 to 20 million Americans (Geller *et al.*, 1996).

B. ENHANCING GENETIC PRIVACY

Protecting the privacy of genetic information is challenging and difficult. For example, if an applicant for health insurance responds honestly to the question of whether he or she has a genetic or hereditary illness, this could eliminate any chance of obtaining health insurance. If genetic information is withheld or concealed from the insurance company, coverage for associated problems may be denied. Either way, whether a person decides to respond truthfully or withholds or conceals information, coverage can be denied.

To attempt to keep genetic information as private as possible, people should instruct their physicians and other medical providers in writing not to disclose their genetic information to anyone without prior verbal or written consent. People who apply for insurance and respond affirmatively to the question that asks "if you have been advised of any genetic or hereditary illnesses, condition or diseases" should know that the insurance company can send a copy of the application to the Medical Information Bureau. This means all future insurers will have access to those individuals' genetic information (Morelli, 1992). People may check the accuracy of the information in their MIB file and can file a statement of dispute if they disagree with any information in the file. If the information was accurate when reported, but has changed and is no longer accurate, a statement of additional information can be submitted describing the improvement or correction.

States are busy proposing or adopting confidentiality laws. Most such laws would prohibit insurance companies, health maintenance organizations, and employers from requiring genetic screening or using genetic information in deciding whom to insure, how much to charge, and what diseases to cover. Critics of the laws believe that insurance companies at least are entitled to have the same information as individuals do. Otherwise, people who know their risk factors will decide to purchase particular types of insurance coverage, knowing they will benefit. Insurers argue that, if they cover people who buy extra coverage at regular rates and incur disproportionately higher expenses, insurers will make up the difference by raising rates for all (Gollaher, 1998).

C. IMPORTANCE OF INFORMED CONSENT IN TESTING AND RESEARCH PARTICIPATION

Given the current concerns about lack of privacy of genetic information and risk of genetic discrimination, it is very important that families who consider having children tested or adults who consider genetic tests for themselves understand the risks. It is also important that anyone considering participation in a genetic research study also understand the risks (National Bioethics Advisory Committee, 1998). Informed consent is a term explaining the process by which information given to a patient by a physician or other health care provider about a test, treatment, or research study is adequately understood. Signing a consent form indicates a voluntary willingness on behalf of the participant or patient to submit to a procedure with an awareness of its inherent risks, benefits, and alternatives. Informed consent is usually obtained through a written document that a person signs before a procedure. Obtaining informed consent is required by law for research studies (Wertz, 1997a). The NIH–DOE Task Force on Genetic Testing (1997) recommends clinicians obtain informed consent before offering genetic testing.

Individuals and families must recognize that, if they choose to participate in a research study, they are engaging in a form of public service that may involve risk. Genetic research that studies pedigrees, identifies genes, and develops genetic tests may involve risks of psychological and social harm. Research subjects may learn information about their own genetic status that can provoke anxiety and confusion in themselves and affected family members. Their insurance and employment status may be compromised if genetic information is disclosed to insurers or employers. Even though these studies may not involve physical risks of harm, researchers must be aware of and disclose the social and psychological risks. Gene therapy research, on the other hand, requires special safety precautions because it attempts to treat genetic conditions by inserting properly functioning genes into the individual's somatic (body) cells (see Chapter 11). At the time, researchers are still learning how to control the genes inserted for the treatment. And there may be risks of physical injury (National Institutes of Health, 1993).

The risks of participation in many research studies are similar to those facing individuals who obtain genetic tests. Genetic studies typically involve families. One of the first steps in most genetic research studies is to draw a family tree (a pedigree) that also contains some medical information. Highly sensitive information may be revealed about a person's health and the health of family members. Individuals may learn information about their own genetic status, such as a risk of developing symptoms of a genetic disorder. This information is typically limited to probabilities. Many factors determine whether the person will develop the disorder. Participants are subjected to the stress of receiving such information and may experience emotional distress. Other participants may be grateful to learn they will not develop a disease that runs in the family, or if they do have the gene, be glad they know their risk and can plan accordingly for the future (The Arc, 1998).

Some family members do not want to participate in research or know about certain information that could be found during the research project. Special privacy and confidentiality protections should ensure that such individuals do not learn by chance about genetic information affecting them.

Persons other that the research team may learn information about a participant in genetic research. While researchers strive to protect confidential health information, there is no absolute guarantee that at some point other researchers, insurance companies, employers, or other people will not find this information. Participants should ask for assurance that this information will not be put in their medical record. However, it is important for participants to realize that insurance companies will learn about it if an individual files a claim for any costs associated with the research project.

D. RISK OF PHYSICAL INJURY IN GENE THERAPY STUDIES

Any genetic research involves social and psychological risks related to learning about one's genetic condition. Gene therapy involves the additional risk of possible physical injury. One hurdle is to get the therapeutic genes into cells without causing harm to the body. Researchers also need to control the specific types of cells a therapeutic gene enters. For example, if the condition affects liver function, the therapeutic genes will be targeted to reach the liver cells. Once the genes are inside the cell, scientists need to be able to control the level of activity needed to correct the problem. This means the new gene must function normally in the cell (Orkin & Motulsky, 1995).

Because of the risks that something can go wrong in each of these functions, gene therapy research proposals submitted to the National Institutes of Health undergo stringent review. Researchers must justify the gene therapy research techniques against alternative methods and state the risks and benefits of the research. They must also address how subjects will be selected for the research, how their informed consent will be obtained, and how their privacy and confidentially will be protected (National Institutes of Health, 1993.)

Although families and researchers have been confident that gene therapy may result in treatment of a number of genetic conditions, only one apparently successful cure through gene therapy has been documented (Weiss, 2000). Recently, a gene therapy study that underwent rigorous government review resulted in the death of an 18-year-old man (Weiss & Nelson, 1999). Usually, gene therapy studies include people who are seriously affected and have a poor prognosis because there is no effective treatment. In this situation, the young man, who had ornithine transcarbamylase (OTC) deficiency, was doing well with current treatment. The study has been halted, and more than 100 researchers conducting gene therapy research have been warned and asked to report any evidence of trouble.

Many people believe that gene therapy holds great potential for treating conditions that have severe effects on individuals, but there are others who question whether it should be pursued as a form of treatment. They are concerned about its misuse, recalling the eugenics movement of the 1920s through the 1940s, when people with mental retardation and others considered undesirable were involuntarily sterilized. Many candidates for gene therapy are likely to be children who are too young or too disabled to understand the ramifications of the treatment. There is also concern about the potential expense of gene therapy. If only the wealthy can afford it, the distribution of biological traits will widen the differences among various socioeconomic groups. In spite of these concerns, a survey of members of The Arc (1999) revealed that 87% of respondents, primarily family members, believed The Arc should pursue funding for gene therapy research.

IV. CONCLUSION

Unraveling the mystery of the human genome holds great promise for people affected by genetic disorders and for those who have a gene or genes placing them at risk for a future genetic disease or condition. Unfortunately, many people are unaware of the research moving forward and the issues being discussed by scientists, ethicists, and some policymakers. Families affected by a genetic condition and providers of services may not be familiar with the risks associated with lack of genetic privacy. Families, in particular, may hold unrealistic hope for gene therapy as a cure for a genetic condition. It is important for everyone to be informed about the issues. People need to make informed personal choices about genetic testing and participation in research. Providers need to be able to inform and guide families in such decisions. Finally, we must all continue to advocate for acceptance of individuals with genetic conditions and their fair treatment as citizens.

REFERENCES

Alper, J. S., & Natowicz, M. R. (1993). Genetic discrimination and the public entities and public accommodations titles of the Americans with Disabilities Act. *American Journal of Human Genetics, 53*, 26–32.

Alpert, S. (1993). Smart cards, smarter policy: Medical records, privacy and health care reform. *Hastings Center Report, 6*, 13–23.

Baker, C. (1997). *Your genes, your choices: Exploring the issues raised by genetic research.* Washington, DC: American Association for the Advancement of Science.

Collins, F. S. (1995). Evolution of a vision: Genome project origins, present and future challenges, and far-reaching benefits. *Human Genome News, 7*(3&4), 3, 16.

Council for Responsible Genetics. (1995). *Genetic privacy: A discussion paper on DNA data banking.* Cambridge, MA: Author.

Equal Employment Opportunity Commission (EEOC) (1995). Directives transmittal. *Executive Summary: Compliance Manual Section 902, Definition of the Term Disability.* Washington, DC: Author.

Geller, L. N., Alper, J. S., Billings, P. R., Barash, C. I., Beckwith, J., & Natowicz, M. R. (1996). Individual, family, and societal dimensions of genetic discrimination: A case study analysis. *Science and Engineering Ethics, 2*, 71–88.

Gollaher, D. (1998). The paradox of genetic privacy. *The New York Times* [online]. Jan. 7. Available: http://personal.ecu.edu/schumachere/gentest.htm.

Kotval, J. S. (1994). *DNA-based tests: Policy implications for New York State. LCST Report No. 94-1.* Albany, NY: Legislative Commission on Science and Technology.

McGoodwin, W. (1996). Genie out of the bottle: Genetic testing and the discrimination it's creating. *The Washington Post*, May 5, p. C3.

Mohammed, A. (1999). Clinton proposes patient privacy. *Reuters Limited on America Online*, October 29.

Morelli, T. (1992). Genetic discrimination by insurers: Legal protections needed from abuse of biotechnology. *Health Span, 8*(9), 8–11.

National Bioethics Advisory Committee (1998). *Research involving persons with mental disorders that may affect decision-making capacity* [online]. Available: http://bioethics.gov.

National Cancer Institute (undated). *Understanding gene testing.* U.S. Department of Health and Human Services, Public Health Service, National Institutes of Health.

National Institutes of Health. (1993). *Biomedical and behavioral research: An overview.* Human subject protections: Institutional Review Board. Office for Human Subject Protections [Available: Http://ohrp.osophs.dhhs.gov/irb/irb_guidebook.htm].

NIH–DOE Task Force on Genetic Testing (1997). *Promoting safe and effective genetic testing in the United States: Principles and recommendations.* Washington, DC: NIH–DOE Working Group on Ethical, Legal and Social Implications of Human Genome Research.

Office of Technology Assessment, U.S. Congress (1991). *Medical monitoring and screening in the workplace: Results of a survey-background paper.* Washington, DC: Government Printing Office.

Orkin, S. H., & Motulsky, A. G. (1995). *Report and recommendations of the panel to assess the NIH investment in research on gene therapy.* Washington, DC: National Institutes of Health.

Reilly, P. R. (1997). Fear of genetic discrimination drives legislative interest. *Human Genome News, 8*(3&4), 1–3.

The Arc (1997). Protecting genetic privacy. *Genetic Issues in Mental Retardation, 2*(1), 1–4.

The Arc (1998). Participating in genetic research: Considerations for people with mental retardation and their families. *Genetic Issues in Mental Retardation, 3*(1), 6.

The Arc (1999). *Final Report: The Arc's Human Genome Education Project.* Unpublished.

U.S. Department of Energy and the Human Genome Project (1996). *To know ourselves.* Oak Ridge, TN: Oak Ridge National Laboratory.

Weiss, R. (2000). Genetic therapy apparently cures 2. *The Washington Post*, April 28, p. A1.

Weiss, R., & Nelson, D. (1999). Teen dies undergoing gene therapy. *The Washington Post*, September 29, p. A1.

Welch, H. G., & Burke, W. (1998). Uncertainties in genetic testing for chronic disease. *Journal of the American Medical Association, 280*(17), 1525–1527.

Wertz, D. C. (1997a). Survey of informed consents. *The Gene Letter* [online]. Vol. 1, No. 4.

Wertz, D. C. (1997b). Privacy: Genetic and otherwise. *The Gene Letter* [online]. Vol. 1, No. 4. Available: http://www.geneletter.org/0197/consent.html.

11

TREATMENT AND PREVENTION

SANFORD E. GERBER

Department of Speech and Hearing Sciences
Washington State University
Spokane, Washington

I. INTRODUCTION

In this final chapter, we come to still more really intriguing notions. Can we treat genetic disorders? How? Can they be prevented? How? These are difficult questions, and they are sometimes controversial. One issue often raised is: Should we treat genetic disorders? Questions about treatment and prevention are not answered with a "yes" or "no." For example, during the preparation of this chapter, the press reported a case of a patient who died in a gene-therapy experiment (Nelson & Weiss, 1999; Weiss & Nelson, 1999; Wheeler, 1999). In this case, genetically engineered viruses were delivered in high doses directly into this young man's liver. Nevertheless, he succumbed after four days. This resulted in the government's Recombinant DNA Advisory Committee to suggest changes in this field (Anonymous, 1999). The committee is concerned that we don't yet have standardized controls and that scientific information is being inadequately shared.

We must be aware of such an event, but also aware that he was the only one among 17 patients to die. On the other hand, there has been a report of successful gene therapy for three children with severe combined immunodeficiency (Seppa, 2000). We must also be determined that serious, untoward events cannot stop progress. There are those, however, who are concerned about the possible dangers. Wright (1998), for example, was concerned about treatment's "social misuse, about the health and environmental hazards of modified organisms, about the ethical problems of using our technical ingenuity on ourselves and other life-forms" (p. 183). Care is always required.

I do have biases. We all know the principle that says "If it ain't broke, don't fix it." It has a corollary, I believe: "If it is broke, and it can be fixed, so fix it." There is place for treatment. Genetic treatment programs for communicative disorders are being developed. The National Institute for Deafness and Other Communicative Disorders (NIDCD) has established a working group to consider the development and implementation of genetic diagnostic tests. The group will study the feasibility of early identification of genetic communicative disorders (Ruben, 1999). Genetic engineering has been called a "key enabling technology" (Coates *et al.*, 1998). This technology can and will be applied to the treatment of communicative disorders. It has been claimed, for example, that "gene transfer is feasible in the cochlea and may in due course become the means of managing certain forms of deafness" (Gibbin, 1999, p. 15).

There is also a place for prevention. I am a strong advocate of the principles and methods of prevention. I once had a doctoral student who commented, facetiously, that "the best way to avoid birth defects is to not have children." He was right, of course, and his comment is not entirely facetious. How about not having it "broke" in the first place? Genetic disabilities, in theory, can be prevented. Treatment and prevention by new genetic engineering means are the issues of this chapter.

II. TREATMENT

Treatment of genetic disorders is an essential part of our ability to deal with unfavorable genetic alterations. The term "genetic engineering" has entered our vocabulary; not only the scientific vocabulary, but the popular lexicon as well. Kmiec (1999) suggested that some of this popularity might have been oversold. Agricultural scientists have been very much publicized as practitioners in genetic engineering. We now have genetically engineered tomatoes, wheat, and corn, for example, and these are considered (by some of us, anyway) to be improvements. Creating crops that are resistant to certain diseases has important implications for the animal kingdom as well as for crop plants. Wolff and Lederberg (1994) reminded us about not only agriculture, but also about dog training, horse racing, or better-smelling roses as well-established examples of genetic engineering. Hapgood (2000) pointed out that genetically engineered organisms are being used—or soon will be used—to clean air and water, to concentrate minerals for mining, as sensors of environmental changes, and to develop new materials.

Would it not also be a good thing to create people who are resistant to certain diseases? There are those who agree and there are those who disagree. We must take the view here that such things can be done and have been done, and we raise the question of how. Doing it, however, is a rather recent idea. It was 1991 when the relevant committee of NIH approved the first experiments in gene therapy in humans. These were to treat metastatic melanoma and adenosine deaminase deficiency (Snow, 1991).

A. GENE THERAPY

Gene therapy has been defined as modifying the structure or function of genes to control or cure disease (Garver, 1996). This implies the alteration of enough somatic cells to ameliorate the disorder. If germ cells are modified by gene correction or addition, then it may be that the alteration can be passed to future generations. Garver listed a number of technical problems that must be resolved in each case: isolating genes and, in some cases, the gene regulatory regions; generating sufficient DNA for treatment; purifying the cell population into which the genes are to be inserted; identifying, modifying, and producing appropriate vectors for transporting the therapeutic genetic material to the cells; inserting the genetic material into patients' cells (usually via a vector); returning the treated cells to the patient; animal testing; and ensuring that the procedure does not carry any serious risks for the patient.

The underlying problem was described by Kmiec (1999): "Abnormal cell behavior is often the result of an altered gene whose expression is either absent or unregulated. A mutation in just one gene can sometimes cause a cell to malfunction. The mutated gene directs the synthesis of a dysfunctional protein, with the consequence that the cell functions marginally or not at all" (p. 240). Not always, however. Wenthold (1980) noted that even a single incorrect amino acid could alter the properties of the protein such that it is totally ineffective, or it may function with limited efficiency. On the other hand, a mutation may cause little or no change either physically or functionally until later generations.

The current guiding ethic is that gene therapies are designed to alleviate symptoms in an individual (somatic). The ongoing effort is to create therapies that address the source of the problem, treat and even cure the problem, a specific gene mutation, provide a correcting gene that acts on the gene itself (Kmiec, 1999). Indeed, there are other more traditional ways to treat genetic diseases: nutrition, modifying enzyme activity, enzyme replacement, chelation, organ transplantation, *inter alia* (Nyhan, 1991). We are concerned here with treating the genes directly and thereby eliminate the adverse effects of certain genes. We examine gene addition, gene replacement, and gene repair.

1. Gene Addition

Adding genes has been done in human patients, but the results have been disappointing (Kmiec, 1999). The point of gene addition as therapy is to deliver a correct version of a given gene in the case where an incorrect version is operating. The expectation is that the presence of the correct version will lead to production of the normal protein and thence to normal function. The correct gene must be delivered to the nuclei of many cells of the target tissue and then maintain tissue vitalization in the person. Gene delivery is by some chemical or electronic means that provides a sufficient amount of correct gene DNA, and this therapeutic DNA is delivered to target tissue nuclei such that at least some of the nuclei are transformed with a correct, functioning gene. Also, to be of benefit, the gene must become a permanent part of the relevant chromosomes by incorporating its DNA directly into chromosomal DNA. The final problem becomes one of getting sufficient and lasting levels of protein expression to cause control of the disordered biology (Dowty & Wolff, 1994). Closer to the present concern is that such therapies are being studied to treat a considerable variety of diseases. There is potential to treat inner ear disorders (Kelly, 1999).

How do genes get added? One needs to add the correct genetic material into defective cells by microinjection or by chemical methods (Friedmann, 1991). Friedmann pointed out that viral vectors must be capable of transferring the foreign genes into the chromosomal DNA, and then having them expressed in a stable manner. He indicated a number of candidates for viral vectors: certain tumor viruses, viruses with DNA genomes (e.g., papovaviruses and papillomaviruses), and some with RNA genomes (i.e., retroviruses). Retroviruses were thought to be especially effective, and they are still used in many trials.

In 1994, Curiel showed that, although a number of viruses can enter cells, the adenovirus has an especially "well-characterized" mechanism of cell entry. It enters the cell and its DNA localizes to a host nucleus to translocate its DNA. Adenoviruses satisfy the criteria indicated by Dowty and Wolff (1994): they produce a sufficient amount of normal DNA to overwhelm the effects of the abnormal DNA. Moreover, adenoviruses can deliver genes to cells without disruption of the normal chromosomal configuration (Kmiec, 1999). And, they can be used to infect a wide variety of cells. Some small success in this area has been seen in the treatment of cystic fibrosis.

2. Gene Replacement

It seems like a good idea to remove or block the problematic genes and replace them with correct ones that function properly. In fact, early in the history of gene therapy, it was expected that the patient's cells would have to be removed in order to be treated with DNA. However, this would limit such treatment to cells that can be removed and then reintroduced, such as blood or bone marrow cells. If gene addition works as we want, it has the effect of gene replacement, that is, the added gene masks the faulty one. In that way, it has replaced a defective gene. Adenoviruses are especially useful for gene delivery.

Liposomes may also be valuable for gene delivery. These are artificial hollow spheres that resemble those that make up the membranes of cells. Because they have the same composition as cell membranes, they can fuse with cell membranes and empty their contents (e.g., corrective genes) into the cell interior. In this way, the genes get delivered and go on to replace faulty genes. Singhal and Huang (1994) considered liposomes to have several advantages in the delivery of drugs or DNA: they can accommodate different materials, they can be targeted to specific cells or tissues, and they can protect DNA (or RNA) from inactivation or degradation. They have been introduced into vascular cells and into tumors. Moreover, there is the potential with liposomes to overcome some of the difficulties encountered with viral vectors such as low levels of gene expression. A major goal of using liposomes for DNA delivery systems, according to Singhal and Huang, is to deliver nucleic acids to the desired sites.

3. Gene Repair

Maybe it is a good idea to try to repair defective genes rather than to replace them or to add new genes. The logic of this idea is quite elegant. Normal chromosomes are made up of two strands of DNA such that the nucleotides of one can bind with the nucleotides of the other. This is very specific: adenine always binds with thymine and guanine always binds with cytosine. Each strand of DNA has a nucleotide sequence that is exactly complementary to the other. Hence, every adenine nucleotide on one strand is matched to the thymine on the other strand, and every guanine nucleotide is matched to the cytosine. If a wrong nucleotide is inserted into some spot, it cannot bind to its partner. Actually, there are DNA repair mechanisms for just such a mismatch, but sometimes they fail. Hence, the point is to get the natural repair mechanisms to do their job. One repair scenario involves recombination of new, correct DNA, replacing a section of original mutated, faulty DNA. This is done by creating an artificial string of nucleotides that is complementary to the faulty one that contains the error. This creates a three-stranded DNA region with a bulge that is detected by the cell's DNA-repair system. The invading correct DNA thereby activates the natural repair cycle. What happens is that the repair enzymes remove the erroneous nucleotide or section and replace it with a correct one. However, Kmiec (1999) reports that clinical trial "has enjoyed few successes and many failures" (p. 245). As he said, "It 'sort of' works" (p. 246). In his patient with familial hypercholesterolemia, the LDL was indeed reduced but not to normal levels. Yet, in other cases, he reported successful correction for seven different chromosomal target genes including the sickle cell mutation.

4. Conclusion

Have these techniques been used for the amelioration of communicative disorders? They have indeed been used to treat complex genetic disorders that have communicative consequences. More is expected, and soon.

III. PREVENTION

Can genetic communicative disorders be prevented? Indeed they can, just as other disorders can be prevented. The not-so-facetious comment, mentioned at the beginning of this chapter, is certainly one way to prevent them: don't have children. The fact is that adoption accomplishes several social benefits. It allows prospective parents who are at unacceptably (to them) high risk for having children with some kind, any kind, of defect to have children. It provides a home for a child who needs one, and it does not add to the world's population. This is primary prevention. Secondary prevention is usually possible, also, as is tertiary prevention.

A. PRIMARY PREVENTION

Primary prevention means that the event or condition didn't happen in the first place. Adoption, as described above, is a form of primary prevention of genetic disease. A family may adopt when the prospective parents are unable or unwilling to add to the population of impaired persons or to care for a disabled child.

Again, primary prevention means that the event or condition simply didn't happen. There are many familiar examples of primary prevention. Inoculations against disease are very effective primary preventers. Seat belts and bicycle helmets are intended to prevent injuries to head and face, and to prevent death; diet often has the capacity to have favorable effects on such things as diabetes and coronary heart disease; prenatal diagnosis and even treatment often work. In fact, because these preventers have been so effective, genetic disease has appeared to become relatively more common in the past few decades. This is not because there has been a worldwide increase in the incidence of genetic disease, but because there has been a decrease in the incidence (and therefore the prevalence) of other disorders.

But how to prevent genetic disease in cases when families decide that they do want to reproduce? Information about risk, genetic counseling, and genetic screening can be excellent forms of primary prevention. Kelly (1986) listed three purposes for genetic screening. These are early recognition in a case in which presymptomatic treatment can be beneficial, identification of individuals at risk for transmission of genetic disease, and for population studies even when identification may not prove to benefit the affected person or family. What do we need to do, however, about presymptomatic treatment? Harrison and colleagues (1984) insisted that first there must be discussion with specialists who are not involved in the case at hand and that opposing viewpoints (where they exist) must be discussed with the patient or family. Of course, informed consent needs to be obtained. They described three aims of genetic counseling—which implies screening. They are, first, to get the relevant information, both medical and genetic; second, to consider the reproductive options that could be available; and, third, to assess the family's emotional state. This last, in fact, may be better done by the primary care provider, the family's physician, or other counselor.

We have two issues here. One is prepregnancy counseling, and the other is prenatal counseling. In the first case, it is the role of the genetic counselor to determine the risks that the couple may have of producing a disabled child (see Chapter 10). In the latter case, the pregnancy has already commenced, and the issue becomes one of determining the risk to an existing embryo or fetus. Prenatal diagnosis is, of course, possible. One can use cytogenetic or biochemical analyses of amniotic fluid, one can examine the mother's blood, and the fetus can be visualized by ultrasonography, by radiography, or (rarely) by fetoscopy (Nora & Fraser, 1989).

Can we prevent genetic disease from appearing in offspring if we treat it in an affected parent? That is, can we prevent a genetic disorder from appearing in children if it is corrected (by any of the means discussed above) in the affected or carrier parent? That is a very attractive notion; however, it usually does not work. Nevertheless, this is an area deserving of intensive investigation.

B. SECONDARY PREVENTION

Secondary prevention refers to early identification and, thereby, early intervention. Primary prevention prevents pathology; secondary prevention prevents pathology from becoming an impairment or prevents an impairment from becoming a disability. An obvious example vis-à-vis communicative disorders is hearing screening of newborns. The National Institutes of Health, in a consensus development report (1993), recommended the hearing screening of *all* births. Note that the recommendation is not for high-risk births only or for only those infants found in the Neonatal Intensive Care Unit; it is for *all* births. Why? The fact is that about half of infants who are eventually determined to have been born deaf were not known to be at risk, or were not in the NICU, or were not examined for other reasons (Elssman *et al.*, 1987). As an example, in one study (Gerber *et al.*, 1994) that uncovered four deaf infants, one of those infants was to have been a control, that is, a child found in the well-baby nursery. More recently, Fonseca *et al.* (1999) found that only 39% of congenitally deaf children were identified in the first year and 19% in the first 6 months. The so-called "Walsh bill" has passed the congress of the United States. Its official title is The Newborn and Infant Hearing Screening and Intervention Act of 1999. It provides new funding to the states for hearing screening. In general, the goal of the Walsh bill is to effect the NIH consensus recommendation, that is, to screen the hearing of all newborns. This has the possibility of achieving primary (or secondary) prevention of the best kind.

Who is a high-risk infant? Rossetti (1986) gave us a very good descriptive definition:

> the high-risk infant is an infant who because of low birth weight, prematurity, or the presence of serious medical complications associated with or independent from birth weight or prematurity, has a greater than normal chance of displaying development delay or later cognitive or motor deficits or a combination of these that can be linked with the high-risk status present in the neonatal or postnatal period. (p. 2)

Pyeritz (1998) defined risk factors as those that could increase one's relative risk to acquire a disease by a certain age. Von Oeyen (1990) described prenatal risk assessment to include medical history, physical examination, and initial laboratory tests. Gerber (1998) discussed amniocentesis, chorionic villus sampling, ultrasonography, and fetoscopy as means to prenatal diagnosis and prediction of risk. The point is that means exist to identify (even prenatally) those infants who are or who may become at risk for communicative impairments, and, of course, this includes those with prospective or actual genetic disorders.

A high-risk register (for anything) is a form of secondary prevention. For example, the state of California mandates a genetic and a metabolic screen. It screens for galactosemia, phenylketonuria, hypoglycemia, hypercalcemia, maple syrup urine disease, biotinadase deficiency, and some others. Note that some of these (e.g., PKU) can have communicative consequences.

C. TERTIARY PREVENTION

Tertiary prevention means habilitation or rehabilitation. Habilitation becomes prevention when the disorder is ameliorated or repaired. Certainly, surgery may come under this heading, even prenatal surgery (Harrison *et al.*, 1984). Moreover, there is an effect of the environment on genetic traits. This has been called genotype–environment correlation (DeFries & Plomin, 1983). People may react differently, and in beneficial ways, to persons of different genotypes. Special education could be an example. Of course, tertiary prevention is also the domain of the speech–language clinician and the rehabilitative audiologist. Research continues to need doing with respect to the measurement and prediction of treatment outcomes. Does tertiary prevention work? How?

REFERENCES

Anonymous (1999). Gene therapy cautions urged. *Knight Ridder*, 10 December.

Coates, J. F., Mahaffey, J. B., & Hines, A. (1998). Genetic engineering could benefit society. In T. L. Roleff (Ed.), *Biomedical ethics: Opposing viewpoints* (pp. 174–181). San Diego: Greenhaven.

Curiel, D. T. (1994). Receptor-mediated gene delivery employing adenovirus–polylysine–DNA complexes. In J. A. Wolff (Ed.), *Gene therapeutics* (pp. 99–117). Boston: Birkhäuser.

DeFries, J. C., & Plomin, R. (1983). Adoption designs for the study of complex behavioral characteristics. In C. L. Ludlow & J. A. Cooper (Eds.), *Genetic aspects of speech and language disorders* (pp. 121–138). New York: Academic Press.

Dowty, M. E., & Wolff, J. A. (1994). Possible mechanisms of DNA uptake in skeletal muscle. In J. A. Wolff (Ed.), *Gene therapeutics* (pp. 82–98). Boston: Birkhäuser.

Elssman, S., Matkin, N., & Sabo, M. (1987). Early identification of congenital sensorineural hearing impairment. *The Hearing Journal, 13,* 7–12.

Fonseca, S., Forsyth, J., Grigor, J., Lowe, J., MacKinnon, M., Price, E., Rise, S., Scanlon, O., & Umpathy, D. (1999). Identification of permanent hearing loss in children: are the targets for outcome measures attainable? *British Journal of Audiology, 33,* 135–143.

Friedmann, T. (1991). Gene therapy. In T. Friedmann (Ed.), *Therapy for genetic disease* (pp. 107–121). Oxford: Oxford University Press.

Garver, K. L. (1996). Gene therapy for genetic diseases. *Genetics in Practice, 3*(1), 1–3.

Gerber, S. E. (1998). *Etiology and prevention of communicative disorders.* San Diego: Singular.

Gerber, S. E., Thornton, A. R. D., Kennedy, C. R., & Kim, L. (1994). *ABRs and OAEs in three groups of infants.* Paper presented to the XXII International Congress of Audiology.

Gibbin, K. (1999). Developments in paediatric otolaryngology. *ENT News, 8*(8), 15.

Hapgood, F. (2000, April–May). Garage biotech is here or just around the corner. *Civilization,* pp. 46–51.

Harrison, M. R., Golbus, M. S., & Filly, R. A. (1984). *The unborn patient.* Orlando: Grune & Stratton.

Kelly, A. (1999, June). The molecular biology of hearing and deafness, *Hereditary Deafness Newsletter,* pp. 12–15.

Kelly, T. E. (1986). *Clinical genetics and genetic counseling* (2nd ed.). Chicago: Year Book.

Kmiec, E. B. (1999). Gene therapy. *American Scientist, 87,* 240–247.

National Institutes of Health (1993). Early identification of hearing impairment in infants and young children. *NIH Consensus Statement, 11,* 1–24. Washington, DC: National Institutes of Health.

Nelson, D., & Weiss, R. (1999). Family's debate mirrored scientists' on gene therapy risk. *Washington Post,* 30 September, p. A07.

Nora, J. J., & Fraser, F. C. (1989). *Medical genetics* (3rd ed.). Philadelphia: Lea & Febiger.

Nyhan, W. L. (1991). Classic approaches to the treatment of inherited metabolic disease. In T. Friedmann (Ed.), *Therapy for genetic disease* (pp. 1–33). Oxford: Oxford University Press.

Pyeritz, R. E. (1998). Family history and risk factors: forward to the future. *Genetics in Practice, 4*(4), 1–3.

Rossetti, L. M. (1986). *High-risk infants.* Boston: College-Hill.

Ruben, R. J. (1999). Hearing the past: Speaking the future. *AAS Bulletin, 24*(2), 22–25, 28.

Seppa, N. (2000). "Bubble" babies thrive on gene therapy. *Science News, 157,* 277.

Singhal, A., & Huang, L. (1994). Gene transfer in mammalian cells using liposomes as carriers. In J. A. Wolff (Ed.). *Gene therapeutics* (pp. 118–142). Boston: Birkhäuser.

Snow Jr., J. B. (1991). International symposium on the genetics of hearing impairment. In R. J. Ruben, T. R. Van De Water, & K. P. Steel (Eds.), *Genetics of hearing impairment* (pp. 1–2). New York: New York Academy of Sciences.

Von Oeyen, P. T. (1990). Optimal prenatal care. In S. M. Pueschel & J. A. Mulick (Eds.), *Prevention of developmental disabilities* (pp. 55–74). Baltimore: Brookes.

Weiss, R., & Nelson, D. (1999). Teen dies undergoing experimental gene therapy. *Washington Post,* 29 September, p. A01.

Wenthold, R. J. (1980). Neurochemistry of the auditory system. *Annals of Otology, Rhinology, and Laryngology, 89*(Suppl. 74), 121–131.

Wheeler, D. L. (1999). Patient dies in gene-therapy trial at University of Pennsylvania Medical Center. *The Chronicle of Higher Education*, 8 October, p. A23.

Wolff, J. A., & Lederberg, J. (1994). A history of gene transfer and therapy. In J. A. Wolff (Ed.), *Gene therapeutics* (pp. 3–25). Boston: Birkhäuser.

Wright, S. (1998). Genetic engineering could be dangerous. In T. L. Roleff (Ed.), *Biomedical ethics: Opposing viewpoints* (pp. 182–190). San Diego: Greenhaven.

BIBLIOGRAPHY

Achenbach, T. M. (1982). *Developmental psychopathology* (2nd ed.). New York: Wiley.

Adam, J., Myat, A., LeRoux, I., Eddison, M., Henrique, D., Ish-Horowicz, D., & Lewis, J. (1998). Cell fate choices and the expression of Notch, Delta and Serrate homologues in the chick inner ear: Parallels with drosophila sense-organ development. *Development, 125,* 4645–4654.

Admiraal, R. J. (1970). Hereditary hearing loss with nephropathy (Alport's syndrome). *Acta Otolaryngologica, Suppl., 271,* 7–26.

Ahlfors, K., Ivarsson, S. A., & Harris, S. (1999). Report on a long-term study of maternal and congenital cytomegalovirus infection in Sweden: Review of prospective studies available in the literature. *Scandinavian Journal of Infectious Diseases, 31,* 443–457.

Alagramam, K. N., Kwon, H. Y., Cacheiro, N. L., Stubbs, L., Wright, C. G., Erway, L. C., & Woychik, R. P. (1999). A new mouse insertional mutation that causes sensorineural deafness and vestibular defects. *Genetics, 152,* 1691–1699.

Alper, J. S., & Natowicz, M. R. (1993). Genetic discrimination and the public entities and public accommodations titles of the Americans with Disabilities Act. *American Journal of Human Genetics, 53,* 26–32.

Alpert, S. (1993). Smart cards, smarter policy: Medical records, privacy and health care reform. *Hastings Center Report, 6,* 13–23.

Alsobrook, J. P., & Pauls, D. (1998). Molecular approaches to child psychopathology. *Human Biology, 70,* 413–432.

Ambrose, N. G., Cox, N., & Yairi, E. (1997). The genetic basis of persistence and recovery in stuttering. *Journal of Speech, Language, and Hearing Research, 40,* 567–580.

Ambrose, N. G., Yairi, E., & Cox, N. (1993). Genetic aspects of early childhood stuttering. *Journal of Speech and Hearing Research, 36,* 701–706.

Anastasi, A. (1958). Hereditary, environment, and the question of "How?". *Psychological Review, 65,* 197–208.

Andrews, G., & Harris, M. (1964). The syndrome of stuttering. *Clinics in Developmental Medicine*, No. 17. London: Spastic Society Medical Education and Information Unit.

Andrews, G., Morris-Yates, A., Howie, P., & Martin, N. (1991). Genetic factors in stuttering confirmed. *Archives of General Psychiatry, 48*, 1034–1035.

Anonymous (1999). Gene therapy cautions urged. *Knight Ridder*, 10 December.

Anson, B. J., & Donaldson, J. A. (1981). *Surgical anatomy of the temporal bone*. Philadelphia: Saunders.

Anson, B. J., Hanson, J. S., & Richany, S. F. (1960). Early embryology of the auditory ossicles and associated structures in relation to certain anomalies observed clinically. *Annals of Otology, Rhinology, & Laryngology, 69*, 427–447.

Aoki, S., & Asaka, A. (1993). *Genetic analysis of motor development, language development and some behavior characteristics in infancy*. Paper presented at the annual meeting of the Behavior Genetics Association.

Arnold, G. E. (1961). The genetic background of developmental language disorders. *Folia Phoniatrica, 13*, 246–254.

Arvystas, M., & Shprintzen, R. J. (1984). Craniofacial morphology in the velo-cardio-facial syndrome. *Journal of Craniofacial Genetics and Developmental Biology, 4*, 39–45.

Aschner, B. (1934). A typical hereditary syndrome: Dystrophy of the nails, congenital defect of the patella and congenital defect of the head of the radius. *Journal of the American Medical Association, 102*, 2017–2020.

Austin, K. D., & Hall, J. G. (1992). Nontraditional inheritance. *Pediatric Clinics of North America, 39*, 335–348.

Avery, T. (1990). *Developmental anatomy* (7th ed.). Philadelphia: Saunders.

Axelsson, A., Ryan, A., & Woolf, N. (1986). The early postnatal development of the cochlear vasculature in the gerbil. *Acta Otolaryngologica, 101*, 75–86.

Bailey, A. (1998). A full genome screen for autism with evidence for linkage to a region of chromosome 7q [on behalf of the International Molecular Genetic Study of Autism Consortium]. *Human Molecular Genetics, 7*, 571–578.

Bailey, A., Phillips, W., & Rutter, M. (1996). Autism: Towards an integration of clinical, genetic, neuropsychological and neurobiological perspectives. *Journal of Child Psychology and Psychiatry, 37*, 89–126.

Baker, C. (1997). *Your genes, your choices: Exploring the issues raised by genetic research*. Washington, DC: American Association for the Advancement of Science.

Baker, O. (1999). Faulty control gene underlies retardation. *Science News, 156*, 214.

Bakwin, H. (1973). Reading disability in twins. *Developmental Medicine and Child Neurology, 15*, 184–187.

Barrett, S., Beck, J. C., Bernier, R., *et al.* (1999). An autosomal genomic screen for autism. *American Journal of Medical Genetics, 88*, 609–615.

Batshaw, M. L. (1997). Heredity. In M. L. Batshaw (Ed.), *Children with disabilities* (pp. 17–33). Baltimore: Brookes.

Becker, A., Geiger, D., & Schaffer, A. A. (1998). Automatic selection of loop breakers for genetic linkage analysis. *Human Heredity, 48*, 49–60.

Behrents, R. G. (1985). *Growth in the aging craniofacial skeleton* (Monograph No. 17). Craniofacial Growth Series. Ann Arbor: Center for Human Growth and Development, University of Michigan.

Bell, A. G. (1880). *On a deaf variety of the human race*. Washington, DC: National Academy of Sciences.

Bell, A. G. (1883). Memoir upon the formation of a deaf variety of the human race. *Proceedings of the National Academy of Sciences*, pp. 1–86.

Bell, C. (1833). *The nervous system of the human body*. Papers presented to the Royal Society on the Subject of Nerves. Stereotyped by Duff Green for the Register and Library of Medical and Chirurgical Science.

Berger, W., Meindl, A., van de Pol, T. J., Cremers, F. P., Ropers, H. H., Doerner, C., Monaco, A., Bergen, A. A., Lebo, R., & Warburg, M. (1992). Isolation of a candidate gene for Norrie disease by positional cloning. *Nature Genetics, 1,* 199–203. [Published erratum appears in *Nature Genetics,* 1992, *2,* 84.]

Bermingham, N. A., Hassan, B. A., Price, S. D., Vollrath, M. A., Ben-Arie, N., Eatock, R. A., Bellen, H. J., Lysakowski, A., & Zoghbi, H. Y. (1999). Math1: An essential gene for the generation of inner ear hair cells. *Science, 284,* 1837–1841.

Bhat, A., Heath, S. C., & Ott, J. (1999). Heterogeneity for multiple disease loci in linkage analysis. *Human Heredity, 49,* 229–231.

Biancalana, V., Le Marec, B., Odent, S., van den Hurk, J. A. M. J., & Hanauer, A. (1991). Oto-palato-digital syndrome type I: Further evidence for assignment of the locus to Xq28. *Human Genetics, 88,* 228–230.

Bibby, R. E. (1979). A cephalometric study of sexual dimorphism. *American Journal of Orthodontia, 76,* 256–259.

Biederman, J., Munir, K., Knee, D., Habelow, W., Armentano, M., Autor, S., Hoge, S. K., & Waternaux, C. (1986). A family study of patients with attention deficit disorder and normal controls. *Journal of Psychiatric Research, 20,* 263–274.

Biesold, H. (1988). *Klagende hande*. Germany: Solms.

Biesold, H. (1999). *Crying hands: Eugenics and deaf people in Nazi Germany*. Washington, DC: Gallaudet University Press.

Bisgaard, M. L., Eiberg, H., Moller, N., Niebuhr, E., & Mohr, J. (1987). Dyslexia and chromosome 15 heteromorphism: Negative LOD in a Danish material. *Clinical Genetics, 32,* 118–119.

Bishop, D. V. M., & Edmundson, A. (1986). Is otitis media a major cause of specific developmental language disorders? *British Journal of Disorders of Communication, 21,* 321–338.

Bishop, D. V. M., *et al.* (1995). Genetic basis of specific language impairment: Evidence from a twin study. *Developmental Medicine and Child Neurology, 37,* 56–71.

Black, G., & Redmond, R. M. (1994). The molecular biology of Norrie's disease. *Eye, 8*(Pt. 5), 491–496.

Blackwelder, W., & Elston, R. (1985). A comparison of sib-pair linkage tests for disease susceptibility loci. *Genetic Epidemiology, 2,* 85–97.

Blangero, J. (1993). Statistical genetic approaches to human adaptability. *Human Biology, 65,* 941–966.

Blum, K., & Noble, E. P. (1997). *Handbook of psychiatric genetics*. New York: CRC.

Bolton, P., MacDonald, H., Pickles, A., Rios, P., Goode, S., Crowson, M., Bailey, A., & Rutter, M. (1994). A case-control family history study of autism. *Journal of Child Psychology and Psychiatry, 35,* 877–900.

Bonet, J. P. (1620). *Reduction de las letras y arte para enseñar a abler las mudos*. Madrid: Francisco Abarca de Angulo.

Borges-Osorio, M. R., & Salzano, F. M. (1985). Language disabilities in 3 twin pairs and their relatives. *Acta Geneticae Medicae et Gemellologiae, 34,* 95–100.

Bouchard, T. J., & Propping, P. (Eds.) (1993). *Twins as a tool of behavioral genetics*. New York: Wiley.

Brancal, B., & Ferrer, M. (1998). Análisis perceptual de las características del habla en personas afectas de ataxias hereditarias. *Revista Logopedia, Foniatría, y Audiología, 18,* 213–224.

Bretos, M. (1980). La morphogenese primordial du ganglion stato-acoustique et de l'oreille interne chez l'embryon de souris, II: Etude de l'evolution des ebauches chez l'embryons de 101/2 à 12 jours. *Archiv Belgique, 91,* 77–113.

Brown, K. A., Leek, J. P., Lench, N. J., Moynihan, L. M., Markham, A. F., & Mueller, R. F. (1996). Human sequences homologous to the gene for the cochlear protein OCP-II do not map to currently known non-syndromic hearing loss loci. *Annals of Human Genetics*, *60*, 385–389.

Bryden, M. P., McManus, I. C., & Bulman-Fleming, M. B. (1994). Evaluating the empirical support for the Geschwind–Behan–Galaburda model of cerebral localization. *Brain and Cognition*, *26*, 103–167.

Byrne, B., Willerman, L., & Ashmore, L. (1974). Severe and moderate language impairment: Evidence for distinctive etiologies. *Behavioral Genetics*, *4*, 331–345.

Capecchi, M. R. (1994, March). Targeted gene replacement. *Scientific American*, 52–59.

Cardon, L. R., Smith, S. D., Fulker, D. W., Kimberling, B. F., & DeFries, J. C. (1994). Quantitative trait locus for reading disability on chromosome 6. *Science*, *266*, 276–279.

Cardon, L. R., Smith, S. D., Fulker, D. W., Kimberling, B. F., Pennington, B. F., & DeFries, J. C. (1995). Quantitative trait locus for reading disability. *Science*, *268*, 1553.

Carrel, R. E. (1977). Epidemiology of hearing loss. In S. E. Gerber (Ed.), *Audiometry in infancy* (pp. 3–16). New York: Grune & Stratton.

Casselbrant, M. L., Mandel, E. M., Fall, P. A., Rockette, H. E., Kurslasky, M., Bluestone, C. D., & Ferrell, R. E. (2000). The heritability of otitis media: A twin and triplet study. *Journal of the American Medical Association*, *282*, 2125–2130.

Castles, A., Datta, H., Gayan, J., & Olson, R. K. (1999). Varieties of developmental reading disorder: Genetic and environmental influences. *Journal of Experimental Child Psychology*, *72*, 73–94.

Chandola, C. A., Robling, M. R., Peters, T. J., Melvill-Thomas, G., & McGuffin, P. (1992). Pre- and perinatal factors and the risk of subsequent referral for hyperactivity. *Journal of Child Psychology and Psychiatry*, *33*, 1077–1090.

Chang, W., Nunes, F. D., De Jesus-Escobar, J. M., Harland, R., & Wu, D. K. (1999). Ectopic Noggin blocks sensory and nonsensory organ morphogenesis in the chicken inner ear. *Developmental Biology*, *216*, 369–381.

Chen, A., Wayne, S., Bell, A., Ramesh, A., Srisailapathy, C. R., Scott, D. A., Sheffield, V. C., Van Hauwe, P., Zbar, R. I., Ashley, J., Lovett, M., Van Camp, G., & Smith, R. J. (1997). New gene for autosomal recessive non-syndromic hearing loss maps to either chromosome 3q or 19p. *American Journal of Medical Genetics*, *71*, 467–471.

Coates, J. F., Mahaffey, J. B., & Hines, A. (1998). Genetic engineering could benefit society. In T. L. Roleff (Ed.), *Biomedical ethics: Opposing viewpoints* (pp. 174–181). San Diego: Greenhaven.

Cohen Jr., M. M. (1997). *The child with multiple birth defects.* New York: Oxford University Press.

Cohn, E. S., Kelley, P. M., Fowler, T. W., Gorga, M. P., Lefkowitz, D. M., Kuehn, H. J., Schaefer, G. B., Gobar, L. S., Hahn, F. J., Harris, D. J., & Kimberling, W. J. (1999). Clinical studies of families with hearing loss attributable to mutations in the connexin 26 gene (GJB2/DFNB1). *Pediatrics*, *103*, 546–550.

Collins, F. S. (1995). Positional cloning moves from perditional to traditional. *Nature Genetics*, *9*, 347–350.

Collins, F. S. (1995). Evolution of a vision: Genome project origins, present and future challenges, and far-reaching benefits. *Human Genome News*, *7*(3&4), 3, 16.

Cotanche, D. A., & Sulik, K. K. (1984). The development of stereociliary bundles in the cochlear duct of the chick embryo. *Developmental Brain Research*, *16*, 181–193.

Council for Responsible Genetics. (1995). *Genetic privacy: A discussion paper on DNA data banking.* Cambridge, MA: Author.

Cox, N. (1988, April). Molecular genetics: The key to the puzzle of stuttering? *Asha*, 36–40.

Cox, N., & Kidd, K. (1983). Can recovery from stuttering be considered a genetically milder subtype of stuttering? *Behavior Genetics*, *13*, 129–139.

Cox, N., Kramer, P., & Kidd, K. (1984). Segregation analyses of stuttering. *Genetic Epidemiology*, *1*, 245–253.

Cox, N., Seider, R., & Kidd, K. (1984). Some environmental factors and hypotheses for stuttering in families with several stutterers. *Journal of Speech and Hearing Research, 27,* 543–548.

Coyle, B., Coffey, R., Armour, J. A., Gausden, E., Hochbatic, Z., Grossman, A., Britton, K., Pembrey, M., Reardon, W., & Trembath, R. (1996). Pendred syndrome (goiter and sensorineural hearing loss) maps to chromosome 7 in the region containing the nonsyndromic deafness gene DFNB4. *Nature Genetics, 12,* 421–423.

Cremers, C. W., & Fikkers-Van Noord, N. M. (1980). The earpits-deafness syndrome. Clinical and genetic aspects. *International Journal of Pediatric Otorhinolaryngology, 2,* 309–322.

Cremers, C. W., & Huygen, P. L. (1983). Clinical features of female heterozygotes in the X-linked mixed deafness syndrome (with perilymphatic gusher during stapes surgery). *International Journal of Pediatric Otorhinolaryngology, 6,* 179–185.

Cremers, C. W., Hombergen, G. C., Scaf, J. J., Huygen, P. L., Volkers, W. S., & Pinckers, A. J. (1985). X-linked progressive mixed deafness with perilymphatic gusher during stapes surgery. *Archives of Otolaryngology, 111,* 249–254.

Cremers, C. W., Marres, H. A., & van Rijn, P. M. (1991). Nonsyndromal profound genetic deafness in childhood. In R. J. Ruben, T. R. Van De Watter, & K. P. Steel (Eds.), Genetics of hearing impairment. *Annals of the New York Academy of Sciences, 630,* 191–196.

Cremers, C. W., Bolder, C., Admiraal, R. J., Everett, L. A., Joosten, F. B., VanHauwe, P., Green, E. D., & Otten, B. J. (1998). Progressive sensorineural hearing loss and a widened vestibular aqueduct in Pendred syndrome. *Archives of Ptolaryngology—Head & Neck Surgery, 124,* 501–505.

Crowe, R. R. (1993). Candidate genes in psychiatry: An epidemiological perspective. *American Journal of Medical Genetics, 48,* 74–77.

Curiel, D. T. (1994). Receptor-mediated gene delivery employing adenovirus–polylysine–DNA complexes. In J. A. Wolff (Ed.), *Gene therapeutics* (pp. 99–117). Boston: Birkhäuser.

Cusimano, F., Martines, E., & Rizzo, C. (1991). The Jervell and Lange–Nielsen syndrome. *International Journal of Pediatric Otorhinolaryngology, 22,* 49–58.

Dale, P. S., Simonoff, E., Bishop, D. V. M., Eley, T. C., Oliver, B., Price, T. S., Purcell, S., Stevenson, J., & Plomin, R. (1998). Genetic influence of language delay in two-year-old children. *Nature: Neuroscience, 1,* 324–328.

D'Amico-Martel, A., & Noden, D. M. (1983). Contributions of placodal and neural crest cells to avian cranial peripheral ganglia. *American Journal of Anatomy, 166,* 445–468.

Daniels, J., McGuffin, P., Owen, M. J., & Plomin, R. (1998). Molecular genetic studies of cognitive ability. *Human Biology, 70,* 281–296.

de Andrade, M., Amos, C. I., & Thiele, T. J. (1999). Methods to estimate genetic components of variance for quantitative traits in family studies. *Genetic Epidemiology, 17,* 64–76.

Dechesne, C. J., & Pujol, R. (1986). Neuron-specific enolase immunoreactivity in the developing mouse cochlea. *Hearing Research, 21,* 87–90.

Dechesne, C. J., Sans, A., & Keller, A. (1985). Onset and development of neuron-specific enolase immunoreactivity in the peripheral vestibular system of the mouse. *Neuroscience Letters, 61,* 299–304.

DeFries, J. C., & Fulker, D. W. (1988). Multiple regression analysis of twin data: Etiology of deviant scores versus individual differences. *Acta Geneticae Medicae et Gemellologiae, 37,* 205–216.

DeFries, J. C., & Gillis, J. (1993). Genetics of reading disability. In R. Plomin & G. McClearn (Eds.), *Nature, nurture, and psychology* (pp. 59–76). Washington, DC: APA Press.

DeFries, J. C., & Plomin, R. (1983). Adoption designs for the study of complex behavioral characteristics. In C. L. Ludlow & J. A. Cooper (Eds.), *Genetic aspects of speech and language disorders* (pp. 121–138). New York: Academic Press.

DeFries, J. C., Fulker, D. W., & LaBuda, M. C. (1987). Evidence for a genetic aetiology in reading disability of twins. *Nature, 329,* 537–539.

DeMeyer, W. (1975). Median facial malformations and their implications for brain malformations. In D. Bergsma (Ed.), *Morphogenesis and malformation of face and brain* (pp. 155–181). New York: Liss.

DeStefano, A. L., Cupples, L. A., Arnos, K. S., Asher, J. H. J., Baldwin, C. T., Blanton, S., Carey, M. L., da Silva, E. O., Friedman, T. B., Greenberg, J., Lalwani, A. K., Milunsky, A., Nance, W. E., Pandya, A., Ramesar, R. S., Read, A. P., Tassabejhi, M., Wilcox, E. R., & Farrer, L. A. (1998). Correlation between Waardenburg syndrome phenotype and genotype in a population of individuals with identified PAX3 mutations. *Human Genetics, 102*, 499–506.

Dibbets, J. M., deBruin, R., & Van der Weele, L. (1987). *Shape change in the mandible during adolescence* (Monograph No. 20). Craniofacial Growth Series. Ann Arbor: Center for Human Growth and Development, University of Michigan.

Dowty, M. E., & Wolff, J. A. (1994). Possible mechanisms of DNA uptake in skeletal muscle. In J. A. Wolff (Ed.), *Gene therapeutics* (pp. 82–98). Boston: Birkhäuser.

Drayna, D. (1997). Genetic linkage studies of stuttering: Ready for prime time? *Journal of Fluency Disorders, 22*, 237–241.

Dunham, I., Shimizu, N., Roe, B. A., & Chissoe, S. (1999). The DNA sequence of human chromosome 22. *Nature, 402*, 489–495.

Durant, J., Hansen, A., & Bauer, M. (1996). Public understanding of the new genetics. In T. Marteau & M. Richards (Eds.), *The troubled helix: Social and psychological implications of the new human genetics* (pp. 235–248). Cambridge: Cambridge University Press.

Eaves, L. J., Eysenck, H. J., & Martin, N. G. (1989). *Genes, culture, and personality: An empirical approach.* San Diego: Academic Press.

Elssman, S., Matkin, N., & Sabo, M. (1987). Early identification of congenital sensorineural hearing impairment. *The Hearing Journal, 13*, 7–12.

Enlow, D. H. (1973). Growth and the problem of the local antral mechanism. *American Journal of Anatomy, 178*, 2.

Enlow, D. H. (1990). *Handbook of craniofacial growth.* Philadelphia: Saunders.

Equal Employment Opportunity Commission (EEOC) (1995). Directives transmittal. *Executive Summary: Compliance Manual Section 902, Definition of the Term Disability.* Washington, DC: Author.

Erkman, L., McEvilly, R. J., Luo, L., Ryan, A. K., Hooshmand, F., O'Connell, S. M., Keithley, E. M., Rapaport, D. H., Ryan, A. F., & Rosenfeld, M. G. (1996). Role of transcription factors Brn-3.1 and Brn-3.2 in auditory and visual system development. *Nature, 381*, 603–606.

Estivill, X., Govea, N., Barcelo, E., Badenas, C., Romero, E., Moral, L., Scozzri, R., D'Urbano, L., Zeviani, M., & Torroni, A. (1998). Familial progressive sensorineural deafness is mainly due to the mtDNA A1555G mutation and is enhanced by treatment of aminoglycosides. *American Journal of Human Genetics, 62*, 27–35.

Fagerheim, T., Raeymaekers, P., Tonnessen, F. E., Pedersen, M., Tranebjaerg, L., & Lubs, H. A. (1999). A new gene (DYX3) for dyslexia is located on chromosome 2. *Journal of Medical Genetics, 36*, 664–669.

Falconer, D. S. (1981). *Introduction to quantitative genetics* (2nd ed.). London: Longman.

Faraone, S. V., Biederman, J., Keenan, K., & Tsuang, M. T. (1991). Separation of DSM-III attention deficit disorders and conduct disorder: Evidence from a family genetic study of American child psychiatric patients. *Psychological Medicine, 21*, 109–121.

Fekete, D. M. (1996). Cell fate specification in the inner ear. *Current Opinions in Neurobiology, 6*, 533–541.

Fekete, D. M., Muthukumar, S., & Karagogeos, D. (1998). Hair cells and supporting cells share a common progenitor in the avian inner ear. *Journal of Neuroscience, 18*, 7811–7821.

Felsenfeld, S. (1996). Progress and needs in the genetics of stuttering. *Journal of Fluency Disorders, 21*, 77–103.

Felsenfeld, S. (1997). Epidemiology and genetics of stuttering. In R. F. Curlee & G. M. Siegel (Eds.), *Nature and treatment of stuttering: New directions* (pp. 3–23). Boston: Allyn and Bacon.

Felsenfeld, S., McGue, M., & Broen, P. A. (1995). Familial aggregation of phonological disorders: Results from a 28-year follow up. *Journal of Speech and Hearing Research, 38*, 1091–1107.

Felsenfeld, S., Kirk, K., Zhu, G., Statham, D., Neale, M., & Martin, N. (2000). A study of the genetic and environmental etiology of stuttering in a selected twin sample. *Behavior Genetics*. Submitted manuscript.

Fenson, L., Dale, P. S., Reznick, J. S., Bates, E., Thal, D. J., & Pethick, S. J. (1994). Variability in early communicative development. *Monographs of the Society for Research on Child Development, 59*, 1–173.

Ferguson-Smith, M, Aitken, D., Turleau, C., & de Grouchy, J. (1976). Localisation of the human ABO: Np-1:AK-1 linkage group by regional assignment of AK-1 to 9q34. *Human Genetics, 34*, 35–43.

Field, L. L., & Kaplan, B. J. (1998). Absence of linkage of phonological coding dyslexia to chromosome 6p23–p21.3 in a large family data set. *American Journal of Human Genetics, 63*, 1448–1456.

Fields, H. W., Warren, D. W., Black, K., & Phillips, C. H. (1991). Relationship between vertical dentofacial morphology and respiration in adolescents. *American Journal of Orthodontia and Dentofacial Orthopedics, 99*, 147–154.

Filipek, P. A. (1995). Neurobiological correlates of developmental dyslexia: How do dyslexics' brains differ from those of normal readers? *Journal of Child Neurology, 10*(Suppl. 1), S62–S67.

Finucci, J. M., Guthrie, J. T., Childs, A. L., Abbey, H., & Childs, B. (1976). The genetics of specific reading disability. *Annual Review of Human Genetics, 40*, 1–23.

Fischel-Ghodsian, N., Prezant, T. R., Bu, X., & Oztas, S. (1993). Mitochondrial ribosomal RNA gene mutation in a patient with sporadic aminoglycoside ototoxicity. *American Journal of Otolaryngology, 14*, 399–403.

Fisher, R. A. (1918). The correlation between relatives on the supposition of Mendelian inheritance. *Transactions of the Royal Society of Edinburgh, 52*, 399–433.

Fisher, S. E., Vargha-Khadem, F., Watkins, K. E., Monaco, A. P., & Pembrey, M. E. (1998). Localisation of a gene implicated in a severe speech and language disorder. *Nature Genetics, 18*, 168–170.

Fisher, S. E., Marlow, A. J., Lamb, J., Maestrini, E., Williams, D. F., Richardson, A. J., Weeks, D. E., Stein, J. F., & Monaco, A. P. (1999). A quantitative trait locus on chromosome 6p influences aspects of developmental dyslexia. *American Journal of Human Genetics, 64*, 146–156.

Fonseca, S., Forsyth, J., Grigor, J., Lowe, J., MacKinnon, M., Price, E., Rise, S., Scanlon, O., & Umpathy, D. (1999). Identification of permanent hearing loss in children: are the targets for outcome measures attainable? *British Journal of Audiology, 33*, 135–143.

Forrest, S., Cotton, R., Landegren, U., & Southern, E. (1995). How to find all those mutations. *Nature Genetics, 10*, 375–376.

Folstein, S., & Rutter, M. (1977). Infantile autism: A genetic study of 21 twin pairs. *Journal of Child Psychology and Psychiatry, 18*, 297–321.

Fowler, K. B., Dahle, A. J., Boppana, S. B., & Pass, R. F. (1999). Newborn hearing screening: Will children with hearing loss caused by congenital cytomegalovirus infection be missed? *Journal of Pediatrics, 135*, 60–64.

Fraser, F. C. (1970). The genetics of cleft lip and cleft palate. *American Journal of Human Genetics, 22*, 336–352.

Fraser, G. F. (1976). *The causes of profound deafness in childhood*. Baltimore: The Johns Hopkins University Press.

Frenz, D. A., & Liu, W. (1998). Role of FGF3 in otic capsule chondrogenesis *in vitro*: An antisense oligonucleotide approach. *Growth Factors, 15*, 173–182.

Frenz, D. A., & Van De Water, T. R. (1991). Epithelial control of periotic mesenchyme chondrogenesis. *Developmental Biology, 144*, 38–46.

Frenz, D. A., Galinovic-Schwartz, V., Flanders, K. C., & Van De Water, T. R. (1992). TGF₁ is an epithelial-derived signal peptide that influences otic capsule formation. *Developmental Biology*, *153*, 324–336.

Frenz, D. A., Liu, W., Williams, J. D., Hatcher, V., Galinovic-Schwartz, V., Flanders, K. C., & Van De Water, T. R. (1994). Induction of chondrogenesis: Requirement for synergistic interaction of basic fibroblast growth factor and transforming growth factor-beta. *Development*, *120*, 415–424.

Frenz, D. A., Liu, W., & Capparelli, M. (1996). The role of BMP-2a in otic capsule chondrogenesis. *Annals of the New York Academy of Sciences*, *785*, 256–258.

Frenz, D. A., Yoo, H., & Liu, W. (1998). Basilar papilla explants: A model to study hair cell regeneration-repair and protection. *Acta Otolaryngologica*, *118*, 651–659.

Friedmann, T. (1991). Gene therapy. In T. Friedmann (Ed.), *Therapy for genetic disease* (pp. 107–121). Oxford: Oxford University Press.

Froster, U., Schulte-Korne, G., Hebebrand, J., & Remschmidt, H. (1993). Cosegregation of balanced translocation (1:2) with retarded speech development and dyslexia. *Lancet*, No. 8864, 178–179.

Fukushima, K., Kasai, N., Ueki, Y., Nishizaki, K., Sugata, K., Hirakawa, S., Masuda, A., Gunduz, M., Ninomiya, Y., Masuda, Y., Sato, M., McGuirt, W. T., Coucke, P., VanCamp, G., & Smith, R. J. (1999). A gene for fluctuating, progressive autosomal dominant nonsyndromic hearing loss, DFNA16, maps to chromosome 2q23–24.3. *American Journal of Human Genetics*, *65*, 141–150.

Fuller, J. L., & Simmel, E. C. (Eds.) (1983). *Behavior genetics: Principles and applications*. Hillsdale, NJ: Erlbaum.

Fuller, J., & Thompson, W. (1978). *Foundations of behavior genetics*. St. Louis: Mosby.

Fundudis, T., Kolvin, I., & Garside, R. (1979). *Speech retarded and deaf children: Their psychological development*. New York: Academic Press.

Ganetzky, B. (2000). Tracking down a cheating gene. *American Scientist*, *88*, 128–135.

Garrett, H. E. (1961). *General psychology* (2nd ed.). New York: American Book Company.

Garver, K. L. (1996). Gene therapy for genetic diseases. *Genetics in Practice*, *3*(1), 1–3.

Gasser, R. (1967). The development of the facial nerve in man. *Annals of Otology, Rhinology, and Laryngology*, *76*, 37–56.

Gates, G. A., Couropmitree, N. N., & Myers, R. H. (1999). Genetic associations in age-related hearing thresholds. *Archives of Otolaryngology—Head and Neck Surgery*, *125*, 654–659.

Gayan, J., Forsberg, H., & Olson, R. K. (1994). Genetic influences on subtypes of dyslexia. *Behavioral Genetics*, *24*, 513.

Gayan, J., Datta, H. E., Castles, A. E., & Olson, R. K. (1997). *The aetiology of group deficits in word decoding across levels of phonological decoding and orthographic decoding*. Paper presented at the annual meeting of the Society for the Scientific Study of Reading.

Gayan, J., Smith, S. D., Cherny, S. S., Cardon, L. R., Fulker, D. W., Brower, A. M., Olson, R. K., Pennington, B. F., & DeFries, J. D. (1999). Quantitative-trait locus for specific language and reading deficits on chromosome 6. *American Journal of Human Genetics*, *64*, 157–164.

Geis, N., Seto. B., Bartoshesky. L., Lewis, M. B., & Pashayan, H. M. (1981). The prevalence of congenital heart disease among the population of a metropolitan cleft lip and palate clinic. *Cleft Palate Journal*, *18*, 19–23.

Gelderman, H. (1975). Investigations on inheritance of quantitative characters in animals by gene markers, I: Methods. *Theoretical and applied genetics*, *46*, 319–330.

Geller, L. N., Alper, J. S., Billings, P. R., Barash, C. I., Beckwith, J., & Natowicz, M. R. (1996). Individual, family, and societal dimensions of genetic discrimination: A case study analysis. *Science and Engineering Ethics*, *2*, 71–88.

Gerber, S. E. (1990). Review of a high risk register for congenital or early-onset deafness. *British Journal of Audiology*, *24*, 347–356.

Gerber, S. E. (1998). *Etiology and prevention of communicative disorders*. San Diego: Singular.

Gerber, S. E., Thornton, A. R. D., Kennedy, C. R., & Kim, L. (1994). *ABRs and OAEs in three groups of infants.* Paper presented to the XXII International Congress of Audiology.

Gerlach, L. M., Hutso, M. R., Germiller, J. A., Nguyen-Luu, D., Victor, J. C., & Barald, K. F. (2000). Addition of the BMP4 antagonist, noggin, disrupts avian inner ear development. *Development, 127,* 45–54.

Gibbin, K. (1999). Developments in paediatric otolaryngology. *ENT News, 8*(8), 15.

Gilger, J. W. (1995). Behavioral genetics: Concepts for research in language and language disabilities. *Journal of Speech and Hearing Research, 38,* 1126–1142.

Gilger, J. W. (1998). Late talking toddlers may have special genes. *Nature (Medicine), 4,* 7–8.

Gilger, J. W., & Hershberger, S. (1998). Introduction to special issue on human behavioral genetics: Synthesis of quantitative and molecular approaches. *Human Biology, 70,* 155–157.

Gilger, J. W., & Pennington, B. F. (1995). Why associations among traits do not necessarily indicate their common etiology: A comment on the Geschwind–Behan–Galaburda model. *Brain & Cognition, 27,* 89–93.

Gilger, J. W., Pennington, B. F., & DeFries, J. C. (1991). Risk for reading disability as a function of parental history in 3 family studies. *Reading and Writing, 3,* 205–217.

Gilger, J. W., Borecki, I., Smith, S. D., DeFries, J. C., & Pennington, B. F. (1996). The etiology of extreme scores for complex phenotypes: An illustration using reading performance. In C. Chase, G. Rosen, & G. Sherman (Eds.), *Developmental dyslexia: Neural, cognitive and genetic mechanisms* (pp. 63–85). Baltimore: York.

Gilger, J. W., Hanebuth, E., Smith, S. D., & Pennington, B. F. (1996). Differential risk for developmental reading disorders in the offspring of compensated versus noncompensated parents. *Reading and Writing: An Interdisciplinary Journal, 8,* 407–417.

Gilger, J. W., Ho, H-Z., Whipple, A., & Spitz, R. (in review). Gene–environment correlations for typically and atypically developing children aged 2–12 years.

Gillis, J., Gilger, J. W., Pennington, B. F., & DeFries, J. C. (1992). Attention deficit hyperactivity disorder in reading disabled twins: Evidence for a genetic etiology. *Journal of Abnormal Child Psychology, 20,* 303–316.

Godai, U., Tatarelli, R., & Bonnani, G. (1976). Stuttering and tics in twins. *Acta Genetica Medicae et Gomellologiae, 25,* 369–375.

Gollaher, D. (1998). The paradox of genetic privacy. *The New York Times* [online]. Jan. 7. Available: http://personal.ecu.edu/schumachere/gentest.htm.

Gopnik, M. (1990). Feature-blind grammar and dysphasia. *Nature, 344,* 715.

Gopnik, M., & Crago, M. B. (1991). Familial aggregation of a developmental language disorder. *Cognition, 39,* 1–50.

Gottesman, I. I. (1991). *Schizophrenia genesis: The origins of madness.* New York: Freeman.

Gravel, J. S., & Traquina, D. N. (1992). Experience with audiologic assessment of infants and toddlers. *International Journal of Pediatric Otolaryngology, 23,* 59–71.

Gray, M. (1940). The X Family: A clinical and laboratory study of a "stuttering" family. *Journal of Speech Disorders, 5,* 343–348.

Green, G. E., Drescher D. G., & Beisel, K. W. (1994). Identification of a cardiac-type potassium channel expressed in the mouse cochlea. *Abstracts of the Association for Research in Otolaryngology, 17,* 320.

Green, G. E., Scott, D. A., McDonald, J. M., Woodworth, G. G., Sheffield, V. C., & Smith, R. J. (1999). Carrier rates in the midwestern United States for *GJB2* mutations causing inherited deafness. *Journal of the American Medical Association, 281,* 2211–2216.

Grigorenko, E. L., Wood, F. B., Meyer, M. S., Hart, L. A., Speed, W. C., Shuster, A., & Pauls, D. L. (1997). Susceptibility loci for distinct components of developmental dyslexia on chromosomes 6 and 15. *American Journal of Human Genetics, 60,* 27–39.

Grigorenko, E. L., Wood, F. B., Meyer, M. S., & Pauls, D. L. (2000). Chromosome 6p influences on different dyslexia-related cognitive processes: Further confirmation. *American Journal of Human Genetics, 66*, 715–723.

Grobstein, C. (1988). *Science and the unborn.* New York: Basic Books.

Guo, S. (1999). The behaviors of some heritability estimators in the complete absence of genetic factors. *Human Heredity, 49*, 215–228.

Guo, X., & Elston, R. C. (1999). Linkage information content of polymorphic genetic markers. *Human Heredity, 49*, 112–118.

Gustavson, K. H., Anneren, G., Malmgren, H., Dahl, N., Ljunggren, C. G., & Backman, H. (1993). New X-linked syndrome with severe mental retardation, severely impaired vision, severe hearing defect, epileptic seizures, spasticity, restricted joint mobility, and early death. *American Journal of Medical Genetics, 45*, 654–658.

Hadrys, T., Braun, T., Rinkwitz-Brandt, S., Arnold, H. H., and Bober, E. (1998). Nkx5-1 controls semicircular canal formation in the mouse inner ear. *Development, 125*, 33–39.

Hallahan, D. P., & Kauffman, J. M. (1997). *Exceptional learners* (7th ed.). Boston: Allyn & Bacon.

Hallahan, D. P., Kauffman, J. M., & Lloyd, J. W. (1996). *Introduction to learning disabilities.* Boston: Allyn & Bacon.

Hallgren, B. (1950). Specific dyslexia: A clinical and genetic study. *Acta Psychiatrica et Neurologica Scandinavia*, Suppl. 65.

Hapgood, F. (2000, April–May). Garage biotech is here or just around the corner. *Civilization*, pp. 46-51.

Hardy-Brown, K. (1983). Universals and individual differences: Disentangling two approaches to the study of language acquisition. *Developmental Psychology, 19*, 610–624.

Hardy-Brown, K., & Plomin, R. (1985). Infant communicative development: Evidence from adoptive and biological families for genetic and environmental influences on rate differences. *Developmental Psychology, 21*, 378–385.

Hardy-Brown, K., Plomin, R., & DeFries, J. C. (1981). Genetic and environmental influences on the rate of communicative development in the first year of life. *Developmental Psychology, 17*, 704–717.

Harrison, M. R., Golbus, M. S., & Filly, R. A. (1984). *The unborn patient.* Orlando: Grune & Stratton.

Hay, D. A., Prior, M., Collett, S., & Williams, M. (1987). Speech and language development of twins. *Acta Geneticae Medicae et Gemellologiae, 36*, 213–223.

Heath, A., & Madden, P. F. (1995). Genetic influences on smoking behavior. In J. R. Turner, L. R. Cardon, & J. K. Hewitt (Eds.), *Behavior genetic approaches in behavioral medicine* (pp. 45–66). New York: Plenum.

Hier, D. B., & Rosenberger, P. B. (1980). Focal left temporal lobe lesions and delayed speech acquisition. *Journal of Developmental and Behavioral Pediatrics, 1*, 54–57.

Hooker, D. (1939). Fetal behavior. *Association for Research in Nervous and Mental Disease, XIX: Interrelationships of mind and body* (pp. 237–243). Baltimore: Williams & Wilkins.

Howie, P. (1981). Concordance for stuttering in monozygotic and dizygotic twin pairs. *Journal of Speech and Hearing Research, 24*, 317–321.

Hugdahl, K., Synnevag, B., & Satz, P. (1990). Immune and autoimmune disorders in dyslexic children. *Neuropsychologia, 28*, 673–679.

Humphrey, T. (1970). Reflex activity in the oral and facial area of the human fetus. In J. Bosma (Ed.), *Second symposium on oral sensation and perception* (pp. 195–233). Springfield, IL: Thomas.

Hunt, A. R., Collins, J. E., Bruskiewich, R., *et al.* (1999). The DNA sequence of human chromosome 22. *Nature, 402*, 489–495.

Hurst, J. A., Baraitser, M., Auger, F., Grahm, F., & Norcll, S. (1990). An extended family with a dominantly inherited speech disorder. *Developmental Medicine and Child Neurology, 32*, 352–355.

Ingerslev, C. H., & Solow, B. (1975). Sex differences in craniofacial morphology. *Acta Odontologica Scandinavica, 33*, 85–94.

Ingham, R. J. (1987). Stuttering: Recent trends in research and therapy. In H. Winitz (Ed.), *Human communication and its disorders* (pp. 1–63). Norwood, NJ: Ablex.

Ingram, T. T. S. (1959). Specific developmental disorders of speech in childhood. *Brain, 82*, 450–454.

Isaacson, G., & Mintz, M. C. (1986). Magnetic resonance image of the fetal temporal bone. *Laryngoscope 96*, 1343–1346.

Isaacson, G., & Mintz, M. C. (1986). Prenatal visualization of the inner ear. *Journal of Ultrasound in Medicine, 5*, 409–410.

Isaacson, G., Mintz, M. C., & Crelin, E. S. (1986). *Atlas of fetal sectional anatomy*. New York: Springer Verlag.

Israel, H. (1968). Continuing growth in the human cranial skeleton. *Archives of Oral Biology, 13*, 133–137.

Jabs, E. W., Li, X., Coss, C. A., Taylor, E. W., Meyers, D. A., & Weber, J. L. (1991). Mapping the Treacher–Collins syndrome locus to 5q31.3–q33.3. *Genomics, 11*, 193–198.

Jahn, A. F. (1988). Bone physiology of the temporal bone, otic capsule, and ossicles. In A. Jahn & J. Santos-Sacchi (Eds.), *Physiology of the ear* (pp. 143–158). New York: Raven Press.

Jahrsdoerfer, R. A., & Jacobson, J. T. (1995). Treacher Collins syndrome: Otologic and auditory management. *Journal of the American Academy of Audiology, 6*, 93–102.

Johnson, W., *et al.* (1959). *The onset of stuttering*. Minneapolis: University of Minnesota Press.

Johnston, M. C. (1975). The neural crest in abnormalities of the face and brain. *Birth Defects Original Articles Series, 11*, 1–18

Jones, B. C., & Mormede, P. (Eds.) (1999). *Neurobehavioral genetics: Methods and applications*. Boca Raton, FL: CRC.

Jones, M. C. (1988). Etiology of facial clefts: Prospective evaluation of 428 patients. *Cleft Palate Journal, 25*, 16–20.

Jones, M. B., & Szatmari, P. (1988). Stoppage rules and genetic studies of autism. *Journal of Autism and Developmental Disorders, 18*, 31–40.

Jung, J. H. (1989). *Genetic syndromes in communication disorders*. Boston: College-Hill.

Kapur, Y. P. (1996). Epidemiology of childhood hearing loss. In S. E. Gerber (Ed.), *The handbook of pediatric audiology* (pp. 3–14). Washington, DC: Gallaudet University Press.

Kelly, A. (1999, June). The molecular biology of hearing and deafness, *Hereditary Deafness Newsletter*, pp. 12–15.

Kelly, T. E. (1986). *Clinical genetics and genetic counseling* (2nd ed.). Chicago: Year Book Medical.

Kidd, K. (1977). A genetic perspective on stuttering. *Journal of Fluency Disorders, 2*, 259–269.

Kidd, K. (1980). Genetic models of stuttering. *Journal of Fluency Disorders, 5*, 187–201.

Kidd, K. (1983). Recent progress on the genetics of stuttering. In C. Ludlow & J. Cooper (Eds.), *Genetic aspects of speech and language disorders* (pp. 197–213). New York: Academic Press.

Kidd, K. (1984). Stuttering as a genetic disorder. In R. F. Curlee & W. H. Perkins (Eds.), *Nature and treatment of stuttering: New directions* (pp. 149–169). Boston: Allyn and Bacon.

Kidd, K., Kidd, J., & Records, M. A. (1978). The possible causes of the sex ratio in stuttering and its implications. *Journal of Fluency Disorders, 3*, 13–23.

Killackey, H. P., & Belford, G. R. (1979). The formation of afferent patterns in the somatosensory cortex of the neonatal rat. *Journal of Comparative Neurology, 183*, 285–303.

Kmiec, E. B. (1999). Gene therapy. *American Scientist, 87*, 240–247.

Konigsmark, B. W. (1971). Hereditary congenital severe deafness syndromes. *Annals of Otology, Rhinology, & Laryngology, 80*, 269–288.

Konigsmark, B. W., & Gorlin, R. J. (1976). *Genetic and metabolic deafness*. Philadelphia: Saunders.

Korres, S. G., Manta, P. B., Balatsouras, D. G., & Papageorgiou, C. T. (1999). Audiological assessment in patients with mitochondrial myopathy. *Scandinavian Audiology, 28*, 231–240.

Kotval, J. S. (1994). *DNA-based tests: Policy implications for New York State. LCST Report No. 94-1.* Albany, NY: Legislative Commission on Science and Technology.

Krogman, W. (1974). Craniofacial growth and development: An appraisal. *Yearbook of Physical Anthropology, 18*, 31–64.

Kunst, H., Marres, H., Huygen, P., Ensink, R., VanCamp, G., VanHauwe, P., Coucke, P., Willems, P., & Cremers, C. (1998). Nonsyndromic autosomal dominant progressive sensorineural hearing loss: Audiologic analysis of a pedigree linked to DFNA2. *Laryngoscope, 108*, 74–80.

Kurnit, D. M., Layton, W. M., & Matthysse, S. (1987). Genetics, chance, and morphogenesis. *American Journal of Human Genetics, 41*, 979–995.

Lahey, M., & Edwards, J. (1995). Specific language impairment: Preliminary investigation of factors associated with family history and with patterns of language. *Journal of Speech and Hearing Research, 38*, 643–657.

Lalwani, A. K., Mhatre, A. N., San Agustin, T. B., & Wilcox, E. R. (1996). Genotype-phenotype correlations in type 1 Waardenburg syndrome. *Laryngoscope, 106*, 895–902.

Lander, E. S., & Botstein, D. (1989). Mapping Mendelian factors underlying quantitative traits using RFLP linkage maps. *Genetics, 121*, 185–199.

Lander, E. S., & Schork, N. J. (1994). Genetic dissection of complex traits. *Science, 266*, 2037–2048.

Lanford, P. J., Lan, Y., Jiang, R., Lidsell, C., Weinmaster, G., Gridley, T., & Kelley, M. W. (1999). Notch signaling pathway mediates hair cell development in mammalian cochlea. *Nature Genetics, 21*, 289–292.

Latham, R. A. (1970). Maxillary development and growth: The septomaxillary ligament. *Journal of Anatomy, 107*, 471–478.

Lenoir, M., Puel, J. L., & Pujol, R. (1987). Stereocilia and tectorial membrane development in the rat cochlea: An SEM study. *Anatomy and Embryology (Berl.), 175*, 477–487.

Lewis, B. A. (1992). Pedigree analysis of children with phonology disorders. *Journal of Learning Disability, 25*, 586–597.

Lewis, B. A., & Thompson, L. A. (1992). A study of developmental speech and language disorders in twins. *Journal of Speech and Hearing Research, 35*, 1086–1094.

Lewis, B. A., Cox, N. J., & Byard, P. J. (1993). Segregation analysis of speech and language disorders. *Behavior Genetics, 23*, 291–297.

Lewis, E. R., & Li, C .W. (1967). Evidence concerning the morphogenesis of saccular receptors in the bullfrog (*Rana catesbeiana*). *Journal of Morphology, 139*, 351–361.

Li, C. W., Van De Water, T. R., & Ruben, R. J. (1978). The fate mapping of the eleventh and twelfth day mouse ototcyst: An *in vitro* study of the sites of origin of the embryonic inner ear sensory structures. *Journal of Morphology, 157*, 249–268.

Light, J. G., DeFries, J. C., & Olson, R. K. (1998). Multivariate behavioral genetic analysis of achievement and cognitive measures in reading-disabled and control twin pairs. *Human Biology, 70*, 215–237.

Lim, D. J., & Anniko, M. (1985). Developmental morphology of the mouse inner ear: A scanning electron microscopic observation. *Acta Otolaryngologica (Suppl.), 422*, 1–69.

Lina-Granade, G., Kreiss, M., Gelas, T., Collet, L., & Morgan, A. (1998). Cochlear irregularities in obligate carriers of recessive genetic hearing impairment and in control subjects. In D. Stephens, A. Read, & A. Martini (Eds.), *Developments in genetic hearing impairment* (pp. 68–76). London: Whurr.

Lipson, A. H., Yuille, D., Angel, M., Thompson, P. G., Vanderwoord, J. G., & Beckenham, E. J. (1991). Velo-cardio-facial syndrome: An important syndrome for the dysmorphologist to recognize. *Journal of Medical Genetics, 28*, 596–604.

Liu, X. Z., Newton, V. E., & Read, A. P. (1995). Waardenburg syndrome type, II: Phenotypic findings and diagnostic criteria. *American Journal of Medical Genetics, 55*, 95–100.

Locke, J. L., & Mather, P. L. (1989). Genetic factors in the ontogeny of spoken language: Evidence from monozygotic and dizygotic twins. *Journal of Child Language, 16*, 553–559.

Love, J. K. (1896). *Deaf mutism: A clinical and pathological study.* Glasgow: James MacLehose and Sons.

Lubs, H. A., Rabin, M., Feldman, E., Jallad, B. J., Kushch, A., & Gross-Glenn, K. (1993). Familial dyslexia: Genetic and medical findings in eleven three-generation families. *Annals of Dyslexia, 43*, 44–60.

Lubs, M.-L. (1983). In M. J. Krajicek & A. I. Tearney (Eds.), *Detection of developmental disorders in children* (2nd ed.). Austin: ProEd.

Luchsinger, R. (1970). Inheritance of speech deficits. *Folia Phoniatrica, 22*, 216–230.

Ludlow, C. (1999). A conceptual framework for investigating the neurobiology of stuttering. In N. B. Ratner & E. C. Healey (Eds.), *Stuttering research and practice: Bridging the gap* (pp. 63–84). Mahwah, NJ: Erlbaum.

Lykken, D. T. (1982). Research with twins: The concept of emergenesis. *Psychophysiology, 19*, 361–373.

Lyons, M. J., True, W., Eisen, S., Goldberg, J., Meyer, J. M., Faraone, S., Eaves, L. J., & Tsuang, M. T. (1995). Differential heritability of adult and juvenile antisocial traits. *Archives of General Psychiatry, 52*, 906–915.

Ma, Q., Sommer, L., Cserjesi, P., & Anderson, D. J. (1997). Mash1 and neurogenin 1 expression patterns define complementary domains of neuroepithelium in the developing CNS and are correlated with regions expressing notch ligands. *Journal of Neuroscience, 17*, 3644–3652.

Ma, Q., Chen, Z., del Barco Barantes, I., de la Pompa, J. L., & Anderson D. J. (1998). Neurogenin-1 is essential for the determination of neuronal precursors for proximal cranial sensory ganglia. *Neuron, 20*, 469–482.

MacKenzie-Stepner, K., Witzel, M. A., Stringer, D. A., Lindsay, W. K., Munro, I. R., & Hughes, H. (1987). Abnormal carotid arteries in Velocardiofacial syndrome: A report of three cases. *Plastic and Reconstructive Surgery, 80*, 347–351.

Mansour, S. L., Goddard, J. M., & Capecchi, M. (1993). Mice homozygous for a targeted disruption of the proto-oncogene int-2 have development defects in the tail and inner ear. *Development, 117*, 13–28.

Matarazzo, J. D., & Pankeratz, L. D. (1980). Intelligence. In R. H. Woody (Ed.), *Encyclopedia of clinical assessment* (pp. 697–713). San Francisco: Jossey-Bass.

Matheny, A. P., & Bruggemann, C. E. (1973). Children's speech: Hereditary components and sex differences. *Folia Phoniatrica, 25*, 442–449.

Mather, P. L., & Black, K. N. (1984). Hereditary and environmental influences on preschool twins' language skills. *Developmental Psychology, 20*, 303–308.

May, M. (1986). *The facial nerve.* New York: Thieme.

Maynard-Smith, J., & Szathmary, E. (1995). *The major transitions in evolution.* Oxford: Freeman.

McGoodwin, W. (1996). Genie out of the bottle: Genetic testing and the discrimination it's creating. *The Washington Post*, May 5, p. C3.

McGuffin, P., Owen, M. J., O'Donovan, M. C., Thapar, A., & Gottesman, I. I. (1994). *Seminars in Psychiatric Genetics.* London: Royal College of Psychiatrists.

McGuirt, W. T., & Smith, R. J. H. (1999). Connexin 26 as a cause of hereditary hearing loss. *American Journal of Audiology, 8*, 93–100.

McKenna, M. J., & Mills, B. G. (1989). Immunohistochemical evidence of measles virus antigens in active otosclerosis. *Otolaryngology–Head and Neck Surgery, 101*, 415–421.

McKusick, V. (1991). *Mendelian inheritance in man* (9th ed.). Baltimore: Johns Hopkins University Press.

McKusick, V. A. (2000). *Mendelian inheritance in man* [online]. 4-29-2000. Internet Communication.

McPhee, J. R., & Van De Water, T. R. (1986). Epithelial–mesenchymal tissue interactions guiding otic capsule formation: The role of the otocyst. *Journal of Embryology and Experimental Morphology*, *97*, 1–24.

McReady, E. B. (1926). Defects in the zone of language (word-deafness and word-blindness) and their influence in education and behavior. *American Journal of Psychiatry*, *6*, 267–277.

Mendel, G. (1865). *Versuche über Pflantzenhybriden*. Brünn: Verhandlungen des Naturvorschenden Vereins.

Minton, H., & Schneider, F. (1985). *Differential psychology*. Prospect Heights, IL: Waveland.

Mitnick, R. J., Bello, J. A., Golding-Kushner, K. J., Argamaso, R. V., & Shprintzen, R. J. (1996). The use of magnetic resonance angiography prior to pharyngeal flap surgery in patients with velo-cardio-facial syndrome. *Plastic and Reconstructive Surgery*, *97*, 908–919.

Mohammed, A. (1999). Clinton proposes patient privacy. *Reuters Limited on America Online*, October 29.

Molfese, V. J. (1989). *Perinatal risk and infant development: Assessment and prediction*. New York: Guilford.

Morell, R., Friedman, T. B., Asher, J. H. J., & Robbins, L. G. (1997). The incidence of deafness is nonrandomly distributed among families segregating for Waardenburg syndrome type 1 (WS1). *Journal of Medical Genetics*, *34*, 447–452.

Morell, R. J., Kim, H. J., Hood, L. J., Goforth, L., Friderici, K., Fisher, R., VanCamp, G., Berlin, C. I., Oddoux, C., Ostrer, H., Keats, B., & Friedman, T. B. (1998). Mutations in the connexin 26 gene (GJB2) among Ashkenazi Jews with nonsyndromic recessive deafness. *New England Journal of Medicine*, *339*, 1500–1505.

Morelli, T. (1992). Genetic discrimination by insurers: Legal protections needed from abuse of biotechnology. *Health Span*, *8*(9), 8–11.

Morris, D. W., Robinson, L., Turic, D., Duke, M., Webb, V., Milham, C., Hopkin, E., Pound, K., Fernando, S., Easton, M., Hamshere, M., Williams, N., McGuffin, P., Stevenson, J., Krawczak, M., Owen, M. J., O'Donovan, M. C., & Williams, J. (2000). Family-based association mapping provides evidence for a gene for reading disability on chromosome 15q. *Human Molecular Genetics*, *9*, 855–860.

Morsli, H., Choo, D., Ryan, A. L., Johnson, R., & Wu, D. K. (1998). Development of the mouse inner ear and origin of its sensory organs. *Journal of Neuroscience*, *18*, 3327–3335.

Morsli, H., Tuorto, F., Choo, D., Postiglione, M. P., Simeone, A., & Wu, D. K. (1999). Otx1 and Otx2 activities are required for the normal development of the mouse inner ear. *Development*, *126*, 2335–2343.

Moss, M. L. (1962). The functional matrix. In B. S. Kraus & R. A. Riedel (Eds.), *Vistas in orthodontics* (pp. 85–97). Philadelphia: Lea & Febiger.

Munsinger, H., & Douglass, A. (1976). The syntactic abilities of identical twins, fraternal twins, and their siblings. *Child Development*, *47*, 40–50.

Murgia, A., Orzan, E., Polli, R., Martella, M., Vinanzi, C., Leonardi, E., Arslan, E., & Zacchello, F. (1999). Cx26 deafness: Mutation analysis and clinical variability. *Journal of Medical Genetics*, *36*, 829–832.

Murray, J. C., Nishimura, D. Y., Buetow, K. H., Ardinger, H. H., Spence, M. A., Sparkes, R. S., Falk, R. E., Falk, P. M., Gardner, R. J. M., Harkness, E. M., Glinski, L. P., Pauli, R. M., Nakamura, Y., Green, P. P., & Schinzel, A. (1990). Linkage of an autosomal dominant clefting syndrome (van der Woude) to loci on chromosome 1q. *American Journal of Human Genetics*, *46*, 486–491.

Murray, J. C., Buetow, K. H., Weber, J. L., Ludwigsen, S., Scherpbier-Heddema, T., Manion, F., Quillen, J., Sheffield, V. C., Sunden, S., Duyk, G. M., Weissenbach, J., Gyapay, G., Dib, C., Morrissette, J., Lathrop, G. M., Vignal, A., White, R., Matsunami, N., Gerken, S., Melis, R., Albertsen, H., Plaetke, R., Odelberg, S., Ward, D., Dausset, J., Cohen, D., & Cann, H. (1994). A comprehensive human linkage map with centimorgan density. *Cooperative Human Linkage Center (CHLC). Science, 265,* 2049–2054.

Nance, W. E., Sweeney, A., McLeod, A. C., & Cooper, M. C. (1970). Hereditary deafness: A presentation of some recognized types, modes of inheritance, and aids in counseling. *Southern Medical Bulletin, 58,* 41–57.

National Bioethics Advisory Committee (1998). *Research involving persons with mental disorders that may affect decision-making capacity* [online]. Available: http://bioethics.gov.

National Cancer Institute (undated). *Understanding gene testing.* U.S. Department of Health and Human Services, Public Health Service, National Institutes of Health.

National Institutes of Health. (1993). *Biomedical and behavioral research: An overview.* Human subject protections: Institutional Review Board. Office for Human Subject Protections [Available: Http://ohrp.osophs.dhhs.gov/irb/irb_guidebook.htm].

National Institutes of Health (1993). Early identification of hearing impairment in infants and young children. *NIH Consensus Statement, 11,* 1–24. Washington, DC: National Institutes of Health.

Neale, M., & Cardon, L. (1992). *Methodology for genetic studies of twins and families.* Dordrecht, The Netherlands: Kluwer.

Neils, J., & Aram, D. (1986). Family history of children with developmental language disorders. *Perceptual and Motor Skills, 63,* 655–658.

Nelkin, D. (1992). The social power of genetic information. In D. J. Kevles & L. Hood (Eds.), *Scientific and social issues in the Human Genome Project* (pp. 177–190). Cambridge: Harvard University Press.

Nelson, D., & Weiss, R. (1999). Family's debate mirrored scientists' on gene therapy risk. *Washington Post,* 30 September, p. A07.

Nelson, S. E. (1939). The role of heredity in stuttering. *Journal of Pediatrics, 14,* 642–654.

Nelson, S. E., Hunter, N., & Walter, M. (1945). Stuttering in twin types. *Journal of Speech Disorders, 10,* 335–343.

Neyroud, N., Tesson, F., Denjoy, I., Leibovici, M., Donger, C., Barhanin, J., Faure, S., Gary, F., Coumel, P., Petit, C., Schwartz, K., & Guicheney, P. (1997). A novel mutation in the potassium channel gene KVLQT1 causes the Jervell and Lange–Nielsen cardioauditory syndrome. *Nature Genetics, 15,* 186–189.

Niedermeyer, H. P., & Arnold W. (1995). Otosclerosis: A measles virus associated inflammatory disease. *Acta Otolaryngologica, 115,* 300–303.

Nigg, J., & Goldsmith, H. H. (1998). Developmental psychopathology, personality, and temperament: Reflections on recent behavior. *Human Biology, 70,* 387–412.

NIH–DOE Task Force on Genetic Testing (1997). *Promoting safe and effective genetic testing in the United States: Principles and recommendations.* Washington, DC: NIH–DOE Working Group on Ethical, Legal and Social Implications of Human Genome Research.

Nora, J. J., & Fraser, F. C. (1989). *Medical genetics* (3rd ed.). Philadelphia: Lea & Febiger.

Nowak, C. B. (1998). Genetics and hearing loss: A review of Stickler syndrome. *Journal of Communication Disorders, 31,* 437–453.

Nuland, S. B. (2000). The misty crystal ball. *American Scholar, 69*(2), 129–132.

Nyhan, W. L. (1991). Classic approaches to the treatment of inherited metabolic disease. In T. Friedmann (Ed.), *Therapy for genetic disease* (pp. 1–33). Oxford: Oxford University Press.

Office of Technology Assessment, U.S. Congress (1991). *Medical monitoring and screening in the workplace: Results of a survey-background paper.* Washington, DC: Government Printing Office.

Oh, S. H., Johnson, R., & Wu, D. K. (1996). Differential expression of bone morphogenetic proteins in the developing vestibular and auditory sensory organs. *Journal of Neuroscience, 16,* 6463–6475.

Olson, R. K., Forsberg, H., & Wise, B. (1994). Genes, environment, and the development of orthographic skills. In V. W. Berninger (Ed.), *The varieties of orthographic knowledge.* Vol. 1: *Theoretical developmental issues* (pp. 1–31). Dordrecht: Kluwer.

Orkin, S. H., & Motulsky, A. G. (1995). *Report and recommendations of the panel to assess the NIH investment in research on gene therapy*. Washington, DC: National Institutes of Health.

Osborne, R. T., Gregor, A. J., & Miele, F. (1968). Heritability of factor V: Verbal comprehension. *Perceptual and Motor Skills, 26*, 191–202.

Owen, F., Adams, P., Forrest, T., Stolz, L., & Fisher, S. (1971). Learning disorders in children: Sibling studies. *Monographs of the Society for Research in Child Development, 36*, No. 4.

Papadaki, E., Prassopoulos, P., Bizakis, J., Karampekios, S., Papadakis, H., & Gourtsoyiannis, N. (1998). X-linked deafness with stapes gusher in females. *European Journal of Radiology, 29*, 71–75.

Papolos, D. F., Faedda, G. L., Veit, S., Goldberg, R., Morrow, B., Kucherlapati, R., & Shprintzen, R. J. (1996). Bipolar spectrum disorders in patients diagnosed with velo-cardio-facial syndrome: Does a hemizygous deletion of chromosome 22q11 result in bipolar affective disorder? *American Journal of Psychiatry, 153*, 1541–1547.

Parving, A., & Christensen, B. (1996). Epidemiology of permanent hearing impairment in children in relation to costs of a hearing health surveillance program. *International Journal of Pediatric Otorhinolaryngology, 34*, 9–23.

Pauls, D. L. (1990). A review of the evidence for genetic factors in stuttering. In *Research needs in stuttering. ASHA reports 18* (pp. 34–38). Rockville, MD: American Speech–Language–Hearing Association.

Pauls, D. L., Leckman, J. F., & Cohen, D. J. (1993). Familial relationship between Gilles de la Tourette's syndrome, attention deficit disorder, learning disabilities, speech disorders and stuttering. *Journal of the American Academy of Child and Adolescent Psychiatry, 32*, 1044–1050.

Pedziwiatr, Z. (1971). Morphological data for the theory of temporal bone vibrations. *Polish Medical Journal, 10*, 547–563.

Pennington, B. F. (1990). Annotation: The genetics of dyslexia. *Journal of Child Psychiatry and Psychology, 31*, 193–201.

Pennington, B. F. (1991). *Diagnosing learning disorders: A neuropsychological framework*. New York: Guilford.

Pennington, B. F. (1997). Using genetics to dissect cognition. *American Journal of Human Genetics, 60*, 13–16.

Pennington, B. F., & Gilger, J. W. (1996). How is dyslexia transmitted? In C. Chase, G. Rosen, & G. Sherman (Eds.), *Neural and cognitive mechanisms underlying speech, language and reading* (pp. 41–62). Baltimore: York.

Pennington, B. F., Smith, S., Kimberling, W., Green, P., & Haith, M. (1987). Left-handedness and immune disorders in familial dyslexics. *Archives of Neurology, 44*, 634–639.

Pennington, B. F., Gilger, J. W., Pauls, D., Smith, S. A., Smith, S. D., & DeFries, J. C. (1991). Evidence for major gene transmission of developmental dyslexia. *Journal of the American Medical Association, 266*, 1527–1534.

Pennington, B. F., Gilger, J. W., Olson, R. K., & DeFries, J. C. (1992). The external validity of age-discrepancy versus IQ-discrepancy definitions of reading disability: Lessons from a twin study. *Journal of Learning Disabilities, 25*, 562–573.

Penrose, L. S. (1963). *The biology of mental defect* (3rd ed.). London: Sidgwick & Jackson.

Peterson-Falzone, S. J. (1989). Basic concepts in congenital craniofacial defects. In K. R. Bzoch (Ed.), *Communicative disorders related to cleft lip and palate* (3rd ed.) (pp. 37–46). Boston: College-Hill.

Petryshen, T. L., Kaplan, B. J., Hughes, M. L., & Field, L. L. (2000). Evidence for the chromosome 2p15–p16 dyslexia susceptibility locus (DXY3) in a large Canadian data set. *American Journal of Medical Genetics (Neuropsychiatric Genetics), 96*, 473.

Petryshen, T. L., Kaplan, B. J., Liu, M. F., & Field, L. L. (2000). Absence of significant linkage between phonological decoding dyslexia and chromosome 6p23–21.3, as determined by use of quantitative-trait methods: Confirmation of qualitative analyses. *American Journal of Human Genetics, 66*, 708–714.

Pfaff, D. W., Berrettini, W. H., Joh, T. H., & Maxson, S. C. (Eds.) (1999). *Genetic influences on neural and behavioral functions.* Boca Raton, FL: CRC.

Phelps, P. D., Coffey, R. A., Trembath, R. C., Luxon, L. M., Grossman, A. B., Britton, K. E., Kendall-Taylor, P., Graham, J. M., Cadge, B. C., Stephens, S. G., Pembrey, M. E., & Reardon, W. (1998). Radiological malformations of the ear in Pendred syndrome. *Clinical Radiology, 53,* 268–273.

Pierce, R. H., Mainen, M. W., & Bosma, J. F. (1977). *The cranium of the newborn infant.* DHEW Publication No. (NIH) 76-788. Bethesda, MD: U.S. Department of Health, Education, & Welfare.

Pinker, S. (1994). *The language instinct: The new science of language and mind.* London: Penguin.

Piven, J., Gayle, J., Chase, G., Fink, B., Landa, R., Wzorek, M. M., & Folstein, S. E. (1990). A family history of neuropsychiatric disorders in the adult siblings of autistic individuals. *Journal of the American Academy of Child and Adolescent Psychiatry, 29,* 177–184.

Plann, S. (1997). *Silent minority: Deaf education in Spain, 1550–1835.* Berkeley: University of California Press.

Plomin, R. (1986). *Development, genetics, and psychology.* Hillsdale, NJ: Erlbaum.

Plomin, R., & Bergeman, C. S. (1991). The nature of nurture: Genetic influence on "environmental" measures. *Behavioral and Brain Sciences, 14,* 373–427.

Plomin, R., & McClearn, G. (Eds.) (1993). *Nature, nurture and psychology.* Washington, DC: APA.

Plomin, R., & Rende, R. (1991). Human behavioral genetics. *Annual Review of Psychology, 42,* 1–66.

Plomin, R., DeFries, J. C., & Fulker, D. W. (1988). *Nature and nurture during infancy and early childhood.* New York: Cambridge University Press.

Plomin, R., Owen, M. J., & McGuffin, P. (1994). The genetic basis of complex behaviors. *Science, 264,* 1733–1739.

Plomin, R., DeFries, J. C., McClearn, G., & Rutter, M. (1997). *Behavioral genetics: A primer.* New York: Freeman.

Ponder, M., Lee, J., Green, J., & Richards, M. (1996). Family history and perceived vulnerability to some common diseases: A study of young people and their parents. *Journal of Medical Genetics, 33,* 485–492.

Probst, F. J., & Camper, S. A. (1999). The role of mouse mutants in the identification of human hereditary hearing loss genes. *Hearing Research, 130,* 1–6.

Pron, G., Galloway, C., Armstrong, D., & Posnick, J. (1993). Ear malformation and hearing loss in patients with Treacher Collins syndrome. *Cleft Palate and Craniofacial Journal, 30,* 97–103.

Pyeritz, R. E. (1998). Family history and risk factors: forward to the future. *Genetics in Practice, 4*(4), 1–3.

Rabin, M., Wen, X. L., Hepburn, M., Lubs, H. A., Feldman, E., & Duara, R. (1993). Suggestive linkage of developmental dyslexia to chromosome 1p34–p36. *Lancet, 342,* 178.

Randall, D., Reynell, J., & Curwen, M. (1974). A study of language development in a sample of 3–year-old children. *British Journal of Disorders of Communication, 9,* 3–16.

Read, A. P., & Newton, V. E. (1997). Waardenburg syndrome. *Journal of Medical Genetics, 34,* 656–665.

Regehr, S. M., & Kaplan, B. J. (1988). Reading disability with motor problems may be an inherited subtype. *Pediatrics, 82,* 204–210.

Reilly, P. R. (1997). Fear of genetic discrimination drives legislative interest. *Human Genome News, 8*(3&4), 1–3.

Represa, J., Frenz, D. A., & Van De Water, T. R. (2000). Genetic patterning of embryonic inner ear development. *Acta Otolaryngologica, 120,* 5–10.

Reus, V. L., & Freimer, N. B. (1997). Understanding the genetic basis of mood disorders: Where do we stand? *American Journal of Human Genetics, 60,* 1283–1288.

Reyes, M. R., LeBlanc, E. M., & Bassila, M. K. (1999). Hearing loss and otitis media in velo-cardio-facial syndrome. *International Journal of Pediatric Otorhinolaryngology, 47,* 227–233.

Riazuddin, S., Castelein, C. M., Friedman, T. B., Lalwani, A. K., Liburd, N., Naz, S., Smith, T. N., Riazuddin, S., & Wilcox, E. R. (1999). A novel nonsyndromic recessive form of deafness maps to 4q28 and demonstrates incomplete penetrance. *American Journal of Human Genetics, 65*, A101.

Rice, M. L. (1996). Of language, phenotypes, and genetics: Building a cross-disciplinary platform for inquiry. In M. L. Rice (Ed.), *Toward a genetics of language* (pp. xi–xxv). Mahwah, NJ: Erlbaum.

Rice, M. L. (1997). Specific language impairments: In search of diagnostic markers and genetic contributions. *Mental Retardation and Developmental Disabilities Research Reviews, 3*, 350–357.

Richards, M. (1996). Families, kinship, and genetics. In T. Marteau & M. Richards (Eds.), *The troubled helix: Social and psychological implications of the new human genetics* (pp. 249–273). Cambridge: Cambridge University Press.

Richards, M. (1997). It runs in the family: Lay knowledge about inheritance. In A. Clarke & E. Parsons (Eds.), *Culture, kinship, and genes: Towards cross–cultural genetics* (pp. 175-194). New York: St Martin's.

Richards, M., & Ponder, M. (1996). Lay understanding of genetics: A test of a hypothesis. *Journal of Medical Genetics, 33*, 1032–1036.

Riggins-Caspers, K., & Cadoret, R. J. (1999). Detecting and measuring gene–environment interaction in human temperament (aggressivity) and personality deviation (conduct disorder, antisocial personality). In B. Jones & P. Mormede (Eds.), *Neurobehavioral genetics: Methods and applications* (pp. 163–186). New York: CRC.

Risch, N. (1990). Linkage strategies for genetically complex traits, I: Multilocus models. *American Journal of Human Genetics, 46*, 222–228.

Robinson, L., Morris, D. W., Turic, D., Duke, M., Webb, V., Milham, C., Hopkin, E., Pound, K., Fernando, S., Easton, M., Hamshere, M., Williams, N., McGuffin, P., Stevenson, J., Krawczak, M., Owen, M. J., O'Donovan, M. C., & Williams, J. (2000). *Dimensions of reading disability.* Unpublished paper.

Rollnick, B. R., & Pruzansky, S. (1981). Genetic services at a center for craniofacial anomalies. *Cleft Palate Journal, 18*, 304–313.

Rossetti, L. M. (1986). *High-risk infants.* Boston: College-Hill.

Rowe, D. C. (1994). *The limits of family influence: Genes, experience, and behavior.* New York: Guilford.

Rowe, D. C. (1997). A place at the policy table? Behavior genetics and estimates of family environmental effects on IQ. *Cognitive Science, 24*, 133–158.

Ruben, R. J. (1967). Development of the inner ear of the mouse: A radioautographic study of terminal mitoses. *Acta Otolaryngologica, 220*, 1–44.

Ruben, R. J. (1991). The history of the genetics of hearing impairment. *Annals of the New York Academy of Sciences, 630*, 6–15.

Ruben, R. J. (1999). Hearing the past: Speaking the future. *AAS Bulletin, 24*(2), 22–25, 28.

Ruben, R. J., & Fishman, G. (1980). Otological care of the hearing impaired child. In G. T. Mencher & S. E. Gerber (Eds.), *Early management of hearing loss* (pp. 105–120). New York: Grune & Stratton.

Ruben, R. J., & Math, R. (1978). Serous otitis media associated with sensorineural hearing loss in children. *Laryngoscope, 88*, 1139–1154.

Ruben, R. J., Van De Water, T. R., & Steel, K. P. (Eds.) (1991). *Genetics of hearing impairment.* New York: New York Academy of Sciences.

Rubin, P. (1964). *The dynamic classification of bone dysplasias.* Chicago: Year Book.

Rueda, J., Cantos, R., & Lim, D. J. (1996). Tectorial membrane-organ of Corti relationship during cochlear development. *Anatomy and Embryology, 194*, 501–514.

Rusch, A., Lysakaowski, A., & Eatock, R. A. (1998). Postnatal development of type I and type II hair cells in the mouse utricle: Acquisition of voltage-gated conductances and differentiated morphology. *Journal of Neuroscience, 18*, 7487–7501.

Rutter, M., Tizard, J., & Whitmore, K. (1970). *Education, health, and behaviour*. London: Longmans.

Ryan, A. K., Goodship, J. A., Wilson, D. I., Philip, N., Levy, A., Seidel, H., Schuffenhauer, S., Oechsler, H., Belohradsky, B., Prieur, M., Aurias, A., Raymond, F. L., Clayton-Smith, J., Hatchwell, E., McKeown, C., Beemer, F. A., Dallapiccola, B., Novelli, G., Hurst, J. A., Ignatius, J., Green, A. J., Winter, R. M., Brueton, L., Brondum-Nielsen, K., Scambler, P. J., *et al.* (1997). Spectrum of clinical features associated with interstitial chromosome 22q11 deletions: A European collaborative study. *Medical Genetics, 34*, 798–804.

Sabouri, L. A., Mahadevan, M. S., Narang, M., Lee, D. S., Surh, L. C., & Korneluk, R. G. (1993). Effect of the myotonic dystrophy (DM) mutation on mRNA levels of the DM gene. *Nature Genetics, 4*, 233–238.

Salminen, M., Meyer, I. B., Bober, E., & Gruss, P. (2000). Netrin 1 is required for semicircular canal formation in the mouse inner ear. *Development, 127*, 13–22.

Samples, J. M., & Lane, V. W. (1985). Genetic possibilities in six siblings with specific language learning disorders. *Asha, 27*, 27–32.

Saunders, A. M., Strittmatter, W. J., & Schmechel, D. (1993). Association of apolipoprotein E allele epsilon4 with late-onset familial and sporadic Alzheimer's disease. *Neurology, 43*, 1467–1472.

Saw, D. J., Steel, K. P., & Brown, S. D. (1997). Shaker mice and a peek into the House of Usher. *Experiments in Animals, 46*, 1–9.

Scarr, S., & Carter-Saltzman, L. (1983). Genetics and intelligence. In J. Fuller & E. Simmel (Eds.), *Behavior genetics: Principles and applications* (pp. 217–335). Hillsdale, NJ: Erlbaum.

Scarr, S., & McCartney, K. (1983). How people make their own environments: A theory of genotype–environment effects. *Child Development, 54*, 424–435.

Schulte-Korne, G., Grimm, T., Nothen, N. M., Muller-Myshok, B., Cichon, S., Vogt, I. R., Propping, P., & Remschmidt, H. (1998). Evidence for linkage of spelling disability to chromosome 15. *American Journal of Human Genetics, 63*, 279–282.

Seider, R., Gladstein, K., & Kidd, K. (1983). Recovery and persistence of stuttering among relatives of stutterers. *Journal of Speech and Hearing Disorders, 48*, 402–409.

Seppa, N. (2000). "Bubble" babies thrive on gene therapy. *Science News, 157*, 277.

Shankweiler, D., Liberman, I. Y., Mark, L. S., Fowler, C. A., & Fischer, F. W. (1979). The speech code and learning to read. *Journal of Experimental Psychology: Human Learning and Memory, 5*, 531–545.

Shaywitz, S. E., Shaywitz, B. A., Fletcher, J. M., & Escobar, M. D. (1990). Prevalence of reading disability in boys and girls. *Journal of the American Medical Association, 264*, 998–1002.

Sheehan, J., & Costley, M. (1977). A reexamination of the role of heredity in stuttering. *Journal of Speech and Hearing Disorders, 42*, 47–59.

Sheffield, V. C., Kraiem, Z., Beck, J. C., Nishimura, D., Stone, E. M., Salameh, M., Sadeh, O., & Glaser, M. (1996). Pendred syndrome maps to chromosome 7q21–34 and is caused by an intrinsic defect in thyroid iodine organification. *Nature Genetics, 12*, 424–426.

Sherman, S. L., DeFries, J. C., Gottesman, I. I., Loehlin, J. C., Meyere, J. M., Pelias, M. Z., Rice, J., & Waldman, I. (1997). ASHG Statement: Recent developments in human behavioral genetics: Past accomplishments and future directions. *American Journal of Human Genetics, 60*, 1265–1275.

Shprintzen, R. J. (1982). Palatal and pharyngeal anomalies in craniofacial syndromes. *Birth Defects Original Articles Series, 18*(1), 53–78.

Shprintzen, R. J. (1988). Pierre Robin, micrognathia, and airway obstruction: The dependency of treatment on accurate diagnosis. *International Anesthesiology Clinics, 26*, 84–91.

Shprintzen, R. J. (1991). The fallibility of clinical research. *Cleft Palate Journal, 28*, 136–140.

Shprintzen, R. J. (1994). A new perspective on clefting. In R. J. Shprintzen & J. Bardach (Eds.), *Cleft palate speech management: A multidisciplinary approach* (pp. 1–15). St. Louis: Mosby.

Shprintzen, R. J. (1997). *Genetics, syndromes, and communication disorders*. San Diego: Singular.

Shprintzen, R. J., & Goldberg, R. B. (1985). Multiple anomaly syndromes and learning disabilities. In S. Smith (Ed.), *Genetics and learning disabilities* (pp. 153–174). San Diego: College Hill Press.

Shprintzen, R. J., & Singer, L. (1992). Upper airway obstruction and the Robin sequence. *International Anesthesiology Clinics*, 30, 109–114.

Shprintzen, R. J., Goldberg, R. B., Lewin, M. L., Sidoti, E. J., Berkman, M. D., Argamaso, R. V., & Young, D. (1978). A new syndrome involving cleft palate, cardiac anomalies, typical facies, and learning disabilities: Velo-cardio-facial syndrome. *Cleft Palate Journal*, 15, 56–62.

Shprintzen, R. J., Goldberg, R. B., Young, D., & Wolford, L. (1981). The velo-cardio-facial syndrome: A clinical and genetic analysis. *Pediatrics*, 67, 167–172.

Shprintzen, R. J., Siegel-Sadewitz, V. L., Amato, J., & Goldberg, R. B. (1985). Anomalies associated with cleft lip, cleft palate, or both. *American Journal of Medical Genetics*, 20, 585–596.

Shprintzen, R. J., Siegel-Sadewitz, V. L., Amato, J., & Goldberg, R. B. (1985). Retrospective diagnoses of previously missed syndromic disorders amongst 1,000 patients with cleft lip, cleft palate, or both. *Birth Defects Original Article Series*, 21(2), 85–92.

Shute, N. C., & Ewens, W. J. (1988). A resolution of the ascertainment sampling problem. III: Pedigrees. *American Journal of Human Genetics*, 43, 387–395.

Singhal, A., & Huang, L. (1994). Gene transfer in mammalian cells using liposomes as carriers. In J. A. Wolff (Ed.). *Gene therapeutics* (pp. 118–142). Boston: Birkhäuser.

Smalley, S. L., Asarnow, R. F., & Spence, M. A. (1988). Autism and genetics: A decade of research. *Archives of General Psychiatry*, 45, 953–961.

Smith, R. J. H., & Schwartz, C. (1998) Branchio-oto-renal syndrome. *Journal of Communication Disorders*, 31, 411–421.

Smith, S. D., Kimberling, W. J., Pennington, B. F., & Lubs, H. A. (1983). Specific reading disability: Identification of an inherited form through linkage analysis. *Science*, 219, 1345.

Smith, S. D., Pennington, B. F., Kimberling, W. J., Fain, P. R., Ing, P. S., & Lubs, H. A. (1986). Genetic heterogeneity in specific reading disabilities. *American Journal of Human Genetics*, 39, 169a.

Smith, S. D., Pennington, B. F., Kimberling, B. F., & Ing, P. S. (1990). Genetic linkage analysis with specific dyslexia: Use of multiple markers to include and exclude possible loci. In G. T. Pavlidis (Ed.), *Perspectives on dyslexia*, Vol. 1: *Neurology, neuropsychology, and genetics* (pp. 77–89). West Sussex: Wiley.

Smith, S., Gilger, J., & Pennington, B. (1996). Genetics of learning disorders. In D. Rimoin, J. M. Connor, & R. Pyeritz (Eds.), *Emery and Rimoin's principles and practice of medical genetics* (pp. 1767–1790). New York: Churchill Livingstone,.

Smith, S. D., Kelley, P. M., & Brower, A. M. (1998). Molecular approaches to the genetic analysis of specific reading disability. *Human Biology*, 70, 239–256.

Smith, S. D., Kimberling, W. J., Schaefer, G. B., Horton, M. B., & Tinley, S. (1998). Medical genetic evaluation for the etiology of hearing loss in children. *Journal of Communication Disorders*, 31, 371–389.

Snik, A. F., Hombergen, G. C., Mylanus, E. A., & Cremers, C. W. (1995). Air-bone gap in patients with X-linked stapes gusher syndrome. *American Journal of Otology*, 16, 241–246.

Snow Jr., J. B. (1991). International symposium on the genetics of hearing impairment. In R. J. Ruben, T. R. Van De Water, & K. P. Steel (Eds.), *Genetics of hearing impairment* (pp. 1–2). New York: New York Academy of Sciences.

Sparks, S. N. (1982). *Birth defects and speech–language disorders*. San Diego: College-Hill.

Spitz, R. V., Tallal, P., Flax, J., & Benasich, A. A. (1997). Look who's talking: A prospective study of familial transmission of language impairments. *Journal of Speech, Language, and Hearing Research*, 40, 990–1001.

Stapells, D. R., & Ruben, R. J. (1989). Auditory brain stem responses to bone-conducted tones in infants. *Annals of Otology, Rhinology and Laryngology*, 98, 941–949.

Stausberg, R. L., Feingold, E. A., Klausner, R. D., & Collins, F. S. (1999). The mammalian gene collection. *Science, 286*, 455–457.

Steffenberg, S., Gillberg, C., Hellgren, L., Andersson, L., Gillberg, I. C., Jakobsson, G., & Bohman, M. (1989). A twin study of autism in Denmark, Finland, Iceland, Norway and Sweden. *Journal of Child Psychology and Psychiatry, 28*, 229–247.

Stein, J. F. (1993). Visuospatial perception in disabled readers. In D. M. Willows, R. S. Kruk, & E. Corcos (Eds.), *Visual processes in reading and reading disabilities* (pp. 331–346). Hillsdale, NJ: Erlbaum.

Stein, J. F., & Walsh, V. (1997). To see but not to read: The magnocellular theory of dyslexia. *Trends in Neuroscience, 20*, 147–152.

Stevenson, J. (1991). Which aspects of processing text mediate genetic effects? *Reading and Writing, 3*, 249–269.

Stevenson, J., & Richman, N. (1976). The prevalence of language delay in a population of 3-year-old children and its association with general retardation. *Developmental Medicine and Child Neurology, 18*, 431–441.

Stevenson, J., Graham, P., Fredman, G., & McLoughlin, V. (1987). A twin study of genetic influences on reading and spelling ability and disability. *Journal of Child Psychiatry and Psychology, 28*, 229–247.

Stewart, R., and Prescott, G. (Eds.) (1976). *Oral facial genetics.* St. Louis: Mosby.

Stromswold, K. (1994). *The nature of children's early grammar: Evidence from inversion errors.* Paper presented at the Linguistic Society of America.

Stromswold, K. (1998). Genetics of spoken language. *Human Biology, 70*, 297–324.

Sullivan, P. G. (1986). Skull, jaw, and teeth growth patterns. In F. Falkner & J. M. Tanner (Eds.), *Human growth,* Vol. 2.: *Postnatal growth* (pp. 381–412). New York: Plenum.

Tallal, P., Ross, R., & Curtiss, S. (1989). Familial aggregation in specific language impairment. *Journal of Speech and Hearing Disorders, 54*, 167–173.

Tanaka, T., Ozeki, Y., Aoki, T., & Ogura, Y. (1975). Morphological relation of the vestibular sensory hairs to the otolithic membrane and cupula: A scanning electron microscopic study. In M. Marimoto (Ed.), *The Proceedings of the 5th Extraordinary Meeting of the Barany Society* (pp. 403–409). Kyoto: Barany Society.

Terwilliger, J. D., & Ott, J. (1994). *Handbook of human genetic language.* Baltimore: Johns Hopkins.

The Arc (1997). Protecting genetic privacy. *Genetic Issues in Mental Retardation, 2*(1), 1–4.

The Arc (1998). Participating in genetic research: Considerations for people with mental retardation and their families. *Genetic Issues in Mental Retardation, 3*(1), 6.

The Arc (1999). *Final Report: The Arc's Human Genome Education Project.* Unpublished.

Thompson, M. W. (1986). *Genetics in medicine* (4th ed.). Philadelphia: Saunders.

Tomblin, J. B. (1989). Familial concentration of developmental language impairment. *Journal of Speech and Hearing Disorders, 54*, 287–295.

Tomblin, J. B. (1996). Genetic and environmental contributions to the risk for specific language impairment. In M. L. Rice (Ed.), *Towards a genetics of language* (pp. 191–210). Mahwah, NJ: Erlbaum.

Tomblin, J. B., & Buckwalter, P. R. (1998). Heritability of poor language achievement among twins. *Journal of Speech, Language, and Hearing Research, 41*, 188–199.

Tomblin, J. B., Hardy, J. C., & Hein, H. (1991). Predicting poor communication status in preschool children using risk factors present at birth. *Journal of Speech and Hearing Research, 34*, 1096–1105.

Tomblin, J. B., Freese, P. R., & Records, N. L. (1992). Diagnosing specific language impairment in adults for the purpose of pedigree analysis. *Journal of Speech and Hearing Research, 35*, 832–843.

Torres, M., & Giraldez, F. (1998). The development of the vertebrate inner ear. *Mechanisms of Development, 71*, 5–21.

Torres, M., Gomez-Pardo, E., & Gruss, P. (1996). Pax2 contributes to inner ear patterning and optic nerve trajectory. *Development, 122,* 3381–3391.

Truett, K. R., Eaves, L. J., Meyer, J. M., Heath, A. C., & Martin, N. G. (1992). Religion and education as mediators of attitudes: A multivariate analysis. *Behavior Genetics, 22,* 43–62.

Turic, D., Robinson, L., Duke, M., Morris, D. W., Webb, V., Hamshere, M., Milham, C., *et al.* (2000). Linkage disequilibrium mapping provides evidence for a gene for reading disability on chromosome 6p21.3-22. *American Journal of Human Genetics.* Submitted manuscript.

Turner, J. S. (1970). Hereditary hearing loss with nephropathy (Alport's syndrome). *Acta Otolaryngologica, Suppl., 271,* 7–26.

Tyson, J., Tranebjaerg, L., Bellman, S., Wren, C., Taylor, J. F., Bathen, J., Aslaksen, B., Sorland, S. J., Lund, O., Malcolm, S., Pembrey, M., Bhattacharya, S., & Bitner-Glindzicz, M. (1997). IsK and KvLQT1: Mutation in either of the two subunits of the slow component of the delayed rectifier potassium channel can cause Jervell and Lange–Nielsen syndrome. *Human Molecular Genetics, 6,* 2179–2185.

U.S. Department of Energy and the Human Genome Project (1996). *To know ourselves.* Oak Ridge, TN: Oak Ridge National Laboratory.

Van Camp, G., & Smith, R. J. H. (2000). Hereditary hearing loss homepage [online]. Internet Communication.

Van Camp, G., Kunst, H., Flothmann, K., McGuirt, W., Wauters, J., Marres, H., Verstreken, M., Bespalova, I. N., Burmeister, M., VandeHeyning, P. H., Smith, R. J., Willems, P. J., Cremers, C. W., & Lesperance, M. M. (1999). A gene for autosomal dominant hearing impairment (DFNA14) maps to a region on chromosome 4p16.3 that does not overlap the DFNA6 locus. *Journal of Medical Genetics, 36,* 532–536.

Van der Lely, H. K., & Stollwerck, L. (1996). A grammatical specific language impairment in children: An autosomal dominant inheritance? *Brain and Language, 52,* 484–504.

Van De Water, T. R. (1986). Determinants of neuron–sensory receptor cell interaction during development of the inner ear. *Hearing Research, 22,* 265–277.

Van De Water, T. R. (1988). Tissue interactions and cell differentiation: Neuron–sensory cell interaction during otic development. *Development, 103,* 185–193.

Van De Water, T. R., & Represa, J. (1991). Tissue interactions and growth factors that control development of the inner ear: Neural tube–otic anlage interaction. In R. J. Ruben, T. R. Van De Water, & K. P. Steel (Eds.), Genetics of hearing impairment, *Annals of the New York Academy of Sciences, 630,* 116–128.

Van De Water, T. R., & Ruben, R. J. (1983). A possible embryonic mechanism for the establishment of innervation of inner ear sensory structures. *Acta Otolaryngologica, 95,* 470–479.

Vargha-Khadem, F., & Passingham, R. E. (1990). Speech and language defects. *Nature, 346,* 226.

Vargha-Khadem, F., Watkins, K., Alcock, K., Fletcher, P., & Passingham, R. E. (1995). Praxic and nonverbal cognitive deficits in a large family with a genetically transmitted speech and language disorder. *Proceedings of the National Academy of Sciences, 92,* 930–933.

Vogler, G. P., DeFries, J. C., & Decker, S. N. (1985). Family history as an indicator of risk for reading disability. *Journal of Learning Disabilities, 18,* 419–421.

Von Oeyen, P. T. (1990). Optimal prenatal care. In S. M. Pueschel & J. A. Mulick (Eds.), *Prevention of developmental disabilities* (pp. 55–74). Baltimore: Brookes.

Wadsworth, S. J., DeFries, J. C., Stevenson, J., Gilger, J. W., & Pennington, B. F. (1992). Gender ratios among reading-disabled children and their siblings. *Journal of Child Psychiatry and Psychology, 33,* 1229–1239.

Wagenaar, M. (2000). *The Usher syndrome: A clinical and genetic correlation.* Den Haag: CIP—gegevens koninklijke bibliotheek.

Walker, L., & Cole, E. (1965). Familial patterns of expression of specific reading disability in a population sample. *Bulletin of the Orton Society, 15,* 12–24.

Wang, A., Liang, Y., Fridell, R. A., Probst, F. J., Wilcox, E. R., Touchman, J. W., Morton, C. C., Morell, R. J., Noben-Trauth, K., Camper, S. A., & Friedman, T. B. (1998). Association of unconventional myosin MYO15 mutations with human nonsyndromic deafness DFNB3. *Science, 280*, 1447–1451.

Wang, W., Van De Water, T. R., & Lufkin, T. (1998). Inner ear and maternal reproductive defects in mice lacking the Hmx3 homeobox gene. *Development, 125*, 621–634.

Watkins, K. E., Gadian, D. G., & Vargha-Khadem, F. (1999). Functional and structural brain abnormalities associated with a genetic disorder of speech and language. *American Journal of Human Genetics, 65*, 1215–1221.

Watson, J. D. (1953). Molecular structure of nucleic acids. *Nature, 171*, 371.

Weiss, R. (2000). Genetic therapy apparently cures 2. *The Washington Post*, April 28, p. A1.

Weiss, R., & Nelson, D. (1999). Teen dies undergoing experimental gene therapy. *Washington Post*, 29 September, p. A01.

Weissenbach, J., Gyapay, G., Dib, C., Vignal, A., Morissette, J., Millasseau, P., Vaysseix, G., & Lathrop, M. (1992). A second-generation linkage map of the human genome. *Nature, 359(6398)*, 794–801.

Welch, H. G., & Burke, W. (1998). Uncertainties in genetic testing for chronic disease. *Journal of the American Medical Association, 280*, 1525–1527.

Wenthold, R. J. (1980). Neurochemistry of the auditory system. *Annals of Otology, Rhinology, and Laryngology, 89*(Suppl. 74), 121–131.

Wepman, J. (1939). Familial incidence of stammering. *Journal of Heredity, 30*, 207–210.

Wertz, D. C. (1997). Survey of informed consents. *The Gene Letter* [online]. Vol. 1, No. 4.

Wertz, D. C. (1997). Privacy: Genetic and otherwise. *The Gene Letter* [online]. Vol. 1, No. 4. Available: http://www.geneletter.org/0197/consent.html.

West, R., Nelson, S., & Berry, M. (1939). The heredity of stuttering. *Quarterly Journal of Speech, 25*, 23–30.

Wexler, N. (1992). Clairvoyance and caution: Repercussions from the Human Genome Project. In D. J. Kevles & L. Hood (Eds.), *Scientific and social issues in the Human Genome Project* (pp. 211–243). Cambridge: Harvard University Press.

Whalsten, D. (1990). Insensitivity of the analysis of variance to heredity–environment interaction. *Behavioral and Brain Sciences, 13*, 109–161.

Wheeler, D. L. (1999). Patient dies in gene-therapy trial at University of Pennsylvania Medical Center. *The Chronicle of Higher Education*, 8 October, p. A23.

Whitehead, M. C., & Morest, D. K. (1985). The development of innervation patterns in the avian cochlea. *Neuroscience, 14*, 255–276.

Wilde, S. W. R. W. (1853). *Particle observations on aural surgery and the nature and treatment of diseases of the ear with illustrations.* Philadelphia: Blanchard & Lea.

Williams, C. A., Zori, R. T., Stone, J. W., Gray, B. A., Cantu, E. S., & Ostrer, H. (1990). Maternal origin of 15q11-13 deletions in Angelman syndrome suggests a role for genomic imprinting. *American Journal of Medical Genetics, 35*, 350–353.

Williams, P., and Wendell-Smith, C. (1969). *Basic human embryology* (2nd ed.). Philadelphia: Lippincott.

Willig, S., Moss, S., & Lapham, E.V. (2000). The new genetics: What does it mean to us? *The ASHA Leader, 5*, 4–5.

Wolf, M., & Bowers, P. G. (1999). The double-deficit hypothesis for the developmental dyslexias. *Journal of Educational Psychology, 91*, 415–438.

Wolff, J. A., & Lederberg, J. (1994). A history of gene transfer and therapy. In J. A. Wolff (Ed.), *Gene therapeutics* (pp. 3–25). Boston: Birkhäuser.

Wolff, P. H., Melngailis, I., Obregon, M., & Bedrosian, M. (1995). Family patterns of developmental dyslexia, Part II: Behavioral phenotypes. *American Journal of Genetics, 60*, 494–505.

Wolff, P. H., Melngailis, I., & Kotwica, K. (1996). Family patterns of developmental dyslexia. Part III: Spelling errors as a behavioral phenotype. *American Journal of Medical Genetics, 67*, 378–386.

Wright, A., Carothers, A., & Pirastu, M. (1999). Population choice in mapping genes for complex diseases. *Nature Genetics, 23,* 397–404.

Wright, S. (1998). Genetic engineering could be dangerous. In T. L. Roleff (Ed.), *Biomedical ethics: Opposing viewpoints* (pp. 182–190). San Diego: Greenhaven.

Wu, D. K., & Oh, S. H. (1996). Sensory organ generation in the chick inner ear. *Journal of Neuroscience, 16,* 6454–6462.

Xiang, M., Gao, W.-Q., Hasson, T., & Shin, J. J. (1998). Requirement for Brn-3c in maturation and survival, but not in fate determination of inner ear hair cells. *Development, 125,* 3935–3946.

Yairi, E., Ambrose, N., & Cox, N. (1996). Genetics of stuttering: A critical review. *Journal of Speech and Hearing Research, 39,* 771–784.

Yule, W., & Rutter, M. (1975). The concept of specific reading retardation. *Journal of Child Psychiatry and Psychology, 16,* 181–197.

Zerbin-Rudin, E. (1967). Congenital word-blindness. *Bulletin of the Orton Society, 17,* 47–54.

Zlotogora, J. (1997). Dominance and homozygosity. *American Journal of Medical Genetics, 68,* 412–416.

Zoll, B. (1999, September). Zur Genetik der Sprachentwicklungsstörungen. *Sprach-Stimme-Gehör,* 127–180.

Author Index

SUBJECT INDEX

Basilar membrane, morphogenesis of inner
    ear, 74
Beckwith–Wiedemann syndrome, 142,
    144, 146
Behavioral genetics
    defined, 175–176
    developmental and learning disorders and,
        176–193
Benign polymorphism, 14
Binder syndrome, 145
Bixler syndrome, 145
BMP4 gene, 82
BMP7 gene, 82
Bone formation, 50–51
    abnormal, 54
    morphogenesis of inner ear, 76
Bone growth, 50–52
Bony labyrinth, morphogenesis of inner ear, 76
Branchio-oto-renal syndrome, 17, 93, 94–95
Bravo/NR-CAM, 117
Brn 3.1 gene, 84–85

C

Calvaria, 47, 55
Candidate gene studies, 21–22, 165–166
Cardio–cochlear potassium channel genes,
    21–22
Cell fate specification, inner ear, 80–85
CHARGE, 139
Cheekbones, development of, 47
Chin, development of, 47
Chromosomal inheritance, 17–18
Chromosomes, 14
Clefting
    clefting syndromes, 134–137
    genetics of, 4, 129–148
    multifactorial theory of, 131, 132
    teratogens and, 136–139
Cleidocranial dysplasia syndrome, 146
COCH gene, 100
Cochlea, morphogenesis of inner ear, 71–74,
    79
Cochlear duct, morphogenesis of inner ear, 74,
    77
Cockayne syndrome, 142
COL2A1 gene, 133
Collagen formation, clefting and, 133
Colorado Twin Reading Study, 119–120
Communicative disorders. *See* Genetic
    communicative disorders

Complex diseases, linkage studies of, 166–167
Complex inheritance pattern, 18
Compound heterozygous, 14
Computed tomography (CT), diagnosis of
    genetic deafness by, 106
Computer analysis, locus identification and, 23
Congenital hearing impairment, 5
Connexin 26, 99, 102, 107
Contiguous-gene disorders, 18, 135
Cosanguineous families, 23
Cranial base, flexure of, 34
Craniodiaphyseal dysplasia, prognosis for, 142
Craniofacial anomalies, genetics of, 3–4,
    129–148
Craniofacial complex, 31–33. *See also* Face
    abnormal bone formation, 54
    anomalies. *See* Clefting; Craniofacial
        anomalies
    bone growth, 50–55
    components and structures of, 38–41
    cranium, 55–59
    functions of, 63–66
    growth of, 47–55
    molecular control of development, 45–46
    postnatal development of, 47–62
    prenatal development of, 35–46
Cri-du-chat syndrome, genetics of, 134
Crista ampullares, morphogenesis of inner ear,
    71–73, 77
Crossover, 22
CT. *See* Computed tomography
Cupula, morphogenesis of inner ear, 74
Cytoplasmic inheritance, 16

D

Databases, genetic, 164, 165
dbEST, 164
DDP gene, 102
Deafness. *See* Hearing impairment
del(4p) abnormality, 134
del(5p) abnormality, 134
del(6q) abnormality, 134
del(18p) abnormality, 134
de Lange syndrome, 146
de novo mutations, 16
Dentition, 60–61
Developmental dyslexia. *See* Specific reading
    disability (SRD)